Pregnancy: the Mumsnet Guide

by Morag Preston and the Mumsnet Mums

Illustrated by Charlotte Meyer

BLOOMSBURY

LONDON · BERLIN · NEW YORK

First published in Great Britain 2009

Copyright © 2009 by Mumsnet Limited

Illustrations © 2009 by Charlotte Meyer

Edited by Carrie Longton, Justine Roberts
and Lucy Nicholls

The moral right of the authors has been asserted

Bloomsbury Publishing, London, Berlin and New York

36 Soho Square, London W1D 3QY

A CIP catalogue record for this book is available
from the British Library

ISBN 978 0 7475 9863 3
10 9 8 7 6 5 4 3 2

Typeset by RefineCatch Ltd, Bungay, Suffolk
Printed in Great Britain by Clays Ltd, St Ives plc

The paper this book is printed on is certified by the
© 1996 Forest Stewardship Council A.C. (FSC). It is
ancient-forest friendly. The printer holds FSC chain of
custody SGS-COC-2061

FSC
Mixed Sources
Product group from well-managed
forests and other controlled sources
Cert no. SGS-COC-2061
www.fsc.org
© 1996 Forest Stewardship Council

www.bloomsbury.com/mumsnet

To Mumsnetters everywhere whose intelligence, compassion and wit make parents' lives easier every day.

Foreword

Pregnancy is, somewhat idiosyncratically, the second in our series of Mumsnet Guides, following closely on the heels of *Toddlers*. And truth be told, at no time in our lives do we have quite so many burning questions as when we're pregnant, except maybe when we're three and just learned how to use the word 'why?'; but, as said, that's another book altogether. You pee on a stick and suddenly you are catapulted into a whole, previously unknown, universe of responsibility, not to mention discomfort.

You'd be mightily unlucky to get all the 'minor ailments' that are painstakingly detailed in most pregnancy tomes, but if you got none you'll most likely be preserved for the benefit of scientific research. As one Mumsnet member wrote recently, 'Pregnancy might not be an illness, but if you had half the symptoms and you weren't pregnant you'd think you were dying, wouldn't you?' Whether it's exhaustion, indigestion, constipation, backache, nausea, piles, insomnia, restless leg or carpal tunnel syndrome, everyone seems to have a their own particular bugbear and most will have an unappetising cocktail of them.

And we haven't even mentioned the hormones yet – the ones that will see you weeping uncontrollably at the merest glimpse of an Andrex puppy.

Added to that, these days, it can feel like you need a twenty-four-hour newswire to keep you up to date with the latest guidelines on WHAT PREGNANT WOMEN SHOULD NOT DO. Blink and you'll miss the fact that shellfish are off the menu. Then on again – but only if they are thoroughly cooked and piping hot all the way through... And without a degree in food science you might struggle to establish exactly which cheeses are pregnancy no-nos. If soft ones are off limits, how soft is soft? And what about Feta or, for that matter, the deliciously runny one at the local deli that claims to be pasteurised?

And those are just the first gusts in the hurricane of questions that will engulf you over the next few months. Should you bother with ante-natal classes? How much maternity leave will you need? What tests should you have – and what should you make of them? What kind of birth should you have? What equipment should you buy? Is teal best for a boy or a girl? How will you know if you are going into labour? Or indeed how to ripen your cervix, if you're not? What on earth is a mucus plug anyway?

Every day the Mumsnet community helps a fresh battalion of prospective mothers to navigate the perilous waters of pregnancy, from their first tentative post of 'Could I be pregnant?' to the moment those very waters eventually break (usually over your best Havaianas).

If we at Mumsnet HQ had a pound for every Mumsnetter who'd lamented, if only they'd found the site earlier, when they were pregnant with their first rather than with their third child, I'd no doubt be writing this from a plush Kensington suite rather than a shed in Kentish Town.

Given that you're reading this, we hope you're one of the lucky ones who have discovered this amazing bunch of women (and a few amazing men) right at the beginning of your journey as a parent because, as one Mumsnetter memorably puts it, 'once you deliver the placenta, they insert the guilt.' Rest assured though, Mumsnet will be with you every step of the way.

All of which may leave you wondering why you are reading this book, and not sat in front of a screen chewing the fat in a Mumsnet antenatal club. It's true that to feel the full experience you need to log on and plunge in. But a while ago we realised that, without us ever planning it that way, Mumsnet Talk had turned into the most amazing archive of wisdom. Whereas existing pregnancy manuals offered you the wisdom of a single Stoppard or Kitzinger, Mumsnet could bring you the collected wisdom of a million parents. Just as Wikipedia has rendered almost obsolete the Encyclopaedia Britannica, so we wondered if there was a way to capture the wisdom of this remarkable crowd.

We hope a Mumsnet pregnancy manual might be different from the usual in another way too. If Mumsnet.com is such fun to read that some members have begged us to ban them because they are spending too much of their lives on the boards, might it not be possible, despite the piles and constipation, for a pregnancy book to be a good read too? Even with a thread on the grisliest of subjects, it is not unusual to find yourself chuckling over the keyboard. One member captured the wonderfully batty serendipity of the site a while ago: 'You know, you start a thread about vaginal discharge and within a few posts you find yourself recommending a reasonably-priced shed or telling all about the little hotel you stayed at in the Cotswolds.'

And if traditional pregnancy and parenting guides purport to reveal 'the right way' to give birth, our firm starting point is that there isn't one right way – most of the time – to do the parenting thing. If there were a Mumsnet philosophy it would be something along the lines of 'there's more than one way to skin a cat', so read this as a book of optimistic suggestions, rather than a user's manual. What we provide is a range of options compiled from the hard-won know-how of what has worked for thousands of others; somewhere in here will be answers that work for you and if there's not we hope that at least we'll distract from your varicose veins for a while.

Justine Roberts (Co-founder, Mumsnet.com)

P.S. Huge thanks to Mumsnetter Boco who we found hiding her enormous artistic talents under a bushel somewhere on our vegetable, pulses and wholegrains forum. She translated my frankly incomprehensible briefs into the remarkable illustrations you'll find in this book, and only very occasionally told me I was being unreasonable.

P.P.S. Mumsnetters go by a weird and wonderful array of pseudonyms. JackBauer for instance isn't the real Jack Bauer – or if he is, do bear in mind that you've probably only got twenty-four hours to read this book before some kind of particularly nasty, global catastrophe.

Contents

When Things Go Wrong

Second Trimester: Not Ballooning but Blooming

Health Issues

Tests And Scans

Thinking Ahead

When Things Go Wrong

Third Trimester: OK, Fat Ladies – It's Nearly Time to Start Singing

Health Issues

The Birth

Fourth Trimester: Life After Birth

Appendices

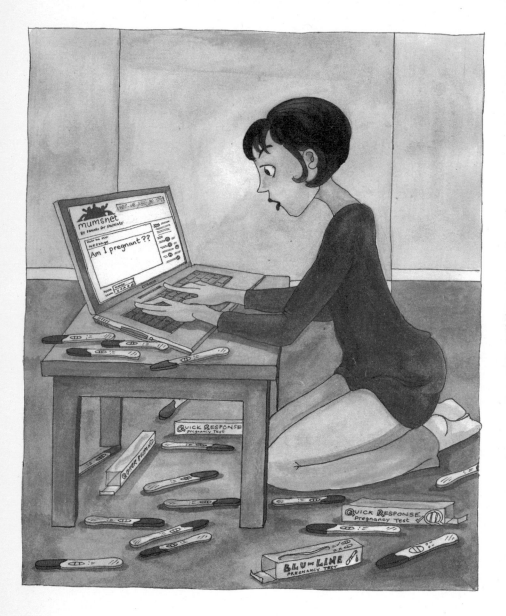

First Trimester:

I'm Not Fat, I'm Just Increasingly Big-Boned

In this chapter ...

The Thin Blue Line

Congratulations – what a result! Not everyone remembers exactly when they actually *got* pregnant or where, but, chances are, you will recall with perfect clarity the finer details of when you first saw that thin blue line. After all, having spent most of your adult life trying to avoid getting knocked up, you have finally hit the jackpot. It's a total heart-stopper; hopefully, in a good way.

But here the confusion starts. It might say 'Rapid Response' on the package but using a pregnancy-testing kit to work out if you really are up the duff suddenly becomes impossible when a news ticker in your head is flashing, 'Life-changing moment alert' while you're thinking, damn it, what do all these lines and pink splodges actually mean? How long is a minute? Is my pee strong enough? Should I wait until morning? It can't possibly be true. The test must be faulty. I knew it – I should have bought the more expensive one ...

It's quite normal at this stage to rush out and buy a few more tests, rather than investing more sensibly in a bumper pack of iron tablets. But one, two, three pregnancy tests later, it will (sort of) sink in that you really are pregnant.

Now how do you feel? Thrilled? Excited? Let us hope so. Totally terrified at the same time? Definitely. Hell, no one has prepared you for this. It's wonderful. And daunting. You're taking a giant leap into the unknown. Even breaking the news to your other half can be a challenge. Will a text message do the job? Should you buy him a T-shirt with 'I'm the Daddy' on it? Should you scream and jump up and down with excitement? Or just sit on the loo in gobsmacked silence until he realises you've been gone for an unusually long time?

Good news is cause for celebration, but life has suddenly become that little bit more complicated. You are starting to think for two. It's not only about what you want any more, but also what's good for your baby. Would he/she/it prefer wine or, perhaps, champagne? Will bubbles make it feel uncomfortable? Should you be drinking at all?

To add to the general confusion, pregnancy maths is a head scrambler (according to doctors, the age of your baby dates from the first day of your last period, not conception) and, for weeks, you will have been going around as normal not even knowing that a storm was brewing inside you. Panic often begins to set in when you start to think about those carefree nights. But pregnancy isn't generally something people get in training for, and if you got completely plastered before you knew you were pregnant, don't worry; you're in the same boat as many, many Mumsnetters.

'My daughter wasn't planned. I was drinking and partying like a mad woman, out on the major lash every weekend. I shared wine with my partner over dinner every night. I also came off a jet ski at high speed and couldn't move my arm for days. But my daughter is a healthy, happy child. I conceived my second daughter around New Year after some wild partying. Again, she is fine.' TeeCee

What can make it all so much harder is that at the very moment you are bursting to tell someone, anyone, the biggest news of your life, caution tells you to keep a lid on it, at least until your 12-week scan. It's not an easy task, especially if you're looking for empathy. How did you go from being a five-fruit-a-day girl to scoffing Hula Hoops by the six-pack? How can they call it morning sickness when you're down on your knees with your head in the loo and it's almost time for *Emmerdale*? And since when did you start watching *Emmerdale*, anyway? (And why does it make you *cry* every time?)

It's natural to want to reach out at this point for a bit of support and, at times, your partner just won't cut it. Of course, he is as thrilled as you are (at least you hope he is) and you will struggle to talk about anything else except your new creation, but what you are really looking for is some words from the wise, from other females who've recently experienced what you're going through, to explain all this stuff. That said, it won't be long until every mum and her pram will have something to say about your bump, so realise now that your time in the spotlight is nigh: you are now a slowing-ticking due date. Even furtively buying a pregnancy test can be the first step towards coming out of the breeder's closet. Witness one mother's story: 'I bought a pregnancy test and was completely taken aback when the lady at the till asked me if it would be good or bad news, then proceeded to ask how many children I already had, and how sure I was that this was what I really wanted.'

Pregnancy is both a uniquely personal and yet public journey. Everybody's experience is different. And, along the way, your perspective will probably change. What we hope to offer here is a wealth of experience to guide you on your way and to give you confidence. Testing the water, so to speak, is just the beginning.

Now, what to do about that pregnancy stick – the one you just peed on? Some sentimentalists hang on to it. But, then again, some people eat their baby's placenta ...

How pregnant am I? The figures that count

Calculating how pregnant you are can be more complicated than filling in your tax return. Fortunately, however, midwives are generally a bit cheaper than accountants and can do all the sums for you – as long as you can remember when your last period was. So no matter how convinced you are that your pregnancy can be traced back to that office Christmas party, all your midwife really wants to know is when you had your last period.

The idea behind this is that most women are more likely to recall when they started their last period than when they ovulated – although if you have been using Natural Family Planning you might be keeping track of both (make sure you count better next time).

Pregnant women are measured in weeks (not tonnes, even though it might feel like it). A full-term pregnancy lasts 40 weeks and is split into three trimesters. The word 'trimester' literally means 'three months', but in fact, the first trimester is 14 weeks, the second is 12 weeks and the third, which feels like it lasts for about 200 weeks, should be around 14.

Be prepared – on a daily basis, total strangers will want to know just how pregnant you are. Not knowing the answer will make you look air-headed, and possibly feel a tad guilty. So it's best to get it sorted from the start.

What are the first pregnancy signs to look out for?

'Tiredness: I was falling asleep on the sofa at 8.30 p.m. and when my partner woke me to take me to bed, I felt like I had been hit on the head with a hammer.' *flubdub*

'Giant, sore, tingly boobs.' *cece*

'A metallic taste in my mouth.' *MrsJoshLyman*

'An inability to form proper sentences or focus my brain.' *PutThatInYourPipeandSmokeIt*

'Feeling hungover all day despite not having drunk any alcohol.' *petitfilou*

'Wanting to eat cucumber every day when I usually can't stand the stuff.' *BeckyBendyLegs*

'A dry mouth like my husband had put sand in it during the night.' *neveronamonday*

'Going mad eating fruit which is strange for me.' *chocciedooby*

'I felt poking feelings down in my abdomen which turned out to be implantation.' *SoExcited*

'Needing to wee all the time.' *MrsMattie*

'I had a dizzy spell à la Vivien Leigh for no apparent reason.' *alibag*

'Guzzling down a large bag of BBQ Beef Hula Hoops, while hiding in the car wash.' *beakas*

'Being sick twice a day without fail.' *babyontheway*

'Being unable to sleep because I was too warm.' *ellideb*

'Thinking I must be terminally ill. Sick, tired, weepy, achy – and for no apparent reason. It was a relief to find out it was "only" a pregnancy.' *custardtart*

'Looking at a bar of Galaxy and not understanding why I didn't want to devour it.' *ellideb*

'Crying at *EastEnders*.' *BeckyBendyLegs*

'Heightened sense of smell.' *sarahloumadam*

'My bowels slowed right down and my jeans got tight around my bum and thighs.' *PutThatInYourPipeandSmokeIt*

'What I thought was really bad PMT. I threw a glass on the floor in frustration and sobbed uncontrollably when my cat started rubbing round my legs affectionately.' *IceCube*

Doctor! Doctor! There's a Baby in My Tummy ...

After the shock of the thin blue line, you may become very aware that you are carrying around a teeny, weeny baby somewhere in there. And surely such a major biological miracle needs urgent medical attention?

'Book yourself a GP appointment, don't smoke, don't drink, keep taking the folic acid, and avoid soft cheese and pâté. And Congratulations!'

LieselVentouse

You can ring your GP as soon as you like, but they probably won't actually do anything at your first appointment, which can be a bit deflating. They may not even want to see you, and could just take your details over the phone and ask you to book an appointment with a midwife at around eight to ten weeks of pregnancy (that's four to six weeks after your period was due). This is called your 'Booking-in appointment'.

The booking-in appointment may be in your home. Your midwife will have lots of notes to complete and will ask you lots of questions about your family and your own medical history, as well as how you are feeling about things. They may take your blood pressure and possibly ask for a urine sample. You might want to ask how the antenatal care works and whether you will see your GP and your midwife or just your midwife; also what scans and tests they do and when, and whether you will have the option of finding out the sex of your baby – no point agonising over this if the option isn't there. You could also ask about NHS antenatal classes.

Your booking-in appointment should be nice and informal and will probably make you feel 'officially pregnant'. Your midwife may give you your 'Maternity Notes' at this point; these will be updated at every appointment between now and when you are finally handed over into the care of the health visitors, when your baby is a week or so old. You will be responsible for your Maternity Notes, and will be expected to take them to every antenatal appointment and carry them around with you for the duration of your pregnancy (although if you don't have them under your arm at the checkout at Asda, it doesn't mean you are a bad mummy).

'My midwife told me she's only had two women lose their notes. Both were found in pubs and handed back to the surgery …' LynetteScavo

Your midwife may listen to your baby's heartbeat at this first appointment, using a small ultrasound gadget called a Doppler, which she presses to your abdomen. She might not be able to hear anything (and some midwives won't bother trying yet for this reason), but don't panic – this is quite normal because the baby is still very tiny and low down in your abdomen. He is most likely busy checking out your internal organs and working out which he will kick the hardest once he's grown some legs.

'I was so excited about the prospect of hearing my child's heartbeat for the first time, but all the midwife seemed to be able to pick up was something that mostly resembled a radio conversation with the local mini-cab firm. The machine she was using was just useless. After three healthy pregnancies I came to see these "listening" sessions as pot luck – sometimes you hear the heartbeat, sometimes you don't; but the first time you fail to hear it can be really scary. So be reassured – it's nearly always the machine's fault!' Munchpot

You will probably be asked to book appointments to see your midwife every month or so, but most of these appointments will be very low-key and mainly to check that things are progressing OK. You can expect to be measured with a tape measure frequently to check the 'fundal height', i.e. how large your baby/womb is growing. But be reassured that 'other than an obsession with wee and blood pressure, not a whole lot happens at midwife appointments'.

Maternity Notes: What does it all mean?

Your Maternity Notes will include the following about your antenatal care: who your GP is, lots of information about your pregnancy, your birth plans and a plethora of mysterious abbreviations. There should also be a phone number for you to ring with questions or in case of emergency.

You will no doubt pore over all of the scribbles in these notes to try to decipher what everyone is saying about you. Here is a brief guide to help you:

Primigravida A medical term which means a woman in her first pregnancy.

(continued)

LMP Last monthly period. This is the date on which your term of pregnancy officially starts.

Length of pregnancy This is measured in weeks and days (so '10 + 4' means ten weeks and four days pregnant).

Blood pressure This will be recorded each time. Severe high blood pressure in pregnancy can be dangerous to mother and baby.

Urine You will probably get your own personal NHS pee-pot to bring with you to each midwife appointment. Take a mid-stream sample (i.e. start peeing, then shove the pot underneath yourself – this avoids getting bacteria from your genitals in the urine sample; and try to avoid peeing all over your sleeves). Your midwife will probably test the urine there and then and hand the pot back. Try not to look too horrified; just stick it in your handbag, empty it when you get home and wash it out thoroughly ready for the next appointment. Your urine notes will often say 'NAD' which stands for 'no abnormalities detected'.

Height of uterus/Fundal height This is measured from the pubic hairline to the top of your bump. Roughly speaking, the number of centimetres corresponds to the number of weeks you are pregnant, although this is a bit haphazard so don't panic if things don't measure up perfectly. If they do, however, your notes will read '= d', which means that height equals dates.

Heartbeat or activity If your midwife listens to your baby's heartbeat (usually using a Doppler ultrasound) she may note the heart rate (number of beats per minute or BPM). She may also note: FHH (foetal heart heard); FHNH (foetal heart not heard – it's not always easy to find); FMF (foetal movements felt – awww sweet!); or FMNF (foetal movements not felt – i.e. lazy baby is asleep again).

Keeping Mum? Is It Best to Share Your News or Wait for a Few Months?

Deciding when to break the news of your pregnancy will be one of the first decisions you make as a parent. Do you let your partner (if you have one) have a say about this? Or is the decision all your own? Some cosy couples enjoy keeping it a sneaky secret, maximising that brief honeymoon period before going public. Others are straight on the phone before their pee is even dry on the pregnancy stick, spreading the word and booking in potential babysitters. 'In an ideal world, I would have waited three months,' says one cautious Mumsnetter. 'But my husband told everyone from the milkman to the postman as soon as we found out.' Perhaps he was looking for guilty faces.

Many mums-to-be hold back a pregnancy announcement, concerned they might miscarry: 'I was so excited that I was pregnant, and I knew my friends and family would be too, but I didn't want to get their hopes up in case anything went wrong.' As well as the personal pain of a miscarriage, having to explain to people what has happened and to listen to them feel sorry for you can be heartbreaking. Keeping a secret gives you thinking space, whatever the outcome. 'I held off completely,' says another. 'I don't particularly want support if things go wrong; I've had two miscarriages and I felt far more comfortable with it just being me and my husband handling it ourselves. I like having just us know for as long as possible.'

Others, on the other hand, want to make sure that support is available in the event that they do miscarry. A first-timer recalls: 'I was so excited that I told everyone straight away. Then I lost the baby and it was horrible having to "un-tell" everyone. But, I'm glad I did, as they were very supportive and it hit me really hard.' Opening up about your experience can be comforting when you realise how many women have been through something similar. One recently pregnant mum, fearing the worst, went as far as telling her boss, in case she miscarried and would need to take time off.

'My work colleagues were thoroughly fed up with the number of office pregnancies, so I baked them a cake to soften the blow.' MrsBadger

Keeping up the 'What, me? Pregnant?' façade calls for a gargantuan effort, especially at work. Morning sickness is hard to disguise, and the subconscious urge constantly to stroke your slightly rounded belly is a dead giveaway. The first few weeks of pregnancy can be surprisingly lonely when all you want to do is tell someone. You're desperate to explain to your colleagues why it is you keep running off to the loo and falling asleep at your keyboard. But then again, pretending you aren't pregnant may help you stay sane during those early months.

'Both times I only told people once I had a dating scan. Keeping it a secret during the sicky, tired stage actually helped me to cope with those symptoms. I still ate lots of Hula Hoops though, so anyone who was in the know would have clicked.' Bundle

Whatever your decision – to tell or not to tell – chances are that your best-laid plans will be scuppered. One would-be secret-keeper thought she would get away with it when she went to stay with a friend in Scotland, only for her hostess to confront her with: 'Are you up the duff, or what? Look at the size of yer tits!' Witness another mother's outing: 'My husband and I decided not to tell anyone, but a mum friend came round the morning after I did the test and I had left *What to Expect When You're Expecting* out on the sofa, so I was busted!' Others have been caught off guard at work, being asked to take on a heavy workload (literally): 'We were moving offices and I didn't want to do much lifting and packing.' Slowing down your alcohol intake, looking green, fat and busty, and generally acting weird, are all signs that people who know you well will pounce upon immediately. Unless, of course, you are Ursula the Sea Witch.

Some people are useless at keeping secrets and it's easier just to tell the truth.

'I think it is superstitious not to tell – it's not like the telling will cause a problem. If anything, not telling would have stressed me out more. As it turned out, I couldn't help myself and told family first and close workmates at about eight weeks, as well as my boss. I had severe morning sickness more or less straight after that, which meant weeks off work and time in hospital on a drip, so then everyone knew. The passing of the first trimester seems to be like some magic sign, but really I think it's better to assume all is well from the start, be positive and go from there.'

Mollipops

Being first to share the news can get surprisingly competitive. 'I went to tell a friend the news only to find my sister-in-law had beaten me to it,' tells one mum. One approach is to tell only close family and swear them to secrecy. That is, if you can trust them not to blab. Alternatively, take a modern approach and just change your Facebook status to 'Up the duff'.

'I chose only to tell family and close friends when pregnant with my first, as I was a bit wary until after the first trimester. My parents-in-law, however, didn't have any such anxieties and apparently rushed out to their local boozer and announced it to all and sundry – cue round of congratulatory drinks. My husband was very miffed when he strolled in there a few weeks later to break the news, only to be greeted with bored faces.' Snugs

A few women feel self-conscious making the announcement, preferring others to spread the juicy gossip on their behalf. 'I kept it a secret until 12 weeks and then let it leak out,' says one cautious mother. 'I felt quite self-conscious about telling friends. I thought they'd think: "Woah, who is she kidding? Does she really think she's up to this?" To be honest, I wasn't sure myself.'

Mothers and Mothers-in-Law

Sometimes it can seem as though your pregnancy is the moment your mother or mother-in-law has been in training for all her life – her opportunity to hijack the arrival of your first child. Like Margaret Thatcher before her, she will announce to all and sundry that 'We are a grandmother'. She may stake her claim early, bustling in with vanloads of immigrants from the Hundred Acre Wood and unearthing your husband's old christening gown from its mouldering nest in the attic.

'I am 40 weeks pregnant with my first baby, and every time my mother-in-law talks about the little one, she calls it "our baby". Ugh, it's really starting to irritate me in a big way. Yes, it's her grandchild, and I am more than happy for her to be involved, but unless she was involved in the conception or pushing it out, she's not entitled to call it "our baby". I'm not having a baby with her, I'm having it with my husband.' Fragolina

If that doesn't drive you insane, then her enthusiastic antenatal classes just might: 'When we visited my parents-in-law to tell them I was pregnant, it went down very well. Next morning my mother-in-law bustled into the sitting room with a teddy and a baby bath, purchased for existing grandchildren, and proceeded to give me a lesson in how to bathe a baby. "You must support the head like this, do you see?" I was three months pregnant. That has coloured all my doings with her regarding the children, I'm afraid.' Another mum recalls: 'My mother recently told me that labour was easy, "All you need is your husband to give you a little back massage. If it gets painful they give you a little injection anyway." I asked if she meant a little injection in her spine. Of morphine. Obviously 30 years have dimmed her memory.'

Or maybe one or other of them has some ideas about breastfeeding she would like to share with you. 'She keeps telling me that breastfeeding is a waste of time and that she tried for one day and gave up. In fact, if she tells me one more time that she has "very small nipples", I'm going to chop them off.'

One poor mum suffering from morning sickness groans: 'If my mother-in-law tells me once more that my sister-in-law never made this much fuss when she was pregnant, I may just lose the plot completely.'

How you handle your relationships with your grannies-to-be now will lay the groundwork for the future. Do you tackle their behaviour head-on, or develop subtle strategies to cope, in the hope that being a good girl now can be cashed in for childcare and laundry services in the years to come? 'Just bite your lip,' cautions one Mumsnetter. 'It helps if you can laugh about it later with your partner, which can sometimes be tricky where mothers-in-law are concerned.'

It's important to try to be gentle, because although it is you having the baby, this is a really important time for them, too, particularly if life otherwise revolves largely around breeding fuchsias or, perhaps, dusting their husband's miniature railway: 'All mothers and mothers-in-law interfere. I would try to ignore her but also be grateful she loves your child so much, even before it has been born, no matter how irritating that may be.'

This is also a time in everyone's life when the family is being jiggled about and new relationships are beginning. Although you might grind your teeth at Granny's gurning smile as she polishes your dinner plates with her Union Jack tea towel, you have had years to become old and cynical. For your child, on the other hand, everything is new and exciting, and they might (literally) wet themselves with excitement on the days their twinkling Gran visits, brandishing a new Tweenies jigsaw puzzle. 'Just let her enjoy it. She is excited and there may be a time when you are really grateful that she wants to build a fantastic relationship with the baby, and with you too.' Try to find a role for her so that she is involved and feels important: 'I give mine jobs to do, little things to find out about; it helps me and she feels useful.'

'Stick to your guns about what you want to do but don't actually fall out, even if you find her extremely irritating. We eventually settled in, and she babysat, and our relationship improved. Then earlier this year I was hospitalised, and unable to look after my son. My mother-in-law was the one who sent me into hospital; she was the one who brought down my fever, which probably saved my life; and she looked after my son while I was ill and recovering. She was a total star. She still comes out with complete howlers, like, "Aren't you going to do anything about losing that baby weight, dear?", but I have to remember that what she does is kinder than what she says.' thebecster

Some advise to speak out early and not let resentments fester: 'Nip unhelpful behaviours in the bud early. Grin and bear it too long and it becomes much harder to tell her.' Another mum cautions: 'If being a mum has taught me anything it is that you have to be assertive and you really need to stand your ground over what you and your husband want for your own family. Your mother-in-law is going to be part of your family now, not vice versa.' Setting your boundaries now might take more than one go: 'I've tried the quiet word with her. I've tried the row. I've tried the going-through-the-husband approach. I've tried the silent treatment. I've decided she's a half wit and I'm thinking about emigrating. Bear up. It's your baby. Don't take on the "Remember, you'll be a mother-in-law one day" bull, because being a mother-in-law doesn't give you the right to be a royal pain in the a**e.'

Be prepared for her to invite herself to move in with you straight after her baby – sorry, *your* baby – is born, but don't forget that you need your own space too. 'It is annoying enough with your own mother interfering, but a different kind of torture to imagine your mother-in-law being there constantly while you are trying to breastfeed and cope with no sleep.'

Of course, there are plenty of fabulous grannies out there who provide great support at a crucial and stressful time. As one philosophical mum points out: 'As a mum, you need to learn to share. When you have children, the wider family is important. You have to bear in mind that the baby may be more like your mother-in-law than you.' And if your toddler becomes an expert at drying the dishes, you'll probably be rather pleased.

Dos and Don'ts

It is well nigh impossible trying to keep up with the list of all the things that PREGNANT WOMEN SHOULD NOT DO! One minute you are trying to sort the old wives' tale from hard-nosed medical fact, then the next, oops! you realise you've overdosed on tuna again. Sometimes, common sense is the best yardstick. Think about all those pregnant women in France nibbling away on Brie, or those in Japan, who are merrily tucking into sushi by the boatload.

'No one's forcing you to avoid certain things, they are just informing you and leaving you to make your own decision. Personally, I'd much rather have the information. It's only nine months of your life, surely it's not going to kill you to avoid a few things?' Philippat

Should you transgress though, don't beat yourself up. One woman says: 'I used to joke that if they started advising pregnant women not to wear black, I might just risk it. I ate tuna by the bucketload, because it wasn't on "the list" then. Obviously people don't want to harm their unborn babies, but the latest current advice is just that – the latest advice, not the definitive advice!'

For the latest advice on what you are and are not allowed to eat (and drink) visit www.eatwell.gov.uk.

Smoking

This is one of the few topics where we are all agreed: it makes you look common and smell terrible. Oh, and it is not a good thing for pregnant mums or their babies. Smoking increases the risk of your baby having a low birth weight or being born prematurely. It is also linked to miscarriage, respiratory problems and sudden infant death syndrome (SIDS). The thought of nicotine crossing the placenta conjures up a grim image, as does the sight of you puffing away outside the pub, but giving up can still be a struggle.

'I am going to be like a lamb to the slaughter writing this – it's embarrassing and I am deeply ashamed of myself. I have smoked for 17 years, heavily (30 a day). On finding out I was pregnant I immediately booked in to see the NHS smoking nurse determined to quit for my baby. However, being such a heavy smoker, the pathetically low nicotine patches that you are allowed while pregnant didn't touch me. I have tried the inhalator and gum, all to no avail. Instead, in the last three weeks, I have cut down to around 10 and am working on reducing this much more over the next few weeks. My carbon monoxide levels on testing weekly have more than halved.' Kezza7779

The good news is that every cigarette you cut back on is better for your baby. A Danish study found that smokers double the risk of stillbirth and infant mortality, but if you quit in your first trimester this risk is reduced to that of a non-smoker.

Morning sickness can be a boon to pregnant women trying to give up. And if that doesn't quash your cravings, here's what worked for one Mumsnetter: 'I put a huge poster on my wall saying, "I DO NOT NEED A CIGARETTE". It also helped to shout it out loud when I felt like giving in.' Another says: 'Every time I craved a cigarette, I would imagine holding my baby in my arms and forcing him to smoke one.' Keep busy, without making yourself stressed. If you get a craving, distract yourself for 10 minutes until it subsides; if you give in, try again tomorrow. Think about one craving at a time. A Mumsnetter who successfully quit recommends: 'Smoke what you have and enjoy them, then don't buy any more. Put the money that you would have spent in a jar and buy something nice for you and the baby.' (However, if you have just come off a flight from Ibiza with a suitcase full of B&H, you might want to be generous and give a few away rather than follow this advice.)

Passive smoking Plenty of studies have shown that secondary smoke is bad for us, and therefore damaging to foetal growth, too. Which means that it isn't just the baby incubator that has to give up; Dad needs to stub it out, too. One woman says: 'My husband stopped smoking with me when I was trying to get pregnant and it has been so helpful. It would have been really hard if he hadn't, and I think I would have felt really resentful too. Also, you will be more tempted to start again once bambino comes if he is still puffing, and you don't want to be a smoker when you have kids for so many reasons.' If he can't go cold turkey, make sure he doesn't smoke near you and keep your house a smoke-free zone.

If your parents or friends smoke, it can be awkward when they start prodding your belly with their yellowed talons, although your maternal instinct to protect your baby might give you the confidence to tackle smokers who are breathing their nasty smoke over your precious newborn. 'I dare say it will claw at my heart when I see my mum holding my new, precious, sweet-smelling baby with those faggy hands,' one mum admits. For another mum, the firm approach worked: 'Telling my mum that she wouldn't be seeing her grandchild unless she gave up smoking was one of the hardest things I had to do. It was a risk, but, so far, it has paid off.'

Dope

Studies have shown that women who use marijuana during pregnancy, even occasionally, are more likely to suffer complications. Marijuana crosses the placenta, putting your child at risk of serious abnormalities. It's quitting now that matters, not how much you have smoked in the past. That just makes you a pot-head, rather than a bad mum. (See your GP for advice on quitting.)

Cocaine

Continue to use cocaine – even once – and you are at serious risk of harming your baby. As cocaine crosses the placenta, it reduces the amount of oxygen reaching the foetus. It is linked to miscarriage, premature birth and low birth weight, as well as long-term problems for your child. Your baby could be born with an addiction and would have to go through withdrawal after it was born. This goes for any other illegal drug substance as well. (See your GP for advice.)

Painkillers

Being transformed from super-lithe babe to sumo wrestler in the course of a few months puts a lot of strain on your body, and pregnancy can be a painful ordeal, particularly for women who experience pelvic, back and hip pain as their ligaments loosen up in preparation for birth. Unfortunately, most painkillers are best avoided during pregnancy. Aspirin and non-steroidal anti-inflammatory drugs (NSAIDs) such as ibuprofen, ketoprofen, naproxen are thought to increase the risk of miscarriage. However, current evidence suggests that occasional use of paracetamol does not increase the risks to your baby. Keep usage to a minimum – two or three times a week maximum. And check with your pharmacist or GP before taking all painkillers and other over-the-counter medicines during your pregnancy.

Paint

The nesting instinct probably hasn't kicked in yet, but chances are, in your eighth or ninth month you will be shilly-shallying over whether to pick up a paintbrush or not. Not because you can't decide between Dulux Celestial Blue or Farrow & Ball Cinder Rose, but because you are concerned about breathing in toxic fumes which may increase your risk of having a baby with birth defects. One keen *Elle Decoration* reader advises: 'There are non-toxic paints, which are more expensive, but, in my opinion, easier to use.' Always read the side of the tin, wear protective clothing, keep the room well ventilated and steer clear of paint removers which are toxic too. And don't go stripping down old paint as it might contain lead. Being up the duff and up a ladder is also a bad idea, and will cause old ladies to faint clean away in horror. Just this once, you are allowed to get a man to do it. He's bound to be positively gagging to get his hands on that Winnie the Pooh border ...

Cleaning products

Hard as we have tried, we have been unable to unearth a study to show that a bit of passive Pledge-inhaling will harm your baby. It is probably best to avoid powerful oven cleaners though. If you can't persuade your partner that cleaning is far too risky, read the labels on the side of products, and wear your Marigolds for extra protection. Pump sprays are less likely to drown you in a toxic cloud than aerosols.

Insecticides

You want to avoid areas where spraying is under way because of the chemical fumes. A Mumsnetter tip: 'Use a DEET-free insect repellent (the sort they advertise as for children), or citronella soap, and light citronella candles.'

Saunas and jacuzzis

Although you would have to work up quite a heat before it becomes dangerous, these are perhaps best avoided. Most health clubs will have warning signs advising you against it, and you don't want to get told off in a public place.

Hair dye

While the rest of your body heads far south, it's understandable
that you might want to keep your hair looking presentable.
Studies show that it is safe to colour your hair during pregnancy.
Only enormous doses of the chemicals used in semi-permanent
and permanent hair dyes would be likely to cause harm. But if you
are concerned, it might be best to wait until after the first 12 weeks
of pregnancy. Otherwise, use a vegetable dye. If you are doing it
yourself at home, wear gloves and open a window for ventilation.
And as your hormones are all over the place, you might be more
susceptible to an allergic reaction from a dye, so it is best to do a
patch test on the bend of an arm or behind an ear 24 hours before
application.

'I coloured my hair all through my pregnancies.
There might be a tiny chemical risk, but I always
figured that my unborn child was more at risk
if he came out to find a mad, dishevelled
mother." fisil

Hair removal cream

The use of hair removal creams has not been formally studied on
pregnant women. But some doctors advise against using them
during pregnancy and breastfeeding as they contain strong
chemicals, which can be absorbed through the skin. Always read
the instructions on the packet, and don't use on broken skin. Do
a patch test on a small area first, as your skin can become more
sensitive during pregnancy. Otherwise, use a razor or an electric
shaver (and possibly some strategically placed mirrors) if you want
to keep your hairy bits and lady garden trimmed and presentable.
You can always go with waxing instead as there seem to be no
ill effects reported (other than that your skin may be a bit more
sensitive than usual). Probably best to visit a spa or therapist
though: waxing 'blind', as it were, could have rather disastrous
consequences. A final word on lady gardening – please don't be
upset if the midwife who is sewing it all back together doesn't
admire your work.

Dental X-rays

Make sure you tell your dentist that you are pregnant – for a start, you'll get free dental treatment on the NHS. If an X-ray is needed, they will probably suggest waiting until after your baby is born to do it, although they are thought to be safe.

Underwired bras

Pregnancy hormones are pumping up your boobs, getting them ready for breastfeeding and your jubblies are growing as fast as marrows in super-dung. You've got to put them somewhere, but you want to be comfortable and look halfway respectable at the same time. At the back of your mind, you may recall something about underwired bras being bad for pregnant women because they can interfere with milk production. But, as one mother says: 'I think the advice is that, whatever bra you wear, you should make sure that it fits well and it's supportive. As long as the wires aren't digging in anywhere, you should be fine.'

'I have worn underwired bras throughout both my previous pregnancies. I breastfed both boys for 10 months. I have just got back from the shops where I picked out a new bra at a large department store, which looked great. I got to the till and the lady said: "Oh, are you pregnant? Well, I'm sorry Madam, I am not allowed to sell that bra to you." My response was: "Please don't be so daft, and take my money." She wasn't happy, but she grudgingly sold me the bra, without calling the bra police, thank goodness. My boobs are increasing at a rate of knots – from 38C to 38F, already – and I am spending rather a lot on bras. But quite frankly I need to feel good and I hate the thought of my boobs sitting slackly either side of my bump.' CharleyF

Toxic foods and drink

It often turns out that the very thing you crave has a big label slapped on it saying: 'Pregnant women: hands off!' Well, sometimes it can feel like that. Is it OK to eat smoked salmon? What about mozzarella? And Greggs' sausage rolls? So much of the advice given to pregnant women is conflicting, and little short of terrifying. The French don't say no to wine and liver pâté, so why should we? But it's hard to be casual when there is so much at stake. Some women prefer to draw their own limits: 'My view, while I was pregnant, was to eat and drink what I liked in moderation, as I figured that's what people have done since the beginning of time and before we had doctors who told us what we couldn't do.' Others find it easier to go cold turkey until the end of their pregnancy: 'I made my husband go out after my daughter was born and find a shop with Stilton and bring me some into the recovery room.'

Caffeine Some women go off coffee when they become pregnant, so caffeine is less of a concern for them, although it is also found in fizzy drinks, tea and chocolate. Too much caffeine has been linked to an increased risk of miscarriage, cleft palate and low birth weight. But small amounts are not thought to be harmful. No more than four average size cups of instant coffee (three if it's fresh), or six cups of tea a day. Or you could try a Mumsnet tip: 'If you are trying to cut back on tea when you are pregnant, try red bush herbal tea. It's naturally caffeine-free but still has the richness of ordinary tea, plus you can have milk in it.' Remember, it's not for ever: once you've had the baby you will probably go back to snorting espressos just to stay awake beyond the six o'clock news.

Alcohol Ideas change about how much alcohol, if any, is acceptable for pregnant women to drink. In 2008, Government guidelines went from suggesting that one or two drinks once or twice a week was fine, to recommending total abstinence. Nobody is in any doubt that heavy drinking over a long period of time is very bad for foetal health – it can cause serious birth defects, including foetal alcohol syndrome, a term used to describe a number of serious foetal abnormalities like brain damage, abnormal facial features and growth deficiency. But many believe the occasional drink probably does no harm. The reality is that many women don't know that they're pregnant for the first few weeks and carry on drinking during that period of their baby's development with no apparent ill effects. As long as you moderate your drinking as soon as you realise, it's extremely unlikely that your baby will be affected. 'I drank Guinness through both my pregnancies and it put a good head on my breast milk,' claims one mum.

Toxoplasmosis and listeriosis

Toxoplasmosis is an infection caused by a parasite most commonly found in raw or undercooked meat, unpasteurised milk and cheeses and cat poo – so you are best off not eating any of them! It can also be caught through contact with lambing, so if you regularly hang out with the local shepherds, you might want to avoid this too. In fact, you can get toxoplasmosis from anything that grows in the ground or eats plants from the ground. Infection in pregnancy is rare but it can lead to serious complications including miscarriage, birth defects and stillbirth. You can minimise your chances of catching it by avoiding unpasteurised products, washing all fruit and vegetables and cooking your food thoroughly. Wash your hands well after handling raw meat and make sure that someone else changes the cat litter tray (hurrah!).

'I was concerned about toxoplasmosis because we have two cats and they used a litter tray. So when I had my routine blood tests I asked to be tested for it. The test confirmed that I'd had it before my pregnancy. I don't know when, where or how I caught it, but a lot of people catch it in childhood. The symptoms are hard to spot – many people don't get any and if they do, they are flu-like. Once you've had it, you can't get it again – so, if you're worried, have a blood test; at least it might put your mind at rest. *Pamela1*

(continued)

Listeriosis is a relatively rare bacterial infection that is transmitted through foods and can make you sick at any time, but pregnant women are particularly susceptible. Symptoms are flu-like and, if not treated, can lead to premature labour or miscarriage. High-risk foods include undercooked meat, eggs, shellfish, bagged salads, pâtés, and unpasteurised dairy products, especially soft cheeses such as feta, blue-veined cheese and Camembert. So pretty much anything you might fancy, then. 'You can eat shellfish if it is thoroughly cooked and piping hot all the way through,' says one mum. 'The same goes for everything really. No piping hot food can contain listeria. And hard cheeses are all safe too.'

Food hygiene is an important factor. Sheep are also carriers, so once again, no hanging out with any woollies while you're pregnant. And avoid the cut-price sushi cabinet at your local Tesco Express on a Friday night. Although that's good advice for life, not just pregnancy.

Peanuts The jury is still out on whether or not eating peanuts while pregnant increases the risk that your baby will be born with an allergy. Some studies suggest that avoiding peanuts may actually increase the risk of allergy, but there is no conclusive research either way, so it's as clear as mud. Nevertheless, Government advice remains that women should avoid peanuts and peanut products in pregnancy if there is a history of allergies in the family. 'When I was pregnant, we didn't have the same warnings, and I have a nut-allergic child, which is certainly worth a bit of pain to avoid,' says a mum. Our best advice is to keep abreast of the latest research and recommendations from the Food Standards Agency (www.eatwell. gov.uk) and NHS Choices (www.nhs.uk).

Liver It's not everybody's favourite food, but pregnant women with a taste for liver are advised to curb their cravings and avoid it. Liver and liver products are a rich source of vitamin A which, in excess, can harm your unborn baby.

Oily fish Experts advise that pregnant women eat no more than two portions of oily fish a week (for example, mackerel, trout or fresh tuna) or more than four tins of tuna, due to risk of contamination with environmental pollutants.

Marlin/shark/swordfish These are all to be avoided during pregnancy due to risk of contamination with heavy metals such as lead and mercury. They are also highly poncey.

What supplements should I be taking?

Folic acid You are encouraged to start taking folic acid as soon as you decide to become pregnant, and to continue taking it for the first three months of your pregnancy. It can reduce the chances of your baby developing a neurological defect such as spina bifida. It is found in green vegetables (for example, asparagus, broccoli, sprouts and spinach), wholegrain cereals and fortified breakfast cereals, but it is recommended that you take a daily supplement rather than eat 20 bowls of Coco Pops a day.

Iron Pregnant women often need extra iron to keep up their levels of haemoglobin (red blood cells) which carries oxygen around the body. If you are feeling tired, and worn out it could be that you are iron deficient; the placenta gives the baby what it needs first, leaching it from your blood. You are more likely to become anaemic if you are pregnant with multiples, a vegetarian or if you have been vomiting from morning sickness. 'Try liquid iron supplements like Floradix or Spatone if the iron tablets that your doctor prescribed have left you constipated,' says a mum. 'An iron-rich diet, including spinach, tofu, red meat, dried apricots, eggs and dark chocolate, washed down with a juice rich in vitamin C, such as orange juice, should boost absorption. Don't take iron with caffeinated drinks because it will have the opposite effect.' And if you have a terrible urge to suck on old rusty nails, try a handful of apricots and a glass of orange juice instead.

Twins and Multiples: Buy One Get One (or Two, or Three) Free!

It's twins – what happened?

Identical twins (known as monozygotic) come from one fertilised egg that splits into two separate embryos. Each of these has its own amniotic membrane and umbilical cord, but they usually share a placenta, depending on when the egg divides. They are the same sex and will be hard to tell apart. Their conception is a lottery!

Non-identical or fraternal twins (dizygotic) develop from two eggs being fertilised at the same time, by different sperm. They each have their own amniotic membrane, placenta and umbilical cord. They tend to run in families and are more common among older mums or if you have had fertility treatment.

Two in the oven – the emotional and physical fallout

You thought that the moment the scanner asks, 'Do twins run in your family?' was the stuff of bad Hollywood movies. So when it happens to you, to suggest that you'll be shocked is an understatement. 'I wasn't planning even ONE baby let alone TWO!' shrieked one mum-to-be of twins.

'We found out at the 12-week scan that we were expecting twins. I promptly phoned in sick and went home to bed for the rest of the day – I went between shock, excitement and sheer terror.'

SuzyFelts

It can be horrifying and bewildering, but, believe it or not, the word from the 'multiple' Mumsnetters (a friendly and terrifyingly prolific bunch), is that it is the best thing that will ever happen to you. It's just that you don't know it yet.

Even though the number of multiple births is on the increase – in 2006, out of 741,067 pregnancies in the UK, 11,165 were twins – few parents are prepared for the bomb-dropping moment when they are told that they're getting rather more than they bargained for on the baby front. According to a National Birth and Motherhood survey, 92 per cent of women would rather do one child at a time, with only 7 per cent preferring twins. Children are scheduled to arrive years apart, not minutes.

'When I was told I was carrying my trio, I didn't stop crying once it sank in. I remember it hitting me while I was cooking the tea for me and my husband and getting two plates out and looking in the cupboard and realising I would soon have to have five plates on the table. I felt the blood drain from my face and I just sank down to the floor and sobbed, rocking back and forth looking like a true loony! I don't think I stopped for at least two hours, and the tea burned and the smoke alarms went off, and I just sobbed! I cursed and screamed!' Tripletsandtwins

It's natural to feel mixed emotions, not least guilt. 'Don't you feel half the time you're crying at the disappointment, but then crying even harder at what a bad person you are for feeling that way in the first place?' asks a multiple mum-to-be. What pregnancy gives you is time to settle into the idea. Better to find out now than in the delivery room.

The trick is to strike a balance – preparing yourself for what is to come, without terrifying yourself silly. 'I read so much and was told so many "facts" by well-meaning professionals that I ended up not coping very well during the first six months, as I was waiting for disaster to strike,' says a mother of triplets.

You'll also find that as a mother of multiples, you are an instant celebrity. Everyone will have something to say on the subject – 'Oooh you're in for trouble, how will you cope?' – and it's unlikely that they will make you feel any better. 'People often say things without thinking, so take it with a pinch of salt, because they probably don't have experience of what you're going through,' says a mother of triplets *and* twins.

Experienced mums of multiples are quite confident that although the early days will be bloody hard work, in the long run, you will have the last laugh over your friends who are popping a paltry one at a time:

'I found it quite hard to come to terms with the things I couldn't do as a mother of twins, and I wasted a lot of time and energy comparing myself bitterly to people with one baby. I would be wrestling my giant pram which didn't fit into coffee shops and staring with undisguised hatred at people dreamily sipping coffee with their tiny prams. I got over that though and started to concentrate on all the positives instead. There are things that are much harder with two babies but you will find a way round them. You do cope, you do get organised and you find a way that works for you. You get lots of support and admiration, which won't help you when it's 4 a.m. and one won't feed and the other has a dirty nappy, but it will bolster you through the early days when you need it most. Now I'd choose twins over and over. When they start playing together and don't need mummy's attention so much, that's when your friends with one baby will start to envy you.' Kitstwins

Three's a crowd: pregnancy with more than one

Aside from the emotional maelstrom, your pregnancy symptoms are, unfortunately, likely to be twice as trying. As one mum puts it: 'Having twins without being pregnant would be the best combination.' The wave of pregnancy hormones that washes over a pregnant woman is more of a tsunami with a multiple pregnancy, leaving increased symptoms of fatigue and nausea in its wake. As well as eating for three, you will probably be vomiting and sleeping for three.

As time goes on, you will start to wonder just how much extra weight a human belly can contain. But don't worry – it isn't just cake. If your twins are fraternal (non-identical), some of the extra weight will be an additional placenta and amniotic fluid; although this knowledge may not reassure you a great deal as you watch a map of the underground emerging on your abdomen as the weeks tick by.

To take some of the pressure off your pelvis, one Mumsnetter suggests getting down on all fours, resting your head on a cushion, and sticking your bum in the air. It is probably best to do this in the privacy of your own home, rather than in the Post Office or during the Family Service on a Sunday morning. Others recommend wearing a maternity support band (or 'belly bra'), but check with your GP first, who might want to refer you to a physiotherapist for further advice.

The aches and pains of pregnancy are hellish enough when you are carrying a solitary baby; when you are carrying more than one, the strain on your bones and ligaments can feel unbearable. And while your pregnant friends are shrieking with horror at the sight of ankles and hands pummelling the underside of their belly, you will be in a state of shock watching eight little limbs fighting for each bit of territory. You might find that one baby is more active than the other: 'The grouchy one would kick like mad if I lay on his side,' says one mum.

Extra pairs of hands (for that extra pair of hands): sources of support

On a practical level, there are support groups to help you cope with a multiple pregnancy and the years to follow. First, of course, there are Mumsnet's multiple birth forums, and as one Mumsnetter wrote: 'We'll be here to help you through everything and at least one mum on here will have advice for your situation.'

You can also try the Twins And Multiple Birth Association TAMBA (www.tamba.org.uk) and its network of registered Twins Clubs.

Financially, you will be entitled to child benefit for each baby. However, you will receive the higher 'firstborn' rate only for your first twin; the second will receive the lower, 'subsequent child' rate. There are no other additional benefits or grants for multiples, although if you have triplets or more, you may receive extra help from local social services. Other sources of free help include the charity Home-Start (www.home-start.org.uk), which has trained volunteers who can help families with pre-school-aged children for a couple of hours a week. Final-year nursery nurse (NNEB) students are always looking for placements. They cannot be left in sole charge of babies, but might be useful as an extra pair of hands, so you might want to contact your local college and ask about availability.

And remember, never turn down an offer of help.

BOGOF – what to buy for multiples

When it comes to shopping for equipment, some baby stores offer good discounts for multiples. There is a wide range of double and triple buggies that are constantly being updated, and even double slings. You might struggle to stay on top of the laundry, so it makes sense to ensure you have plenty of the basics – sheets, vests, sleepsuits, babygros – rather than spending on 'proper' clothes or outfits.

Instead of two (or more) Moses baskets, you might want to consider buying one cot that two babies can share. This will almost certainly last you through the Moses basket stage and maybe even longer. Some hospitals put twins together when they are born (feet to feet). One Mumsnetter advises: 'You need compact stuff and as little as possible when you have to fit in two of everything.'

Giving birth and what comes after

Multiple births have a tendency to come early – and quickly – so you will be monitored more closely than a 'singleton', which means more hospital visits and extra scans. The phrase 'high risk' will be bandied about rather a lot, but try not to let that stress you out too much. Water births and home births are usually ruled out – but that doesn't necessarily mean that your birth has to be a hospital drama. If your pregnancy is normal, there is no reason why your twins shouldn't be born vaginally: 'I had a quite easy and fairly "pleasant" birth with my twins. It was no worse than the birth of my son, except for the thought of having to push another one out. In the end, I didn't even feel the second one come out! I was worried I would need a C-section and was even tempted to ask for one so I didn't have the uncertainty, but am glad it all worked out naturally in the end.'

Many women successfully breastfeed twins, and some have successfully breastfed triplets. There are special feeding cushions for twins if you prefer to feed them at the same time. The main thing you will need though is lots of back-up and good advice. 'Breastfeeding my twins needed support and determination in the early days because they were small,' says one mother of twins. 'They were losing weight the first couple of days and I had no energy to feed. But soon they were feeding well and I didn't find it a problem at all. I would have hated to organise bottles.'

It's a steep learning curve but you will find your own ways of coping. And the rewards are double: 'Getting two lots of "I love you, mummy", two hugs and two kisses every night makes up for the extra work,' says a mother of twin boys. If Mumsnet is anything to go by, you might be surprised by the number of mums with twins who would like to go on and have another set. 'It's heaven and hell in one big bundle,' says one mum of twins. 'And you will never regret it.'

Looks Like It's Just You and Me, Kid – Being Single and Pregnant and How to Cope

Maybe you became pregnant as the result of too many chocolate-flavoured vodka shots and some naughty behaviour at a hen night in Romford (hopefully not your own). Maybe you never had a partner in the first place and chose to go it alone with a sperm donor. Perhaps your partner fled the country after you brandished the thin blue line in his horrified face. Or maybe your partner passed away during your pregnancy, or, for complicated reasons, he is just not able to be there for you now. It could be that you never want to see him again, or, more than anything, you want him to return. Whatever the reason for your situation, it's probably not the cosy domestic setting that you had imagined for the birth of your baby. But take heart; you might be a lone parent, but you are definitely not alone. One in four children in the UK now lives in a lone-parent family, according to the Office for National Statistics.

Working out what's best isn't easy, especially when your hormones are starting to wreak havoc. It's natural to feel, like other pregnant and single Mumsnetters: 'scared', 'broken-hearted', 'resentful', or 'guilty'. 'It can be a very lonely experience when you have no one to share the kicks with, no one to help you choose the names and the clothes,' says a mother whose partner left after she caught him cheating. You have no idea what the future holds, only the reality of your baby growing inside you.

Some fathers aren't meant to be, particularly if you are in a destructive relationship. So how will it feel loving a baby whose father you have no respect for? What if he tries to get involved? How much will he help? Will he help at all? Your feelings are all over place and it can be hard to think rationally. You might just want to run screaming through the streets and impale the errant father through the heart with your positive pregnancy stick. Now is a good time to try to step back from your emotions a little and seek wise counsel, whether from loyal friends and family or from someone more impartial, such as a counsellor:

'I gave up the fight at 12 weeks pregnant, changed all my phone numbers, so I could get on with my pregnancy alone. When the due date came and went without a word I knew in my heart that I'd done the right thing. I gave birth to my daughter on my own (well, with two midwives) and it was a wonderful experience. Try not to get into the "If only" frame of mind, although it's difficult not to feel envious. I had some counselling earlier this year and the best thing it taught me was to identify and concentrate on those things I could control.'

Divastrop

Whatever you do, don't feel guilty; it's a wasted emotion. 'Don't feel bad about choosing the wrong guy; you've had the courage to get rid of him – many women who have made the wrong choice don't,' says a woman who left her partner after she caught him having an affair. 'Take comfort from the thought that your tiny tot won't be in the middle of two warring parents.'

Whatever path you choose, the overall message from single Mumsnetters is that being pregnant and alone is 'very tough, but do-able' – and worth every struggle. 'It may be difficult dealing with him as the father of your child but it will all feel less painful when you're holding your beautiful baby.'

Bear in mind that although 'the man who got you pregnant may not be a good *partner* for you he may well be a good co-parent to his child', and while some men might put their knickers back on and run for the hills at the news of a pregnancy, others will rise to the challenge of their new role:

'Our son is now nearly four and sees his dad at least twice a week. His dad and I are on very amicable terms, though we are not and never will be a couple. Even if the father's initial reaction is, "Nothing to do with me," or worse, try to keep the door open.' Solidgoldbrass

Pregnancy is one of the most challenging stages of lone parenthood: 'I feel resentful of everyone who's got a nice supportive partner. Pregnancy yoga, which I started as a "be nice to myself" thing, is turning into a nightmare because everyone is talking about their husband massaging their feet and how they're wearing their husband's clothes. Sometimes I just want to scream.' Antenatal classes can be equally depressing when you end up partnering the teacher every week. 'I loved being pregnant,' says a single mum. 'The only thing was antenatal classes and all those happy couples.' There are some consolations of course: 'I was just sitting there thinking that half of them will be divorced in a few years!' One single mum laments: 'It would drive me mad, in every baby magazine I read, if I saw anything about fathers mentioned. Just silly things like: "Get your partner to give you a back rub."' But console yourself with the thought that most partners are probably just dribbling over their PlayStation and leaving socks with unimaginable stains down the side of the bed.

Of course, there are practicalities as well as emotions to deal with. Before the birth, you could start looking at your outgoings and work out what sort of budget you will have for you and your baby, and how you will cope financially once it's born. Will the father provide financial support willingly or will you have to fight for it? See www.csa.gov.uk for advice on what you are entitled to. In terms of the hospital visits and the birth do you have close friends or family who could go with you? If you know that you'll find it difficult sitting alone among couples as you wait for your scans, rope a friend in – most would be honoured. You might also want to ask your mum/sister/friend to be there for the birth. Or you might want to think about hiring a doula (for more on doulas, see p. 186), or even doing it without a birth partner – you can make your own rules!

Once the baby is born, prepare yourself for handsome husbands turning up at the hospital with flowers for their neatly coiffed wives, and new mums complaining that their partners only have four weeks off work. Remember that everyone has their problems, and most of the mums in perfect marriages are probably lying in bed fantasising about Colin Firth while the handsome other halves are drooling over their 19-year-old secretaries.

Overall, the feeling from single Mumsnetters is that 'things can get better':

'Once you've got over the shock (and sadness) of being a single mother, in practical terms, it's not that much more difficult. It's easier to get into a routine on your own. You don't have to answer to anyone else. You can have a close relationship with your baby with no third party to worry about.' Lizita

Post birth, could you stay at your parents' house or a friend's place for the first couple of weeks/months? If that works, you might want to think about booking your baby in for a return visit every so often, so that you can catch up on some sleep. Or you could invite your mum or another friend or relative you get on well with to stay for a few nights after the birth, to help you settle in to your new life.

The main message is: forget trying to be a superhero. Adopt the motto of a single Mumsnetter who survived: 'There's no shame in asking for help.' Make sure you discuss your concerns with your GP, community midwives, or health visitor, and let them know your situation. They will be able to advise you about any extra help that is available.

Gingerbread (www.gingerbread.org.uk) is an organisation for lone parents that can put you in touch with local people in similar situations; you might even find a group that meets up near you. Or Home-Start (www.home-start.org.uk) can also help: a volunteer can visit you at home on a regular basis, offering friendship and support. You can be referred via your GP or health visitor. And, of course, there's always Mumsnet's lone parents' forum (www. mumsnet.com/talk/lone_parents).

What worries some single pregnant mums is the thought that they might never find another partner: 'Will anyone want me with a baby? A relationship is the last thing I have time for right now but I'm thinking about the future and having someone to be with.' A reassuring voice replies: 'Anyone worthwhile will not be put off by the fact that you've got a child.' Another single mum agrees: 'I've been told there's nothing more off-putting than a single, childless woman desperately trying to track down a man to provide her with a child. At least if you already have a child you've got time to get to know prospective mates without thinking you need to hurry up and get pregnant quick!' According to one mum who was single throughout her first pregnancy, and is now pregnant again and in a steady relationship: 'To be honest, I am finding things harder this time round with a partner to consider. I liked the fact that before it was just down to me what name to choose, whether I wanted to find out the sex, how I would feed her. So there are some bonuses to doing it alone.'

'I'm now so stuck in my ways that I can't bear the thought of someone else messing up my routine and my way of bringing up my daughter. I actually like being a single parent.' Faeriemum

One Mumsnetter eventually got back together with her child's father for a Disney-style happy-ever-after:

'I found out I was pregnant a few weeks after my fiancé called off our wedding. I was gutted; he was gutted. But I was determined I wasn't going to have a termination. (I'd had one as a student and I didn't want to put myself through that again.) I had a good job and I decided he could be as involved as he wanted to be. We didn't speak for several months. We made contact again when I was six months pregnant and he

agreed to support the baby financially. In the end, he was there for the birth and stayed with me afterwards for a couple of weeks. He fell in love with our son from the start and visited every month (he lived 200 miles away), then every three weeks, then every other weekend. When our son was two and a half years old, we decided that we would give our relationship another go and have since married and are expecting our number two. I realise that this sort of happy ending might not happen for everyone but if anyone had told me when I was pregnant that we would end up here I wouldn't have believed them.' DaisysGotABigBump

So you might find that you actually meet bad-boy Daddy in 20 years on a beautiful Greek island and sail off into the sunset together in his private yacht. Or you might find, as one single mum did, that he comes back to try and burn your house down, big-bad-wolf style. Either way, there will be good times and bad times, and one consolation that will see you through all of them:

'I adore my daughter so much, I feel that would sustain me through anything.' Lucsnowe

HEALTH ISSUES

Morning Sickness (and Early Afternoon Sickness and Late Afternoon Sickness and Evening Sickness ...)

The first thing you learn about morning sickness is that it isn't the cheery sort of appetite-suppressing sickness that you experienced when you were too drunk to properly reheat that microwave fish pie, but is instead, 'This weird feeling of having two stomachs – one that wants to throw up and burp constantly, and another that is ravenous and thinking about food all the time.'

This is the time in your life when you feel you should be fuelling your body with the purest nutrition available, but instead you are unable to fight the urge to drive to the truckers' café on the A303 and order a full double breakfast bap to go.

'I can't remember the last time I ate fruit or veg other than potatoes,' says a mum in the throes of morning sickness. 'I just need stodge. My poor baby will be born in a pastry case.' Morning sickness is miserable, and it can lay any woman low for weeks, or even months. And the name is misleading – some women are more prone to evening sickness and for some poor souls it's an all-day affair. It affects about 70 per cent of pregnant women and it can hit at any time during your pregnancy (even the third trimester). But for most women, it usually begins after the first month and lingers until just after the third.

'The whole experience is so debilitating,' says one greenish mother. 'I can't remember what normal feels like.' It is incredibly draining, as you suddenly find you are a miserable heap on the sofa. And you are as picky as a wheat-free, dairy-free princess, refusing old favourites, turning up your nose at meal suggestions and certainly not above declaring: 'It has to be Volvic – Evian makes me feel sick.'

Why pregnant women get morning sickness is still an unsolved mystery. It could just be those pregnancy hormones again. You are more likely to get it if you are having a multiple pregnancy. According to an old wives' tale, if it's particularly bad, then you are going to have a girl, but sufficient evidence from Mumsnetters suggests that the only firm rule is that if it's particularly bad, you are going to have a baby.

'I am waiting until I can "go public" with this pregnancy, but meanwhile I am exhausted and feel sick constantly, and have to keep up appearances. My husband knows that his life would be in serious danger if he told me that I need to think positive and the sickness will subside. But he isn't above asking me why I don't smile. I try to explain that it's hard to smile when you're exhausted and sick, but I don't think anyone really understands unless they've been through it. Maybe when he has his next hangover – which will be in quite a while because we're so boring at the moment – I'll ask him to smile.' MrsTittleMouse

If you are truly off your food completely, then any food is better than none, even if it is only crisps and crackers. You may lose some weight, but no doubt you will make up for it when your appetite returns. (And you can keep taking a prenatal vitamin supplement; but take it with food, and at a time when you are least likely to vomit!) At the end of the day, even if you spend a few weeks living on Corn Flakes and Haribos, your baby will be all right. A baby is a very efficient sort of parasite. Take it from one mum who worried all through her morning sickness: 'Babies are amazingly resilient. I was convinced I had starved my daughter before she was even born. But, she was fine and, in the end, she was 3.5kg.'

For some women, morning sickness is the worst part of pregnancy. 'I dread being pregnant again,' says one woman. Never let anyone underestimate how you feel. 'I swear I am not having any more, for no other reason than how I feel at the moment.

I can do birth, sleepless nights, no problem. But this sickness ... NO THANKS!' says a second-time mum.

Some women do not actually vomit, but experience very strong nausea. Although feeling sick can be worse than actually vomiting, being sick isn't very pleasant either, especially if you are trying to carry on a normal life. As the sickness becomes routine (what fun), you will find some ways to cope. You can ask frequent-flyer friends to grab a handful of sick bags for you as a holiday souvenir, instead of your usual litre of duty-free grappa. One practical suggestion for public transport emergencies is: 'Take a plastic carrier bag everywhere you go, and line it with kitchen roll so the sick doesn't come out the holes at the bottom.' Or, you could be like this mother, and think on the spot:

'I had terrible sickness with all three pregnancies. With my first son I projectile vomited a litre of water mixed with ginger biscuits (fat lot of good they did!) all over my work desk, keyboard and monitor. It was so bad my boss told me just to bin the keyboard. With my daughter, I was driving along in the car and, out of the blue, I was violently sick all over myself, the windscreen, the dashboard and steering wheel. It came on so suddenly that I had to keep driving while retching everywhere. But the worst time was with my second daughter during the January sales. I hadn't felt sick that week so went shopping with my family. We treated ourselves to a Starbucks and I felt fine until we got to the car park. I knew it was going to happen, so I grabbed my handbag off the bag of the buggy. People stopped to watch me retch into my handbag. Then it started seeping out the bottom, steaming in the cold air. I took everything out of my bag and just dumped it in a bin.' Mummyvicky

If your morning sickness is so severe that you are unable to keep food or drink down and are vomiting several times a day, you might have hyperemesis (see p. 54) for which your doctor may need to prescribe medication. But for run-of-the-mill morning sickness, there is unfortunately no magic cure.

You can, however, take some steps to alleviate your symptoms. 'Lots of early nights' is a popular recommendation. 'You have to sleep when you can. If you have other children, nap when they do.' For fighting all-day nausea, eating 'little and often' seems to be the best advice: 'Don't worry about set meals, just snack all day long. Baby-food portions: literally a spoonful of rice or mashed potato per hour.' Heed the warning: 'Never get cocky and take normal swallows. You have to sip so little that you fool your body into thinking nothing's happening, but you have to do it all day long.' Eating something like a bowl of porridge last thing at night and an oatcake before you get out of bed in the morning might also help.

'Try to eat before you start to feel nauseous, otherwise it becomes a vicious circle. Try to distract yourself while eating, and make the experience as pleasurable as possible. Change the food you eat every day, if possible, so don't buy a lot of one thing. And don't worry – you may lose weight but your baby will be fine, and you'll soon put back those pounds.' Eulalia

Some women find that specific foods make things bearable; they might not stop the nausea completely, but will keep the worst of it at bay: 'I find high-sugar things work best,' says one mum – 'Lucozade, Haribo sweets, doughnuts ...' High-fat foods do the job, says another: 'I have to start the day with a fried breakfast, eat a fried-egg sandwich mid-morning and have a fry-up for lunch,' she writes. 'My colleagues are looking a bit sceptical because I am stuffing myself with food all day despite bleating on about how sick I feel.' One mum's advice is, 'It doesn't matter how unhealthy it is – just eat it if it makes you feel better!' You might find that you have put on two stone by the end of your first trimester, which is a bit depressing when your midwife cheerfully informs you that your foetus now weighs 10 grams, but anything is an option when you are fighting morning sickness.

You must keep drinking because dehydration is bad news both for you and baby; try a smoothie or soup to keep up your liquid intake. 'I found it easier to take tiny sips through a straw,' says one experienced pregnant mum. Another says: 'Fizzy water makes me burp and that seems to take away the sicky feeling.' Melon, sorbet and ice lollies – 'the colder the better' – all provide fluid. 'Ice pops have a kind of stomach-numbing effect but they dribble a little liquid into you, too. It does mean blue puke though.'

Food shopping might be a bit too much of an assault on the senses if you are in the grip of morning sickness, and no one wants the indignity of vomiting into their trolley in the fresh fish aisle at Sainsbury's. It is not unusual to consider giving up shopping and cooking altogether, so horrible is the experience. 'I struggled to get round the supermarket without retching, so in the end starting ordering online,' admits one mum. 'It might seem expensive, but I think it's worth it if it makes you feel less tired.' Ready meals will give a respite from the cooking smells, even if it is just for a few weeks.

A brisk walk in the fresh air would be a good tip, if only the air was fresh, and morning sickness hadn't turned your nose into a supersonic sniffer device. Pregnancy hormones endow you with the power of super-olfactory sensitivity, although this is not very useful in saving people's lives unless you happen to be an investigator for Transco. 'One of the worst things is changing my daughter's nappies,' complains one mother. 'Sometimes even the smell of people's breath makes my stomach turn,' says another. 'Bad smells always bring on a volley of gagging. A woman's perfume at the bus stop had me gagging in full view this morning.'

'Wear a polo-necked top – they make good smell-excluding face masks when required,' advises one mum. Some recommend sniffing something that you find strong, but pleasant, to take your mind off nasty pongs: 'As soon as you start feeling queasy, dig your nail into a lemon and have a good sniff,' recommends one mum, while another swears by spearmint: 'My friend who works at a health-food shop gave me spearmint essential oil to sniff. It smells gorgeous, and is like a talisman in my pocket.'

Some women swear by travel bands, or sea-bands, that work using the principles of acupressure (similar to acupuncture). Others argue for alternative and complementary therapies, such as hypnotherapy and acupuncture – even hardcore sceptics will be sticking pins in themselves after a few weeks of 24/7 nausea. Many recommend audiotherapy, such as a CD called *Morning Well* (a blend of music, frequencies and pulses that allegedly relieve symptoms). Homeopathic remedies you could try include Nux Vomica and Sepia.

You should avoid herbal remedies that may not have been properly tested on pregnant women; ask your doctor for advice if you are unsure. Commonly used herbal teas may relieve symptoms though – mint-based ones in particular – although, again, you should check they are safe for use during pregnancy before you start brewing.

In the meantime, there is not much you can do, but try to take things easy and tick the weeks off the calendar. Hopefully, once your first trimester is over, you will be shouting, 'WOO-HOOO my morning sickness is over!' your nausea will be forgotten and you will be able to tuck into platefuls of cream cakes and sausage rolls without fear that their valuable nutrients may not nourish your precious baby. Bon appétit!

Morning sickness: things you can try, in a nutshell

- Constant eating – little and often is the name of the game
- Sucking on boiled sweets – lollipops are popular and some brands are even marketed at pregnant women
- Ginger – ginger biscuits, ginger snaps, ginger tea, ginger sweets, crystallised ginger, the Gingerbread Man (if you can catch him); only be warned, 'Since I've had the baby I feel fine, but I feel waves of nausea whenever I see a bloody ginger nut!'

(continued)

- Travel-sickness type acupressure bands
- Hypnotherapy
- Acupuncture
- Audiotherapy
- Aromatherapy – sprays or oils
- A day at a health spa (worth a try)

'I never found any remedies which worked for the multitude of pregnancy ailments I have suffered except for a deep, warm bath, which cured everything – but only for the duration of the bath.'
Jasper

Note: with all alternative and complementary therapies, don't forget to check that they are safe to use during pregnancy.

Tiredness

There is something utterly, bone-crushingly exhausting about being pregnant. Your body is working round the clock in the first trimester, knocking together the crucial foundations that should bring your building project in on schedule. All you want to do is to sit back and let your body get on with it. Too bad then, that you have a job to hold down, money to earn and a home to keep clean. Did I mention a partner to keep happy? No, we're not living in the 1950s. In fact, that might have been easier, with only the dusting to do, a trifle to make and, perhaps, a fashionable new hair ribbon to buy.

Juggling a job, a baby on the way and, in some cases, the child you made earlier, is a significant challenge. 'I am 12 weeks pregnant and still so tired,' says one weary mum. 'My doctor signed me off last week because I am – literally – falling asleep on the job. It is also making me feel overwhelmed and tearful.' It can feel so bad, it's not uncommon to fear the worst: 'Before I had the pregnancy confirmed I was thinking of asking the GP if I had a terminal illness as I just feel so tired all the time.' It can be harder at the beginning if you haven't announced your pregnancy;

colleagues may assume it's a case of too much clubbing and that you need to pull yourself together. Even partners struggle to be sympathetic sometimes. 'I don't think he realises that pregnancy makes you tired. He'll only think it's an issue when I'm the size of a house, and that's way down the line.'

'I felt knackered for the whole of my pregnancy, and just had to take it as easy as possible, which was difficult with a toddler. I think that as long as your iron level is OK, you just have to rest as much as you can and accept that this is how pregnancy is. I can honestly say that from two weeks after the birth I felt much less tired than the whole of my pregnancy even though I was being woken up frequently for feeds.' Maxbear

'Trust your body,' advises one mum. 'If it's telling you to slow down, do.' No one is in any doubt that rest helps, it's just getting some that's the hard part. As one Mumsnetter explains: 'I spent most of my pregnancy half-woman-half-couch. I found the trick was to succumb when you can, then you don't fall asleep standing up, as I did a few times.' If you can find a handy snooze spot at work, use it: 'They used to tease me at work when I was pregnant with my daughter. There was a little box room off the toilets, and I would curl up in a chair and sleep there.' Another tip is to put your feet up on a few books or files under your desk. If you can get away with a nap at lunchtime, even if you're just slumped over the steering wheel in Morrison's car park, then grab the opportunity. And be creative with your annual leave if you've got any left: 'I used some of my annual leave and took every Wednesday off; it really made a difference.'

You will no longer feel embarrassed about what one Mumsnetter refers to as 'back-to-front-lie-ins' (in other words, early nights). In fact, by late afternoon, you will be positively looking forward to curling up under the duvet, even though pregnancy sleep is usually interrupted by frequent forays to the loo. 'I was falling asleep by about 8 p.m. for the first three or four months,' says one mum. 'I used to get waves of absolute exhaustion, like I'd been drugged. I'd be half-asleep at my desk, which meant I made lots of silly mistakes.' If you're lucky, your boss might be persuaded to let you work from home the odd day, just try not to sound as if you've just woken up if they call – even if you have!

A little, gentle exercise might help to perk you up. Keep drinking lots of water and review your diet. Make sure that you are eating well and getting enough of the right calories; lots of fruit, iron-rich vegetables, protein and slow-release carbs. Try not to give in to the urge to refuel on Mars bars as you will only get bigger dips (and hips) later. Supplements might also help. And, if this is your first child, lie in at weekends – while you still have the chance.

If you are looking after a toddler at home, you will need to come up with some tactics to get through the days. 'This is the start of them learning to share Mummy albeit with an unborn sibling!' It might be an ideal time to settle your toddler into pre-school or nursery. 'I enrolled my daughter in nursery two afternoons a week,' wrote one mum. 'I used to come home, set my alarm for two hours and sleep.' Call on family for help if they are nearby and arrange play dates with good friends: it will keep your toddler occupied and exercised, while you lounge on the sofa with a cup of tea and a biscuit or two. And remember: CBeebies is your friend: 'If your toddler is watching his favourite television programmes then he is probably happy – and a few weeks of watching more television than he should is certainly not going to have any long-term detrimental effects (that's my excuse and I'm sticking to it!).'

Mumsnetiquette: Pregnant with a toddler – how do you do it?

- 'When pregnant, I shared a book with my four-year-old showing him how big the baby was at each stage. By the time she was born he was so excited to meet her there was no jealousy.' *kazmumto3*
- 'Get your partner involved, taking your toddler to the supermarket or out to the park. Anything that gets them out the house and gives you a break.' *ceedee*
- 'Being pregnant, I avoid steep flights of stairs, even if that's where the kids' loos are. To avoid accidents, I take a travel potty with me wherever I go.' *olivebranch*

- 'My toddler talks and sings to my tummy, and even puts plasters on it.' *weathervain*
- 'LOADS of childcare!' *custardtart*
- 'If you're lucky enough to have a toddler who still naps, join them. Then get them to "help" you do all the housework you should have been doing when you both wake up.' *Biza*
- 'Get your toddler their own baby doll to practise with. This works for both boys and girls, and you can teach them how to look after it, like they are going to look after their new baby brother or sister.' *Munchpot*
- 'It helps if you know someone who is pregnant and also has a toddler so you can take turns to look after each other's little ones and get an occasional break.' *toodlepip*
- 'Towards the end of your pregnancy, arrange for your toddler to be looked after so that you and your partner can spend a long weekend together, eating, talking and sleeping without interruption.' *MoonRiver*
- 'Get your toddler to make a personalised present for the baby: decorate a babygro or make a picture for the wall of the nursery.' *pearlgem*
- 'Try to avoid big changes in your toddler's life around the same time that the baby is born: get things done now, or wait until the baby is a little older. Trying to get them potty-trained, settled at pre-school or out of the cot as well as coping with a new sibling is a recipe for stress all round. OFSTEDoutstanding
- 'I wouldn't advise taking a toddler to any of your scans. What could be a wonderful bonding experience can turn into a nightmare scenario if they discover bad news.' *ceedee*
- 'Think about the routine you already have with your toddler – and make any changes that you need to make now. Our son used to have bedtime stories in our bed before going to his own bed. We changed this, knowing the baby would be asleep in our room. Encourage your toddler's independence as much as possible, e.g. dressing themselves, getting bowls and cutlery out for breakfast, etc.' *puddle*
- 'When you're talking to your toddler about its new sibling, refer to it as "your baby", as in, "What will we do with your baby?" or, "Shall we get this for your baby?"' *Twiglett*
- 'CBeebies.' *Sallie*

Bleeding

Vaginal bleeding (or 'spotting') is one of the more frightening problems associated with pregnancy, but it is also a common one. Spotting is more frequent in the first trimester, but it can happen at any time. There are many reasons for blood other than the one that everyone fears – miscarriage.

'It was a nightmare in the beginning. I'd said goodbye to my baby so many times in my head, and then found I was still pregnant. The bleeding stopped at 12 weeks, and I didn't have any problems after that.' Oops

Lots of women experience implantation bleeding, which is light spotting, usually a week or two after conception, when the egg has been fertilised and implants into the lining of the womb.

It is also thought that some early pregnancy bleeding may be caused by hormonal changes at the time when you would normally have had your period.

'If you are not having cramps or pain, then it is likely to be implantation bleeding. It is very common and generally nothing sinister. I had spotting at around six weeks which lasted for almost three weeks, and thankfully all has been fine. I had an internal scan at seven weeks but they could not tell what was causing it. It's very stressful when this happens. Try to stay calm.'
Lemmiwinks

Another possible cause of vaginal bleeding can be cervical ectropion, or what used to be called 'cervical erosion'. This means that some cells that are more normally seen on the inside of the cervix have 'migrated' to the outside. These cells are rather delicate and may bleed when touched, for example during penetrative sex (you may also notice heavyish and possibly slightly bloody mucus). If you have been getting down to some serious jiggy-jiggy you may notice some bleeding if you are susceptible to cervical ectropion, but it is not an indication of anything untoward.

'I had cervical erosion during my last pregnancy. I was scared stiff as my previous pregnancy ended in miscarriage and I thought that was what was happening again, but the GP assured me that it was cervical erosion and explained that it's to do with the changes in the cervix and hormonal levels throughout pregnancy. I went on to have my son with no problems.'

BettyBatShapedSpaghetti

It's important that you tell your doctor about any bleeding. 'I had bleeding a lot through my first pregnancy, which turned out to be nothing, but I would give your midwife or maternity unit a ring to be on the safe side, or if only to give you peace of mind,' says one mum. Go to your doctor armed with details: make a note of how long you have been bleeding for, whether it is spotting or if there is a heavier flow, what colour it is (it could be anything from bright red blood to dark brown/blackish), if it has an unusual smell and if there is anything in the blood. If possible, take a sample to your doctor, either on a sanitary pad or in an unused plastic bag. Don't use a tampon or have penetrative sex until you get the all-clear from your doctor.

If you are miscarrying, the bleeding usually gets heavier and contains clots. You will probably feel discomfort in the abdomen or lower back; you might also feel weak or feverish. Vaginal bleeding coupled with abdominal and shoulder pain can be a sign of an ectopic pregnancy, which occurs when the fertilised egg implants outside the womb, usually in the Fallopian tubes.

'In my first pregnancy I had a small bleed and some spotting at around six to seven weeks. All was fine. At six weeks into my second pregnancy I had the same kind of thing and, sadly, this time it was a miscarriage. I don't want to sound like the prophet of doom because there's a good chance all will be well.' Spub

Light bleeding in the second or third trimester is also common, but again, it is still best to have it checked out because it could be symptomatic of underlying problems.

The Enemy Within (At Least That's What It Feels Like): Hyperemesis

Hyperemesis, meaning literally 'excessive vomiting', is the extreme version of morning sickness (see also p. 42). You know you have got it if you are vomiting several times a day, you are dehydrated (look out for dark yellow urine), you start to lose weight during your pregnancy and you have ditched your favourite handbag for a caretaker's bucket. Fortunately, it is not very common. Untreated, however, it could harm you or your baby, so it's best to get it checked out.

'I left it until nine weeks with my first child as I didn't really know what "normal" morning sickness was like, and ended up in hospital on drips for two weeks. Quite often, rehydrating the body will alleviate a lot of the symptoms. Tell the midwife exactly what you are eating and drinking and keeping down. If you just tell most doctors/midwives that you are being sick, they'll just tell you it is a feature of your pregnancy and it will wear off. You need to stress how bad it is. Unfortunately, mine didn't really go away until I'd had the babies, but on a positive note, I felt much better after the pregnancy than my friends who had sailed through!' Debsb

If that doesn't encourage you to go and see your GP, consider the potential implications for your marriage: 'I had severe hyperemesis and was in and out of hospital several times. I lost two stone and, when I finally started eating again, my insides had stopped functioning. I was all blocked up. My husband had to insert pessaries up my backside so I could finally poo again.'

If your hyperemesis is not too severe, you may be able to cope at home with the same remedies that folks use for regular morning sickness, which focus on getting you hydrated and keeping down enough fluids to keep you and baby healthy. Failing that, you may be admitted to hospital to be put on a drip and given an anti-emetic (a drug to minimise vomiting). Your urine will be tested for the presence of ketones to see if your body is in need of extra minerals which can be added to your drip.

Here's one Mumsnetter's recollection of the hyperemetic experience:

'I had hyperemesis from week five of my pregnancy, which included very strong aversions to most smells. My husband couldn't wear deodorant and I couldn't go to the supermarket because fresh fruit and veg smelled awful, and I would be sick. It may sound odd but the best times were when I was admitted to hospital as the loneliness of having to stay at home being so physically incapacitated was unbearable. I went through most anti-nausea drugs, most of which had horrible side effects, until I found one which worked. I came off it at 24 weeks and had a fabulous second half of my pregnancy. I didn't put on any weight until about 22 weeks but they kept telling me not to worry – the sickness was a sign of a very healthy pregnancy and I had a lot of scans to reassure me that everything was OK. I now have an exceptionally healthy baby so no harm was done. It's not conventional morning sickness and none of the usual remedies (ginger, etc.) helped at all – it does need proper medical intervention. It is miserable; there were days when I didn't think that I would make it through the next hour, let alone to the next day, and far less an entire pregnancy. Now I can say I love my baby more passionately than I could ever have imagined, but at the time of being ill it wasn't something I was able to focus on. I didn't cope very well at all until I got the medication I needed.' Harrysmum

Hormones and Weepiness

Fed up and pregnant? You're not alone. If PMT turns you into a snarling monster wanting to push your husband off a cliff for leaving the toilet roll facing the wrong way round, it will come as no surprise to discover that the rampaging hormones of pregnancy will possibly turn you into a hysterical banshee out of a Freudian case study.

'I'm nine weeks pregnant and way more emotional than I ever have been before. I was feeling dreadful the other night and cried when my partner gave me a blanket. Last night, we were watching *Gordon Ramsay's Kitchen Nightmares*, and I started sobbing when he told the chef that his meal was nice!' PocketTasha

Few of us bounce through pregnancy without occasionally feeling miserable. Tears will flow – sometimes for no apparent reason. 'I was very weepy until about 14 weeks, which really took me by surprise as I'm not normally like that,' says one mum. Another agrees: 'I spent most of my pregnancy crying at the drop of a hat. It was like nine months of PMT.' For some, this might be a red flag for antenatal depression, in which case, you should consult your GP. But for many, there is no need to despair; it's hormones on overdrive, and it's to be expected.

'There is a Kentucky Fried Chicken advert where one KFC bucket gets left outside in the rain, gets kicked, then finally gets impaled on railings, as the family sit inside eating out of another KFC bucket. I used to bawl over the poor bucket, and yes, my partner thought I was batso.' Louii

Sometimes, there is a specific trigger. A pregnant Mumsnetter admits to having sobbed because Waitrose didn't have the pasta sauce she wanted, another because a lone banana in the fruit bowl didn't have any friends. Certain songs can reduce you to floods ('Two words of "Away in a Manger" and I had to be taken away with a bag over my head!'), and even the most innocent of comments can sound like criticism ('My sister told me I was starting to waddle; she meant it affectionately, but I burst into tears and was still sobbing 20 minutes later'). But when you are a whirlpool of hysterical hormones there doesn't have to be a reason: 'I am tetchy with everyone and frosty with midwives who pat me knowingly. My husband thinks I've lost the plot.'

Those pregnancy hormones don't just make you blub like the big girl's blouse you are shoe-horning yourself into every morning, though. You are also probably worrying more than normal, and your natural and understandable worries will take on scary Godzilla-like proportions that stalk you in the middle of the night:

'I hate being pregnant. I worry all the time about every little thing possible, and feel that whatever I do there will be something wrong with the baby, or something terrible will happen. When I was pregnant with my first child, I felt like something terrible would happen to my husband, and that he would never get to see his baby. Now, pregnant with my second, I feel that something will happen to our first child. It's an awful feeling, and totally consuming.' Sweetbean

Mentally and physically, you are under a lot of pressure. It's stressful being in charge of an unborn baby 24/7. You're going through a period of huge change, and your hormones are fluctuating like the FTSE in the credit crunch. You have no idea what the future holds for you, or your partner. 'I went to see my boss as I am feeling a bit down at work, and I blubbed buckets,' a mum says. 'Poor guy. He had no tissues, so I was sat there wiping snot on the back of my hand, as I gulped for air and tried to explain why I was pissed off. I hate myself for being so emotional.'

The best advice is to just go with the flow (of tears) and let it all out. Everyone is forgiving of a pregnant bloater, sitting away in the corner sobbing into her godawful maternity jumper. 'Just go with it and have a good cry,' advises one mum. 'Don't bottle it up. Talk to your husband, or a friend who can give you a boost. It's perfectly normal to be affected by your hormones, and what you need is some support to get you through it.' And don't forget to stuff your handbag with a prodigious supply of tissues.

Cravings: She's Gotta Have It (But She Probably Shouldn't!)

You know you're pregnant when you eat a whole bar of chocolate without stopping to breathe. Oh, OK, so you did that pre-pregnancy. But now, to get the chocolate bar, your partner had to climb out of bed, dress and drive in the middle of the night to the nearest 24-hour garage. Oh, the lengths men will go to, to satisfy a pregnant woman's cravings. Long live cravings! Studies show that up to 90 per cent of pregnant women will experience a craving (usually for something sweet, but sometimes you might have a terrible urge to lick the damp floor of your shed), and more than half will go off at least one food so badly that they can't even look at it without wanting to heave. Cravings are usually most acute during the first trimester.

No one really knows why we get them, but it could be to do with the wild hormonal changes during pregnancy; the same hormonal changes that leave some women with a strange metallic taste in their mouth. Mumsnetters have admitted to having yearnings for marinated anchovies, steak fat, strawberries dipped in coleslaw and washing powder (note that some of these are OK to indulge; others are not). Sometimes the desire can be overpowering: 'I'm a vegetarian but I think I can smell one of those bad little burger vans calling me.' Sadly, there is usually nothing glamorous about cravings. They are rarely for pomegranates or sugared almonds: 'I used to crunch ice cubes and went through a huge bag from the supermarket one hot afternoon.'

It's not only about what you want, but when you want it. Usually, 'Now'! And just like a fried breakfast after a night on the tequilas, the need to have whatever it is becomes ferocious. 'I had to have a banana in the middle of the night. My partner woke up and muttered about being in bed with a ruddy chimp.' The quantity required is often as astonishing as the urgency: 'My craving was fizzy cola-bottle sweets. I used to get through bags of them a day. The paper shop started making bags up for me before I even got there.' Manners also go out the window: 'I wanted milk so badly I walked to the local shop, but couldn't wait until I got home, so – very embarrassingly – chugged a good pint in the street from a two-litre carton.'

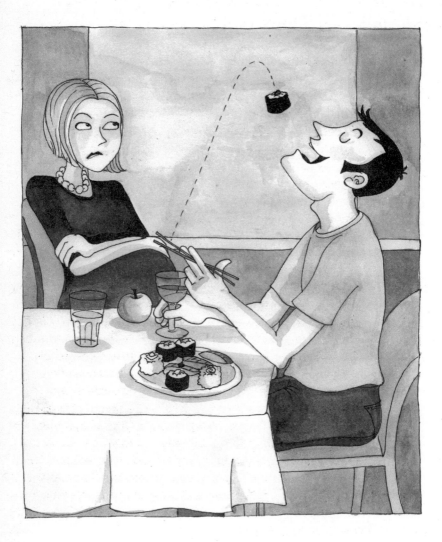

'My once healthy diet went to pot in the first 20 weeks. Forcing myself to eat good things just made me feel worse, so I went with what I felt like and figured the baby would get what it needed. I also took multivits.' BigBertha

One theory is that certain cravings may be meaningful. So, if you are craving meat, for example, it may mean that your body needs protein. This provides you with a handy justification to explain yourself to any bystanders with the virtuous claim, 'Clearly the baby needs a Müller Corner/White Chocolate Magnum.'

This approach does not really work though if you have the urge to gnaw off bits of a bicycle tyre. 'I can't get enough of the smell of rubber and I'm even tempted to steal one of my daughter's dummies to suck and bite on,' one mum confessed, but no, she's not craving contraception. She has a food disorder known as 'pica' (from the Latin word for magpie, a bird that will reputedly eat anything). Pica can affect pregnant women, making them crave non-food substances such as soil, paper, toothpaste or, brace yourself, poo. 'With me, it's synthetic bath sponges,' one woman says. 'I tear them into bits, then chew them. My husband refused to believe that this was a proper craving during my first pregnancy, but this time he just buys them without comment.'

If swallowing your craving – such as washing powder or plasticine – is unwise, shoving your snout in a trough of the stuff might do the trick. 'I remember making excuses to go to the stationery cupboard at work when I was pregnant, as I loved sniffing the rubber bands,' says a sufferer. Others have found themselves touring the aisles of Halfords or Wickes, nuzzling wellies: 'I used to get the hump with my son if he forgot to bring his PE bag home from school every night because I wanted to sniff his plimsolls.' But if you can't lay your hands on a pair, a hot-water bottle will do just as well: 'It's heaven. I sit and sniff it while watching telly of an evening.'

Safe Medicines and Home Remedies

What is and is not a safe medicine for pregnant women is one of those grey areas, so it's best to tell your doctor about any medication you are taking as soon as you think you might be pregnant. Some women, who, at one time, would have quite happily hoovered up a line of cocaine on a Saturday night, come over all puritanical during pregnancy, refusing to touch any medication whatsoever. They feel it's preferable to sit out skull-splitting headaches rather than run the risk of their child being born with three heads and five tails. But thankfully, there are medicines that have been approved for use during pregnancy, so that you don't have to retire to your chamber with nothing but a wet flannel (though of course you can always use that excuse if you fancy it).

Having said that, official NHS advice is: 'Generally, you should not take any medicines while you are pregnant.' So you should certainly consult your GP or midwife before you pop any pills – even before taking herbal teas and nutritional supplements.

The problem with the safety of medication during pregnancy is that it is not generally allowed to trial drugs on pregnant women, the ramifications of buggering about with foetal development being rather serious for drug companies. For this reason, very few medicines are 'licensed for use during pregnancy', and our knowledge about the effects of drugs on foetal development tends to be from retrospective studies on women who have either taken medication before knowing they were pregnant, or for whom medication was the only option.

But the important message here is not to put on a brave face if you're feeling lousy; call your doctor and see if they have anything in their black bag that's OK for you to take. You don't want to run the risk of your symptoms developing into something more serious.

Urinary tract infection (UTI)

Painful enough when you're not up the duff, UTIs can be particularly trying when you are juggling some of the other joyous side effects of pregnancy. Cystitis, the most common form, tends to creep in during pregnancy because pregnancy hormones cause the tubes from your kidneys to your bladder to relax, so your urine flow slows down, giving the bacteria longer to multiply. Symptoms include a need to pee frequently, pain or a burning sensation when you pee and cloudy or smelly urine that might contain blood. You need to visit a doctor to get it diagnosed and sorted out with an antibiotic approved for use during pregnancy. It might help to take a urine sample with you. Untreated, a bladder infection can lead to a kidney infection, which is more of a threat to mother and baby.

One seasoned sufferer advises: 'Drink shed loads of water on a daily basis. Steer clear of tea, coffee, alcohol and fizzy drinks. Wear 100 per cent cotton underwear and stay away from tight clothes. Even sleep without something on your bottom half. Don't use bubble bath and soap, only warm water to wash your bits. Empty your bladder fully before and after getting jiggy.' You could also lean forward on the loo to empty your bladder totally. Wipe from front to back to reduce the chance of transferring organisms from the anus or vagina to the urethra and bladder. Some people swear by drinking cranberry juice or lemon barley water. Others prefer live yoghurt or onions, garlic and chives – all traditional remedies. If that doesn't sound tempting, you could try another Mumsnet tip: 'Sit in a warm bath, drink masses and pee in the water. I know it sounds gross but it really helps the pain.' Just don't try it if your husband is sitting on the loo seat next to you, recounting his work problems.

Hay fever

Sneezing with a growing baby sitting on your bladder is no fun at all. Neither are the runny nose or itchy eyes that come with hay fever. Nasal congestion is more common during pregnancy as a result of the hormone oestrogen, so your symptoms might be worse. Be particularly wary of modern antihistamines (such as loratidine and cetirizine), which haven't been given the all-clear for pregnant women. Some of the old-fashioned antihistamines (such as chlorpheniramine) can be used after the first trimester – but with caution. Saline nasal sprays and eye drops are perhaps a better option, and they have the added bonus of being free on

NHS prescription during pregnancy. If you haven't used eye drops before, try a little at first as some people are allergic to them. Or you could follow this mum's tip: 'I can vouch for Vaseline in the nose. Keep it with you and re-apply.' As always, discuss your options with your doctor before taking anything.

'I keep the bedroom windows closed during the day, otherwise I wake up in the morning after a night of breathing in pollen which has drifted in.' Giraffeski

Fever

During the first few months of your pregnancy a big jump in your body temperature can, occasionally, cause birth defects. It is usually the sign of an infection and should be reported to your GP pronto if it is running above 37.8 degrees Centigrade. Paracetamol can be used in moderation. A cool bath or shower and changing into light clothing can help to bring your temperature down, as can sucking on a Magnum (the ice cream, rather than the firearm, which is to be discouraged for health and safety reasons).

Coughs and colds

Colds can drag on during pregnancy as your immune system is suppressed to stop your body from rejecting your baby. There's no medication really on offer for colds during the first trimester, but Mumsnetters recommend hot water with lemon and honey, and, as always, good nutrition. Some cough mixtures are safe for use later on in pregnancy, but always check the label and speak to a GP or pharmacist before using these. Cough sweets (but again, check the label) or even plain old boiled sweets can sometimes help. Rest, as always, and keep your head elevated with some pillows while you are lying down. 'Hot blackcurrant squash always seemed to make me feel better,' says one mum. Although traditional essential oil remedies for colds (juniper, eucalyptus and pine needle oils) might seem safe for use during pregnancy, they are not recommended, and should be avoided.

Headache

You may be feeling more headachy than usual because of all the hormonal changes going on, which will make you miserable enough, without having to think twice before opening your medicine cabinet. Nevertheless, you should avoid aspirin – which has been linked to miscarriage and neonatal heart defect – unless prescribed by your GP for a particular medical condition.

Paracetamol are out for the first trimester, but you can try gentle exercise, drinking plenty and not waiting until you're starving hungry before you eat. Your ligaments are soft and your spine is curving to accommodate a growing baby, so sitting and standing properly will help to stave off aches and pains. Other helpful hints: 'I had headaches at around 18 weeks in my last pregnancy and they stopped when I got some iron tablets,' says one mum. 'Avoid tea – it really helps.' Oh yes, and find time for some quiet rest – you haven't heard that one before, have you? Tell your doctor immediately if you are experiencing what feels like a migraine as this can be a sign of pre-eclampsia. If you've never had one this might be hard to spot, of course, but suffice to say, if you've got an unusually throbbing pain, with sensitivity to light, sound and movement, visual disturbances and possibly a feeling that your head is actually going to break in two, it sounds like a migraine.

'I had never had a migraine until my first pregnancy, and then had a couple of whoppers with flashing disco lights before my eyes. I didn't think to tell the midwife or doctor but later on I got pre-eclampsia, and they were definitely related. However, I think headaches in general are quite common in pregnancy, so don't leap to terrible conclusions, but it is worth mentioning to your midwife and getting your blood pressure checked as soon as you can.' Bun

Some Mumsnetters swear by osteopathy or acupuncture for recurrent headaches that no amount of brisk walks or even paracetamol will shift. As always, make sure you use an experienced and registered practitioner. Some may prefer to wait until you are out of your first trimester before giving you treatment.

Homeopathic remedies

Some Mumsnetters, desperate for something safe to ease their pregnancy symptoms, become devotees of homeopathic remedies. Derived mostly from plant and mineral sources, these remedies are massively diluted in water or alcohol, and some people claim that they are useful in treating all sorts of conditions. Others claim they are effective only in quashing a healthy, empirically based rationalism about the need for a scientific basis to medicine. But who's going to argue with a pregnant woman with a headache?

Note: approach homeopathic remedies with the same caution as anything else in the medicine cabinet during pregnancy and consult your doctor first. If you want to use them during labour, ask your midwife first. And remember that although Rescue Remedy might be effective, if you find you are drinking 80 bottles a day that's because it's preserved in 27 per cent grape alcohol. Stick to the recommended dose of a couple of drops in a mug of water.

Cimicifuga To calm you down.

Nux Vomica For indigestion, heartburn, stomach pain and constipation during pregnancy. 'Try this for morning sickness,' says one mum. 'It's not a complete cure, but it makes you able to function normally.'

Sepia For poor circulation, nausea, constipation, pains in the cervix and rectum and a general feeling of sluggishness. (Sounds like a must for a pregnant lady.)

Exercise – What to Do (and How Much Is Too Much?)

'I'm 11 weeks and feeling fat. For the last six weeks I have eaten all the time, otherwise I'd feel sick or get a headache. I don't know if I'm feeling fat because of all the food or because of the baby. Given it is only the size of a jelly bean, I expect it's the cake and chocolate. What sort of exercise are other people doing? I used to be really fit but I haven't done anything, except walking, for about four months. I don't want to turn into a huge fat unfit blob, but I care about the baby more than my figure.' Izzzie

Some people love it, some people loathe it, but we all know that exercise is good for us. Or most of us do: 'Forget the gym. It's not like you're going to get to the gym once the baby is born, you may as well give up now. Exercise is overrated. Sleep, on the other hand, is to be treasured.' That's one view, but the consensus is that now is not the time to hang up your trainers and settle into the sofa like a bear in hibernation. Unless, of course, you are in a high-risk category and under doctor's orders to rest. Or if you are a bear – in which case, hurrah! You'll give birth in your sleep.

Even if you weren't particularly fit before you conceived, keeping up your strength and energy levels will help immensely during your pregnancy, labour and after-the-birth life as a busy mum. Remember: you're not ill or dying; it just feels like you are.

Don't worry if you are in your sixth month and the only exercise you have considered is a few rounds with your pelvic floor when you suspect things are getting a bit slack. Start now and your body will thank you later. Staying active will help keep stiffness, sickness, weariness, bloating, constipation and those extra pounds at bay. It will also help circulation and prevent varicose veins. You might have admitted defeat in the battle against cellulite some time in the late 1980s, but varicose veins and a vagina around your knees are definitely *not* very yummy mummy.

Even if you are incredibly fit, exercising for two is different. Oh to be a carefree gym bunny again, wowing the boys as you pound the jogging machine in your skimpy unitard. Now your body is working harder than ever before; just climbing a set of stairs puts extra demands on your heart which is busy pumping blood to uncharted parts of your belly. So, take it steadily, listen to your body and use common sense.

Studies show that even vigorous exercise doesn't increase the risk of pre-term delivery, but there are precautions you can take. For starters, if you've never so much as run for a bus, now is not the time to start training for the next 10K charity race; on the other hand, if you've been used to exercising, unless your doctor advises otherwise, you can carry on – with small amendments. Whatever you do, don't exercise on an empty stomach. Dress appropriately in a well-fitting bra that gives you support (you don't want to have anyone's eye out). Be kind to your joints, they're soft right now due to changes in your hormones. Wear the right shoes and if you're going to continue to run, try not to run on hard surfaces and avoid hills. Keep cool when exercising. Also stay out of saunas, steam rooms and hot tubs post workout. And know when to stop: grunting, breathlessness and a heavy sweat are all warning signs that you are pushing yourself too hard (and looking a bit scary). If in doubt, wear a heart rate monitor.

If the hardcore aerobic stuff isn't your style now that you're carrying extra baggage, or if you've never exercised much at all, it's still worth investing some time in gentle walking, swimming aqua aerobics or antenatal yoga, all of which are easy on the body. 'Swimming is worth it just to feel weightless,' suggests one mum.

Stretch Marks

The French for stretch marks is *les marques disgracieuses*. Enough said. The medical term is *striae gravidarum* and if you haven't seen them before (they don't often appear in *Vogue* modelling shoots) then just imagine: 'the impression of being clawed by a savage tiger' or even 'a wrinkled elephant's scrotum'.

Stretch marks appear when the skin is 'stretched', for example by putting on five stone in as many months (ahem). The middle layer of your skin (the dermis) is made from strong interconnecting fibres, which normally allow your skin to stretch as your body changes shape: but sometimes, these fibres are over-stretched and become thin, and some may break. Where they break, the blood vessels that lie underneath your skin show through, which is why stretch marks first appear red in colour.

Stretch marks usually appear on the breasts, stomach, and thighs. 'It looks like someone has drawn on me in red pen,' shrieked one distraught mum. If you haven't got them, don't start boasting yet, as they tend to appear in the last three months of pregnancy. And in some cases in the last week (rumour has it that is why celebs have C-sections a few weeks early – to avoid a sudden nasty outbreak of stretch marks on the front of *Grazia*).

'I cringe when I think about how long into my pregnancy I patted myself on the back that I had no stretch marks, only to find one night when undressing at my mum's (she has a low-level light in one of the bedrooms) that they were all hiding under my bump where I couldn't see them. It looked like someone had painted a roadmap on my stomach.' SueW

Or even after you've given birth ...

'I didn't have a single stretch mark all the way through my pregnancy. I was so proud that my tummy would return to normal! Gave birth, looked down ... and I was covered in the sodding things. I have a pic of me that was taken a few days before I had my baby – there was no way they were hiding anywhere – and then, wumph, there they were. I was not impressed, but I did get a scrummy, yummy little baby so I say the swap was OK. Just don't think I can ever wear a bikini again and I'm only 20.' Charlotte121

Around 75–90 per cent of women get stretch marks during pregnancy: 'I had flames rising out of my pants – and not in a good way.' 'My stretch marks are HORRIFIC,' chirps another mum. 'I have a massive one on my fanjo area. It looks like I have been hit with an axe.'

But can anything be done to prevent them? 'I faithfully massaged nutritious oils into my tummy every day during pregnancy but still ended up with enough stretch marks to leave me with a postnatal concertina tum. And, as if that weren't bad enough, I have stretch marks at the tops of my thighs and around my sides – really bad ones, like I've never seen before,' says a disconsolate Mumsnetter.

Before you start investing in expensive oils, look to your mother. Some studies have shown that you're more likely to have them if they occur in your family: 'If you're gonna get stretch marks, you're gonna get them and there's absolutely sweet FA you can do about it!' What oils and lotions can do is to make your skin feel softer; they retain moisture, and massage is good for your circulation. If your tight skin feels itchy, try after-sun lotion with cooling agents. Stretch marks will not miraculously disappear after the birth, but they will lighten, turning a silvery colour; this is because the red blood vessels beneath the skin slowly contract and the fat shows through instead. Sexy, eh? Some women consider them a 'badge of honour'. Others consider them more a badge of horror.

'I had the most dreadful stretch marks with my first son. My tummy looked like red zebra stripes all over, from about an inch above my navel to just above my pubic bone. I found them very upsetting – pregnant women in magazines never looked like they'd been whipped. They've faded away now and, while my tummy still looks pretty grim, I would never show it off in public anyway, so they don't really bother me now.'

Marthamoo

Where stretch marks are concerned, there isn't a lot you can do except to accept that they are just part and parcel of bringing babies into the world. As one Mumsnetter wryly noted: 'The only miracle cure is the air brush.' While another's partner had all the right lines: 'My stretch marks did bother me until one day my husband said, "Why do they bother you? They're marks that show you carried our babies. They're beautiful."' Or, as another mum puts it: 'If a few stretch marks is what it takes to have a beautiful little miracle of my own, then bring it on!'

Varicose Veins

Varicose veins are veins that have become swollen, enlarged and sometimes bumpy and lumpy. You may have noticed them on your granny's legs, because they are quite common in the elderly (and more than twice as common in women than they are in men).

They are yet another of those jolly irritating (and painful) symptoms of pregnancy that no one tells you about beforehand. Like stretch marks, they tend to run in families and are most likely to appear on the lower legs and – we're sorry to say – vulva, but you can also get them on your thighs and around the anus. Symptoms can range from a mild aching to a throbbing or severe pain. In some cases, the skin over the veins is dry and itchy. And it will look like you have the Zambezi river snaking up your inside leg.

The job of your veins is to get blood uphill and back to your heart and this anti-gravity work needs little valves to stop the blood flowing backwards. When these valves don't work so well, blood starts to pool up inside the veins, making your legs look like those of a little old lady who spends too much time queuing in the Post Office.

This is happening because you have more blood than usual flowing around your body, and a big fat baby pressing down on things. Your body is also prioritising blood flow to the baby, rather than to your chubby old pins. Pregnancy hormones have sent your vein walls into a stupor. As the veins expand, the valves that control the flow of blood stretch and don't always close completely, so blood collects.

The good news is that varicose veins present no risk to your baby, other than the shame of having a mummy sporting unattractive support stockings.

Varicose veins in your legs

Speak to your GP about your varicose veins. You may be prescribed support stockings to help with the aching feelings, and these should also stop the veins from getting larger. You are advised to avoid standing and walking about for long periods – so take the weight off your feet whenever you can, and get a comfy footstool to raise your legs too.

'I had varicose veins before I became pregnant but they did get worse with each pregnancy. They didn't hurt very much but were horribly unsightly. I did wear support stockings but found them more uncomfortable than the veins themselves, and they took ages to put on. In the end I decided not to bother with them. I did try to keep active – no standing around – and I always elevated my feet when sitting down. When my fourth child was a year old, I had them removed and my legs look reasonably OK again now.' Robina

However, while you don't want to spend hours walking and standing, flopping on the sofa all day is bad news, too – you need to keep active in order to keep your circulation going. Gentle exercise is the best thing, so a leisurely stroll is good – just not a trek across the Himalayas. Swimming is also good and can feel lovely if the size of your bump is weighing you down (literally).

Other tips are to avoid crossing your legs when sitting, try not to lift anything heavy and wear loose clothing and an abdominal support to help take some of the weight off your legs.

It is rare, but varicose veins can lead to complications. If you have pain in veins that doesn't disappear when you rest, there is a possibility that it could be phlebitis, or deep vein thrombosis (DVT), a rare but potentially life-threatening problem. If you are concerned, always speak to your midwife or GP.

Varicose veins in your legs should gradually resolve themselves after the birth, although they may well reappear in subsequent pregnancies. If they don't disappear, there are some surgical approaches that might help, including foam and laser treatments and complete removal of the affected veins. Surgical treatments will usually only be considered after you've have had your last baby, and if your problems are purely cosmetic, you may not be able to get treatment on the NHS. If you know varicose veins run in your family, the best thing would be to take preventative measures, such as maintaining a healthy weight.

Tiny spider veins, which can make it look as though you are wearing a mauve fishnet body stocking, usually disappear after delivery. If they don't, they can be treated by laser, causing them to collapse and disappear.

Vulval varicose veins

Vulval varicose veins may look a little like tiny blood blisters or you might feel them as little lumps inside the vulva area. Or, to put it more bluntly: 'I had a fanjo like a bunch of grapes when I was pregnant with my daughter, and God they ached. For the last six weeks I was waddling along clutching my fanny.' Ahem.

Before you do anything, talk to your midwife or GP. Most treatments will focus on relieving the discomfort by applying gentle pressure to the area, so support pants and old-fashioned giant sanitary pads are probably your first port of call. There are support pants that are made and marketed to pregnant women for just this purpose. They're probably not stocked in your local branch of Ann Summers, but your GP may be able to advise you further.

'The best info I can supply is: buy a pair of the big support pants and wear them with a big sanitary pad. This will take the pressure off. When they are very painful, Anusol relieves any discomfort. Resting is the only other thing that helps, lying flat with your feet up.' Thailand

'I used to sit on a bag of frozen peas wrapped up on a tea towel – that helped. Also, aloe vera gel can help – leave it in the fridge and put it on a big fat sanitary towel and pop that in your knicks. Then sit down and put your feet up.' Tommy

'What you need is a cold pack and a sanitary towel like six mattresses.' Pelvicfloornomore

'The NCT sell soothing gel pads that you can put in the fridge.' Buckets

Varicose veins should not present any major problems to giving birth. It's normal to be a bit worried that they might erupt, but that doesn't tend to happen: 'My labia were like two tennis balls, but to my profound relief they didn't burst or explode and went back to their normal size.' Post birth, they should resolve themselves very quickly (some brave Mumsnetters got busy with the mirror and said they were gone within an hour or so). If you have very swollen areas, then you may be left with a 'grey, wrinkly, loose scrotum' for a while, but things will tighten back up eventually.

Varicose veins in your rectum

Also known as haemorrhoids or piles (because they sometimes look like a pile of grapes – oh joy!), these are one of the less glamorous aspects of pregnancy. 'I made the big mistake of taking a look recently and I nearly cried because it looked like my bottom had fallen out,' wails a mum. They can cause itching, soreness and bleeding and can sometimes be incredibly painful: 'It feels like you are shitting drawing pins.'

'Unless you've suffered from piles, it all seems a bit of a snigger, but there are few things as painful. I had them when I was pregnant with my second daughter. It got to the stage where I was crying with them, so forced myself to drive to the doctor, while attempting to hover above the seat. By the time I got to the receptionist, I could barely speak. Heavily pregnant and obviously in pain – the receptionist took one look and assumed I was in labour. All hell broke loose. With the whole of the surgery looking on, I had to explain that I wasn't in labour – I had piles. Anyway, lots of Anusol cream and suppositories did the trick.' MarmaladeSun

Sufferers also recommend witch hazel gel ('kept in the fridge'), Germoloids cream, Sudocrem, warm baths and using soft wipes instead of loo roll. 'The only thing that has ever worked for me is Proctofoam, which is available on prescription – it really does give immediate relief,' advises a mother (although always check with your GP first, as it contains hydrocortisone). Others recommend cold compresses: 'A peeled, frozen banana in a condom, wrapped in a soft facecloth' (make sure you aren't expecting visitors) or 'a bag of frozen peas wrapped in a tea towel'. Do everything you can to prevent constipation (see p. 159), keep doing your pelvic-floor exercises, take some weight off the area by sleeping on your side, don't stand or sit for long (try sitting on a rubber ring) and don't strain when you are on the loo, or sit there for too long. 'You might find it helps to rest your feet on a stool – no pun intended – or a pile of phone books when on the loo,' advises one mum. 'I had to have one lanced, which sounds ghastly, but was actually such a relief I could have hugged my GP,' says a sufferer.

'The best tip I've ever had from my GP was to try gently shoving back in any that have popped out while under the shower, because when they are in, they are less inflamed, so hurt a lot less.'

Elibean

Consult your doctor if there is bleeding, as what you have may be an anal fissure (like a little tear), rather than piles.

What concerns some pregnant women is what will happen to their piles during labour. 'The piles won't explode,' says a Mumsnetter who is a midwife. 'But the midwife might cover them with a sterile pad at the time of delivery if necessary. Consider delivering on all fours to take some of the pressure off. Next time you see the midwife, ask for a bit of advice.' They do tend to get worse after pushing in labour, but most disappear not long after you have given birth.

'I had them for my final couple of months of pregnancy. They will probably get worse before they get better. Mine were unbelievably big post delivery. But once all the weight was gone – i.e. the baby – they slowly started to shrink and I don't notice them any more.' Fefifofum

Varicose veins can be rather distressing, particularly when you feel that your body is becoming more and more wrecked by the week. And it can be a blow to your ego if your legs (or indeed your labia) were your best feature before you turned into a veiny pufferfish, but most of the problems should start to improve after the birth. So don't go burning those miniskirts just yet.

Fainting

If your green face and enormous boobs haven't 'outed' you as pregnant yet, swooning into the arms of Julian in accounts might raise suspicions. You might so far have managed to cover up your abstemiousness, exhaustion and perpetual visits to the loo, but there's not much you can do when you sink to your knees mid-sentence. Someone's bound to smell a rat. As happened to one poor mum: 'I was keeping my pregnancy a secret for the first three months and thought I was doing a convincing job, until I fainted at a party. My dress rode right up to my waist and I came round to the sound of my friends whispering conspiratorially: "She must be pregnant!"'

Another mum-to-be was at the Victoria and Albert Museum when she saw stars, hitting the side of a glass cabinet on her way down. 'I came round to a scene of concerned onlookers and museum staff busily mopping up the bloody mess, clearly not quite as concerned for me as they were for the contents of the cabinet.'

In actual fact, you'll be relieved to hear not that many women actually faint during pregnancy, but plenty feel occasionally wobbly as they get used to all the changes going on in their body. Your heart has a lot of extra work to do, pumping blood where no man has gone before, and occasionally it doesn't make it to your head quite fast enough. You might feel dizzy as you get out of the bath or out of bed in the morning. If you do faint it's a good idea to let your doctor know in case it's a sign of something else.

'I keep nearly fainting! This happens when I stand still for more than a few minutes. As I am a vicar, this is proving to be a great problem. I passed out at the altar last Sunday while celebrating communion. I now have a high stool to sit on, but still have to stand up for some bits of the service and had to go out and put my head between my knees during the sermon this morning. My colleague asked me to do a funeral this week and I am panicking! I really didn't expect my pregnancy to impact on my work much, certainly not this early.' Miranda2

Supermarket queues are a popular place to faint for Mumsnetters. 'What helped was wiggling my toes as it contracts the calf muscles, causing the blood to keep moving in the deep veins in your legs, which will hopefully stop your blood pressure from dropping,' advises one mum who was prone to blacking out. Alternatively, you could 'invest in a pair of sexy support stockings', 'buy a shooting stick', 'keep some boiled sweets in your pocket – and don't be ashamed to jump queues'. And, of course, 'Always make sure you are wearing large and dignified knickers.'

Eating protein at mealtimes and snacking between meals will help to lift your blood-sugar levels. And keeping up your fluid intake will prevent dehydration, another cause of light-headedness. Avoid getting overheated – either step outside or strip off a few layers. And, as ever, there's gentle exercise; yoga and massage are the way to go, as they keep the circulation moving.

It can all be a bit scary and upsetting, but the good news is that your blood pressure should return to normal on delivery of your baby. And soon you will be fondly reminiscing at all your hapless fainting stories: 'I remember waiting until the room was clear and anxiously asking my NCT teacher if I was likely to faint while giving birth. She looked at me as if I was mad.'

Hip and Pelvic Pain – SPD U (Don't) Like

During pregnancy a hormone called 'relaxin' (fat chance of that) loosens the pelvic ligaments to allow the pelvis to open slightly when you give birth; but sometimes things seem to be 'over-relaxed' and you get the very painful feeling that your pelvis might actually be falling into little pieces. There are a few conditions that affect pregnant women that are probably caused by this hormonal change, one of which is Symphysis Pubis Dysfunction (SPD), which causes pain in the pubic and groin area from the end of the first trimester onwards. We're talking proper pain here:

'I'm 25 weeks and already in eye-watering pain; I had no idea that pregnancy had this nice element to it.' Auntylisa

Because of your bun in the oven, you can't knock back the really stonking drugs that might take the pain away, and most sufferers scowl at the offer of a paracetamol, so ask your GP to refer you to a physiotherapist – ideally one with experience in women's health. This is free on the NHS and shouldn't take too long to process – you might even be seen within a few days. The physiotherapist will probably teach you some exercises to keep your tummy and back muscles in trim which will help to support your growing body and teach you the best ways to move (e.g. getting up from a bed) in order to help reduce the pain. A good physio will also advise you to avoid overreaching and stretching, and show you how to move about while keeping your legs together (no sitting like a builder). You might also find it useful to shove a pillow in between your knees in bed, to keep your pelvis 'in line'.

'A physio will be able to advise on exercises and positions that will help, as well as the ones to really, really avoid. The only way to ease the pain is to do absolutely nothing and rest – not easy though. Don't push a heavy shopping trolley either – that's a killer! You may be a little limited for labouring positions too, when the time comes, but if your pregnancy is problem-free, other than the SPD, then a pool would help.'
Mcmudda

A physio might also try you with a 'pelvic girdle' of some sort – a giant elasticated support belt which holds your pelvic bones in place and may provide some relief. It's not La Perla, but you will probably be past caring.

(See p. 274 for advice for SPD sufferers in labour.)

TESTS AND SCANS
Which Tests to Take

Deciding how much you want to find out about your baby before it is born is a modern-day dilemma. Do you want to know the chances of your baby having an abnormality? Would you go as far as having an invasive test if that meant risking miscarriage? What would you do if you found out that your baby was at high risk of having something wrong with it? Would you have a termination?

'The problem with all antenatal tests is that we then have to make choices. It's great if we get the result we want – although nothing's guaranteed – and not so great when we don't. Pregnancy is a very worrying time and I don't think we realise how much we worry until we feel the relief of seeing our newborns.' Cam

Some pregnant women want to know as much as they can and as early as they can, to avoid a late termination. Others choose to have all the tests and scans available – paying to go privately if necessary – even though they have already decided not to have a termination. 'I had a nuchal scan test for chromosomal abnormalities, but I can honestly say, hand on heart, that we would have continued with the pregnancy, regardless of what showed up on the scan,' as one Mumsnetter says. 'Birth is such an emotional time that I didn't want my joy at delivering a live baby tempered by the discovery that my child had a disability. I would have wanted time to prepare myself and perhaps to grieve. I would also, very importantly, want to share the scan news with close family and friends so that when my beautiful baby was born, everyone would feel joy and I wouldn't be greeted with shock, sadness, or worse still, pity.'

'My risk was high (one in 27) after the nuchal
test and indicated a risk of heart problems.
We never had any intention of having a CVS
because we wouldn't terminate but we are
now able to pay close attention to my son's
heart. We have had three scans so far and the
sonographer has ruled out some more serious
heart defects but can still see some spots she
is unsure of. We are just pleased that we will be
able to make an informed decision about where
I should give birth to my son if it turns out he has
anything wrong with his heart.' Hatrick

'I have had two CVSs,' says one mum. 'It's not particularly painful
– when the needle goes in there is a bit of a scratchy feeling and
it's a little uncomfortable. I think it's the process that makes you
nervous, but it only lasts ten minutes at the most. It is well worth
the slight discomfort just to know your babies are OK.'

Tests are not compulsory and a minority of pregnant women
choose not to have any at all. 'What is there to prepare for?' asks
one mother. 'We don't say, "I want to prepare for having a child
that has no disabilities," so why the need to prepare for one that
does? I think it's part of what I'd call a trend towards "pregnancy
insurance" – the desire to protect oneself from anything perceived
as a "risk". And that risk is always centred around Down's
syndrome, and it's all very negative, where in fact, this is the least
worrying syndrome that can be picked up in the scans available to
women.' Another mum says: 'In the olden days, you got what you
got. I worried in all four pregnancies, but didn't have any tests.
What if? How would I cope? Number four's cerebral palsy was a
birth accident so tests would in fact have shown a healthy baby.'

What are the tests for?

It is worth bearing in mind that the tests that are available are not
necessarily there because they can find out the most important

or worst things that might be wrong with your pregnancy. They are just the tests that we have at our disposal. As one mum points out: 'If we could test for other things, most of us would be nervous wrecks throughout pregnancy.'

Some of the tests are for chromosomal disorders, the most common and well-known of which is Down's syndrome (or Down syndrome). People with Down's syndrome have varying degrees of learning disability and a distinctive facial profile. Almost half will have heart defects, some of which are treatable and some of which are not. People with Down's syndrome may also have gut and thyroid gland problems. The incidence of Down's syndrome varies with the age of the mother: at age 30 it affects approximately 1 in 1,000 pregnancies; at age 40 it affects approximately 1 in 100. That is why maternal age is used as part of the calculation during the testing process.

It is worth noting at this point that Down's syndrome has perhaps unnecessarily become the Big Bad Wolf of prenatal testing. Because it *can* be tested for, it often *is*, but the high rate of termination that follows a diagnosis of Down's syndrome is an area that remains controversial. One Mumsnetter, whose daughter has Down's syndrome, explains her feelings about the issue:

'I have struggled with [questions about prenatal testing] many, many times. My daughter is my daughter, no more, no less. She is who she is, she was always going to be Charlotte. She just happened to carry over an extra chromosome and so the person she was destined to be happened to also be one that has Down's syndrome. I know people are terrified of their child having Down's syndrome but I'm here to say there's nothing scary about it! It can be hard work sometimes, but it's never ever scary. It's just about being a mum to your child, a child that turned out to have Down's syndrome. That's all. Nothing scary about it. Just how it is.' Thomcat

Other more severe chromosomal disorders that can be tested for include Patau's syndrome and Edwards' syndrome. The majority of babies with this disorder will die before birth. With these conditions, all systems of the body may be affected and life expectancy is only a few days or, at most, a few months. Both conditions are extremely rare: Edwards' syndrome affects 1 in 6,000 live births, while Patau's syndrome affects 1 in 4,000.

Spina bifida is a physical developmental disorder which occurs when one of the vertebrae in the spine does not form properly in early pregnancy, leaving nerves in the spine unprotected. It can lead to damage of the central nervous system. It is known as a 'neural tube defect' because it results from a failure of the embryo's neural tube to develop normally. Mild forms of spina bifida actually affect up to 30 per cent of the population and don't cause any problems. More severe cases can result in damage to the spinal nerves, affecting physical ability from the point of damage downwards. It is thought to be caused by a combination of environmental factors, such as the mother's diet (this is why you are encouraged to take folic acid when you are trying for a baby and in the early weeks of pregnancy) and genetic conditions (couples with one child affected have a much higher statistical probability of having another child affected). Ninety per cent of cases are identified during ultrasound scans. If the problem is minor, no treatment is usually necessary; if it is more serious, surgery to close the gap may be performed, in order to prevent further damage to the nerves. The type of spina bifida which causes physical damage and ongoing problems affects around 1 in 1,000 live births.

Some other diseases – including cystic fibrosis, sickle cell anaemia and thalassaemia – can be tested for prenatally, but this is generally done only if there is a family history of the conditions.

Which tests are routine and which are not?

The NHS offers routine ultrasound scans at 12 and 20 weeks – and scans at other points during the pregnancy if there are concerns about the baby's development. You should also be offered the choice of having tests for Down's syndrome (nuchal translucency scan and blood tests).

At 12 weeks the baby is only 5–6 cm long and cannot be seen in detail, so this scan is mainly to date the pregnancy and to make sure that the baby's heart is developing properly. Arms and legs can be seen but the purpose of this scan is not to pick up abnormalities, most of which cannot be seen at this stage. However, if you have opted to have the nuchal translucency scan, this may also be done at this point.

The 20-week scan is the one that most mums get excited about, because the baby will look less like an odd ugly prawn and more like an actual cute baby. You might even be given the option of finding out the sex, as long as baby isn't demurely crossing his or her legs to hide the goodies. See p. 176 for more information.

The nuchal translucency scan and blood tests for Down's syndrome are not 'routine' in that it is not assumed that all women will want them, although guidelines recommend that they be offered to all pregnant women. If tests indicate a high likelihood of abnormalities, the only way to have a certain diagnosis is to have an invasive diagnostic test such as chorionic villus sampling (CVS) or amniocentesis (see p. 178), which will be offered if the tests indicate a high probability of diagnosis. Presently, around 5 per cent of pregnant women will be considered higher risk and offered further tests. At no point do you have to have any of these screening tests if you do not want to do so.

Waiting for the results can be nerve-racking: dreading the worst and worrying what the future holds. 'I felt, in a way, that my husband and I were slightly distancing ourselves from the baby while we were waiting for the results – we just stopped talking about plans for it and practical things.'

'Make sure you take someone with you to the scan. My husband went with me for the tests. His hand on my shoulder when we realised something was wrong was so special.' JanZ

Whether you choose to test or not, remember, 'It's your decision. Don't let anyone make up your mind for you, go with what is in your heart.'

Testing, testing, 1, 2, 3: which tests and when, at a glance

Routine tests

Between six and ten weeks: early pregnancy ultrasound scans
These may be offered if you are experiencing bleeding or other symptoms of miscarriage or infection. This may be an ultrasound scan through your belly, or (for very early scans) through a probe inserted into your vagina.

12 weeks: the ultrasound dating scan This is usually given at around this time to check the age of your baby, how many babies there are (hoho), your baby's heartbeat and whether there are any obvious abnormalities.

20 weeks: anomaly pregnancy scan This scan is routinely given on the NHS to all pregnant women and checks the baby's development and growth. Abnormalities may be picked up at this scan because the baby is much bigger and the sonographer can get a very good idea of what is going on in terms of development.

Any time during second and third trimester: growth scans You may have further ultrasound scans during the second and third trimester if your midwife or consultant have any concerns about the baby's development, or if possible problems were picked up during the 20-week scan. Most of these questions resolve themselves as the weeks go by.

Optional screening tests

Prenatal blood tests There are a few slightly different testing procedures, most of which combine blood tests with nuchal scan results to come up with a risk assessment. Blood tests include the Triple Test and the Quadruple Test (both carried out at around 16 weeks). The results of these are combined with other risk factors, such as the mother's age, to give a statistical likelihood of chromosomal abnormalities and other serious conditions.

You can have blood tests but no nuchal translucency scan, and this is called the Serum Integrated Test.

(continued)

11–14 weeks: nuchal translucency (nuchal) scan This is an ultrasound test which measures the amount of fluid at the back of the baby's neck. These measurements are then combined with the results of one of more blood tests and the risks associated with the mother's age in order to calculate a statistical likelihood of the baby having Down's syndrome. If the probability is high, you will be offered further tests such as amniocentesis or CVS.

The combined test The results of a nuchal translucency scan may be combined with the results of a blood test in the first trimester, and a risk assessment given based on these.

The integrated test A nuchal translucency scan result may be combined with a blood test in the first trimester and the Quadruple Test (mother's blood test) around 16 weeks. The results from both sets of tests are combined and a risk assessment is given based on the results.

11–13 weeks: chorionic villus sampling (CVS) You may be offered this test if you are in a high-risk group or if you have had a high-probability result from a nuchal scan and blood test. A fine needle-like instrument is inserted either via the cervix or through the abdomen, and takes a small sample of chorionic villi cells, which are found on the placenta. These are tested for Down's syndrome and other chromosomal disorders. It is a diagnostic test, which means it is nearly 100 per cent accurate. The test is not without risks, however – approximately 1 out of 100 pregnant women will develop complications after the test that result in a miscarriage.

15–18 weeks: amniocentesis Like CVS testing, this may be offered to women in a high-risk group. A fine needle is passed into the womb and a sample of the amniotic fluid is extracted and tested for Down's syndrome and other chromosomal disorders. Like CVS, the amniocentesis is a diagnostic test and is nearly 100 per cent accurate but again, not without risks. It carries a similar risk of miscarriage to CVS.

THINKING AHEAD

Home Birth vs Hospital Birth – How Do You Choose?

When it comes to deciding on the best place to deliver, rare is the pregnant woman who sits on the fence – and not just because she can't get up there.

The number of home births is currently on the increase in the UK where, at the time of writing, three in 100 babies are born at home (up from around one in 100, 15 years ago). Suddenly, it's hip and all the celebrities are at it: Davina McCall, Thandie Newton, Charlotte Church and Jade Jagger are all home-birthing devotees. Of course, long before it was fashionable, home births were the sole option for many women. In the mid-sixties, the number of home births was one in three – but both infant and maternal mortality rates were higher. As medical procedures advanced to make births safer, however, there followed a movement towards medicalised hospital births, which was the central ambition of the Peel Report in 1970.

These days, the movement is towards more choice: so it is up to you to decide what is right for you and your family; whether that is a candle-lit home birth to the sound of your husband crooning on his guitar or a champagne C-section and a tummy tuck (unfortunately your local Primary Care Trust might not cover all of the latter).

So, despite popular misconception, you do have some choices when it comes to deciding the type of birth that you want and where you want it to take place. Bear in mind, however, that a big fat baby is going to have to come out, so there is only a limited amount of fun to be had, even if you are lucky enough to have lots of options at your disposal.

In a perfect world, of course, you would have all the power of a Premier League football manager assembling your best ante- and postnatal team of twinkly-eyed consultants and large-bosomed doulas. (A doula is a trained birth partner.) But the reality is that the options available will depend in part on where you live.

To get the ball rolling, most pregnant women visit their GP. Yours won't be the first pregnancy on their books, so be prepared for them to be wholly underwhelmed just when you're at your most excited. 'I almost ran to my GP's as soon I found out I was pregnant, only to be told that I should come back in another month,' says a red-faced mum.

Nevertheless, you should:

'Go as soon as you can. It isn't very eventful but you get to register as pregnant for free prescriptions and dental care, and get into the system. They also either tell you or give you a list of dos and don'ts which, in my opinion, are a load of patronising rubbish designed as a catch-all, but you'll probably want to at least consider them.' StarlightMcKenzie

Most women are assigned, through their GP, to a consultant at a hospital near by. Don't expect to see much of your consultant during your pregnancy, unless complications arise. You can opt for midwife-only care if you wish, but you can't generally choose to see the same midwife for your care throughout, and might not even see the same hospital midwife more than once.

Hospital births

'I have had two great hospital births – both times needed no intervention, had 1–1 midwife support, and at no time was left on my own. The food is crap though and you get no sleep post birth due to other people's crying babies. I also have two friends who have caught MRSA in hospital. However, this time, now that I own a house, I have decided to have a home water birth.' Cazzybabs

'I'd had one friend who almost died in childbirth and another whose child needed immediate special care, so a hospital birth was a no-brainer for me. Yes, it would be nice to have better food, but my husband just brought me treats in from the organic café. Yes, the loos and showers could be cleaner and the bed could be more comfy, but you just wear flip-flops and take antiseptic wipes and your own pillow. What mattered for me was that my baby had access to first-class medical care and so did I. Oh, and I wanted to marry the lovely midwife who took my baby and cradled her for a couple of hours during the night shift so I could get some much-needed rest.' Zoots

When it comes to choosing between hospitals, your main concern will probably be their distance from your home. If you are weighing the options between the city hospital down the road or the lovely birthing unit an hour's drive away in the country, take into consideration the fact that whoever is driving you to hospital will feel the full force of your labouring rage every time you hit a bump in the road or turn a sharp corner.

'Speed bumps and contractions don't mix!'

ldilemma

Each maternity unit has its own policies for the management of labour, which is something you could ask about – most units and hospitals offer tours of the labour wards, which are a good idea and will familiarise you with the environment. Hopefully, you will be pleasantly assured by the lack of horror-house screaming and medieval torture devices. (Note: don't ask to see the forceps!) 'I found the tour of the hospital labour ward really reassuring,' admits one mum. 'The rooms were clean and dimly lit, there was a birthing-pool suite, and all the staff were friendly and welcoming.' Don't be put off by the pictures of dolphins in the birthing-pool suite: they won't actually be in there with you.

One thing you might want to check is how many births per midwife per year each unit you are considering has, although word of mouth is probably your best recommendation:

'We have chosen the local hospital, despite the fact that the figures suggest overworked midwives, rather than the one which is less overrun, because the former has a good reputation locally, a brilliant Head of Midwifery Services, decent consultants, a "can-do" approach to VBACs [Vaginal Birth After Caesarean] and a proper birthing pool. You can also find out whether there is an anaesthetist 24/7 to do epidurals. I also asked the local NCT branch and their views were unanimous, no matter what kind of birth you were likely to expect or want.' Clare2

To help you make your decision, you can look up various figures from rates of induction to C-section stats at hospitals across the country at www.birthchoiceuk.com and www.drfoster.co.uk. 'Your choice of hospital depends on the type of care you want. I chose my hospital because I thought the care in labour would be more midwife-driven, as opposed to doctor-driven, as it is not a major teaching hospital. You can do a tour of both hospitals in my area, and I would really recommend this as a good way of getting a feel for the sort of care you'll get.'

Even if they can afford it, going private isn't necessarily everyone's first choice. Some people feel more confident opting for a private ward on an NHS site, in case of an emergency. 'I am driving myself crazy trying to decide on a hospital,' one mum confides. 'I went to look at the three main private hospitals, but my husband's best friend works in obstetrics and thinks I should definitely go somewhere that has NHS facilities but still has a private ward.' Bear in mind that some NHS hospitals have 'private' rooms that you can pay an additional sum to stay in after the birth. This is effectively an 'upgrade' in your accommodation; you will still see the same midwives, physiotherapists and paediatricians that you would see on the ward, but you will have a little more privacy, so you won't have to watch the husband of the new mother in the bed opposite eating chips, while you are sucking on your NHS lunch rations. Some of these private rooms are on a first-come-first-served basis, though. There may also be different rules if you end up having a Caesarean:

'I was all excited about having a private room in my NHS hospital, but after an emergency C-section was told I had to have at least one night on the ward so they could monitor me more closely. When I did eventually move into my en suite room, although it was nice to have some privacy and my own loo, it was quite lonely once the visitors had gone, and quite hard sometimes to get a midwife's attention.' Muncher

Be aware that even though you may have a fight on your hands, it is never too late to change your mind about which hospital you want to use: 'I changed hospitals while I was being transferred from home. I simply told the paramedics that this was the place I was going to! It was the same distance, so they took me there.' Another mother says: 'I switched hospitals midway through pregnancy. In my case, it was because I wanted to have a home birth, and only one of the three choices open to me offered these. I changed through my GP, but it wasn't a problem. Remember that as long as you're in the catchment area, it is your choice.'

Birth centres

If it is your first pregnancy and you don't feel confident enough for a home birth, you might prefer the option of a stand-alone midwifery unit, otherwise known as a birth centre. They are NHS-run, entirely by midwives, and you can apply directly. The set-up is more intimate than that of a large hospital – they aim for a home-from-home atmosphere – and because there are fewer midwives, the care may be more personal. Epidurals and Caesarean sections are not available at these centres, so it is only an option for low-risk pregnancies, when everything is looking straightforward. Should complications arise, you may need to be transferred in an emergency. So if you fancy lying in bed with a menu of chocolates and hardcore drugs, this is not the option for you.

'If you are low-risk, then birth centres are a fab option. You are more likely to have a peaceful, non-interventional, midwife-led delivery than in a hospital, but you feel a bit more secure knowing that medical help is more readily available than at home. If there were complications, you might have to be transferred to a hospital maternity unit, but they are used to doing it. I would have preferred a home birth, medical issues allowing, but my partner was nervous. Instead, I went to a birth centre twice and had wonderful water births with no other pain relief both times. The midwives were fantastic.' notacow

If there isn't a birth centre in your area, you might want to opt for a midwifery unit within a hospital. They are usually staffed by the same midwives that work in the consultant unit at the hospital, but the emphasis is on a more natural birth. It is a low-tech option, if you want to give birth with little or no intervention, and you can easily be transferred to the consultant unit – often just down the corridor – in the event of complications.

'There are now a number of NHS midwife-led units that cater for low-risk, "natural" births. The one I attended had a birthing pool, low-sensory room, showers and baths, gas and air and pethidine (or the equivalent) on hand for pain relief. Epidurals are not available but the unit was on the floor below the standard maternity unit so I could have been transferred if necessary. I had my own room with en suite bathroom. The small team of midwives were brilliant at helping me manage without an epidural and really supportive of my choices.'

NickiB

Home births

You either love the idea or it fills you with horror. And no, we're not talking about bumpy rumpy pumpy to fast-forward labour or sautéeing your placenta for a Hugh Fearnley-Whittingstall-style pâté. The hot issue is home births. Is it the ultimate nesting experience? Or is it Russian roulette for lentil-weaving hippies?

Worldwide, around 80 per cent of children are born at home or in local community settings. In developing countries, local tradition and the long distances women have to travel to reach a hospital make home births routine – although, again, infant and maternal mortality rates can be very high in countries with no medical care.

In America, however, just 1 per cent of babies are born at home, and in ten states it is illegal to practise as a home-birth midwife. Rates of intervention in the US are much higher, largely because of the threat of litigation, and one in three hospital births ends in a Caesarean.

Ultimately, although the choice about where you give birth is partly determined by the sort of pregnancy you have, you do have some say and, for low-risk pregnancies, a home birth can be the right option.

'My home birth was brilliant. When my waters broke I had a quick bath while waiting for my midwife. I was totally relaxed. I moved around a lot and gave birth on the edge of the sofa with a beanbag behind me. Gas and air kept the edge off the pain. After the birth I snuggled down on the sofa while my daughter had a feed and the midwives tidied up and made tea. An hour later we were all tucked up in bed.' Hopeful

If you want a home birth, you will, of course, need to get your partner on your side. But this could be less of a problem than you might think: 'My husband found it easier to go along with a hormonal pregnant wife than to object.'

Fans of home births talk about 'trusting' their body to give birth, as well as feeling 'calmer' and more 'in control' delivering their babies in familiar surroundings without the pressure of medical intervention. At home, they are allowed to labour at their own pace.

'In hospital, I felt very much that I was ignored, and that during one of the strangest, most frightening experiences of my life, nobody seemed to do what I asked, or would even tell me what was happening – it was all about hospital protocol and rules. I felt powerless, which added to the fear and stress. I also ended up with a lot of intervention which I could have

done better without. At home I felt I was much more in control. I could decide better somehow.'

FlightAttendant

Most GPs and community midwives will be happy to discuss your options with you, or might recommend that you discuss these with a consultant. You don't need your GP's permission to have a home birth; you can book direct with the supervisor of midwives at your local hospital. It takes preparation though, so talk to them as early as possible. Usually there is a team of midwives in your area who can attend home births. NHS guidelines stipulate that two midwives must be present for a home delivery. You can also hire an independent midwife who will look after you throughout your pregnancy, or a doula.

When considering a home birth you might want to think about the following: how will any complications be managed? What emergency equipment will they bring? If you want a water birth, will your floor take the weight of a pool? How will you fill it and – perhaps more importantly – empty it? You won't be very popular with the neighbours if you are planning to siphon bloody water and poo out of the window of your fifth-floor flat. If you already have children, what are your plans for them? Who will look after them while you are labouring and delivering? If you live a long way from hospital, what happens if you need to be transferred? You can get lots more information from www.homebirth.org.uk.

Home births are not recommended for multiple pregnancies, if your baby is lying in a breech position, if there are complications such as pre-eclampsia or placenta praevia (see pp. 242 and 250) or if you suffer from a health problem such as epilepsy. It is possible after a previous C-section, as long as you agree to a hospital transfer at the first sign of trouble. Women often wait until their second child before they opt for a home birth. 'I personally wouldn't have felt comfortable having a home birth for my first because of the potential for things to go wrong,' says one GP mum.

Of course, not all home births are planned – some babies arrive so fast they leave you with no choice but to clear a space in the dining room and christen the new carpet. But the majority are well thought out and organised.

'My home birth was brilliant! I had two previous hospital births and hated them. Ten minutes after my home birth, my other kids came in to meet their baby brother and were thrilled. Just six hours after the start of it all, everything was cleaned up and the midwives were gone and we were all cuddled up on the sofa together as one big happy family!' Busybee123

One mum says: 'The best way to have a baby safely is with no intervention. During a hospital birth, if you are not "progressing", as they label it in hospital, you might be given an intervention. At home, you go for a little nap, which sometimes gets things going. It is very rare that things need to be done immediately and the midwives who specialise in home births are very experienced and will know in advance if you need to go to hospital.'

Studies suggest that for low-risk pregnancies, home birth is at least as safe as hospital birth, and more likely to be intervention-free (less chance of a forceps or C-section delivery). But plenty of women would still far rather be on the spot, at hospital, should anything go wrong or for access to more powerful pain relief, such as an epidural.

'I would never have a home birth. You do not know what will happen. I had an emergency section with my daughter and if I hadn't been in hospital she would have died. It seems fairly black and white to me. I had my second daughter in hospital, all fine. I had midwives all the way through, was never left alone and, more importantly, had medical care at the end of the corridor to save my daughter's life.' Oliveoil

And for some house-proud women, a home birth would never be their choice, simply because 'I couldn't bear the mess!' If this worries you, be reassured that most home births are not that messy and midwives will cover up any soft furnishings with plastic sheets and disposable coverings and take these away with them afterwards. So it won't look like someone has slaughtered a pig in your front room.

Pain relief for home births

As far as home birth pain relief is concerned, don't worry – your midwife will bring a large leather strap for you to put between your teeth and bite on. Only kidding. Home births are usually, by definition, fairly intervention-free, and that includes intervention in the way of medicalised pain relief. If you long to labour on Class A drugs or pine for a 1960s morphined-up birth where they wake you up when it's all over, then a home birth is not for you.

However, a home birth does not necessarily mean more pain than a hospital birth. Just being at home can help you deal with the pain more effectively, simply because you are more likely to be relaxed and comfortable. Although that might sound a bit lame, and would certainly not cut the mustard at the dentist's, it is amazing how much difference a relaxing environment alone can make for some women.

'I have had one of each – hospital and home – and know which one I prefer by a mile. My home birth was my second. My first was a fast, straightforward labour and birth so I knew I could birth a baby. My second, I had two midwives with me throughout; it was only two hours and 20 minutes start to finish, I got up, had a shower, got back into my clean bed, my partner brought me tea and toast, then we all got into bed for a cuddle, and about an hour later my daughter came in too, to see her new sister. After a little sleep I was downstairs getting on with it all as usual. No stitches, no pain. Being at home contributed to a better labour and after-birth recovery.' Sweetkitty

Labouring and birthing at home is a more natural experience, and in this unique process, the home environment can encourage better management of the event:

'Being able to move, vocalise, rest, eat and drink as you need to will in itself be a big help; and as labour builds, your own endorphins will help you cope with the pain.' Lulumama

You can also have a TENS machine (see p. 307) if you fancy, which you can buy or hire. And of course, you can always pop a couple of, ermm, paracetamol. (Although anyone who suggests this when you are in labour will probably get short shrift.) Aromatherapy is another option, but make sure you check which oils are safe for labouring women.

Some home birthers say that learning hypnotherapy techniques helped them during labour: 'Hypnobirthing "pushing" really helped me – I didn't quite do what I learned, but I was just breathing slowly and not bearing down until the very, very end.' You can buy books and CDs about hypnotherapy, or hypnobirthing (see p. 305), and some practitioners run private classes for pregnant women.

Your midwife will be able to bring along canisters of gas and air (entonox), which will be available to you in the same way as it is in the hospital, although as one home-birth mum bitterly recalled: 'Just make sure she remembers to bring the mouthpiece!'

Some midwives will also provide more heavy-duty medical pain relief in the form of pethidine or Meptid. Be aware that pethidine and similar drugs can have side effects, for example drowsiness, which can impact on your labour. They can also cross the placenta and therefore have an effect on the baby, so make sure you do all your research before you opt for these. (For more information on pethidine, see p. 310.)

The choice of giving birth in water is a popular one for women giving birth at home. Birthing pools can be hired or bought and are filled with warm water. Giving birth and labouring in water are very ancient ideas (Egyptian hieroglyphs show women giving birth in the River Nile) and the warm, relaxing feel of being weightless in the water can help to relieve pain. Bear in mind, though, that you will need to have someone armed with a sieve to fish out any unsavoury deposits that your enthusiastic pushing might deliver: 'I think I delivered nine pounds of poo and eight pounds of baby.' If your partner thinks this might be one devotional duty too far, your midwife should be happy to discreetly assist.

If you have a birth partner, ask them to give you a relaxing massage during your labour. If this is your husband and he is reluctant or just plain lazy, you might want to make it known that in some cultures a rope is tied to the husband's testicles, for the labouring woman to pull on during contractions, so that they can share the joys of the pain of childbirth. That might make a loving massage seem like a more favourable option. If he is still reluctant, hand him the sieve.

A stitch in time

Probably best not to dwell on this in too much detail, but it's worth knowing what will happen if you need to be stitched up due to any vaginal or perineal tearing after a home birth. Simply put, your midwife will probably lay you on a bed, grab the anglepoise from your desk, and get to work on your nether regions. In a hospital it will also (usually) be the midwife that does this bit, so she will have lots of experience and a good idea of what it looked like beforehand – even if it now resembles a choice selection from the meat counter at Asda.

The midwife will offer you pain relief for the stitches – if not, don't feel shy about asking – and you will probably be given a local anaesthetic, as well as gas and air. She might offer pethidine or Meptid, but this varies from one midwife to the next, and you could ask in advance if this is something you would like. If you need a more complex repair (sorry about this) you will be transferred to a hospital, and given a spinal or an epidural for pain relief.

Right then, if by now you are feeling traumatised, we recommend getting out the teeny, tiny sleepsuits and cooing over them for a bit . . .

Hospital transfers

The idea of making an emergency transfer from home to hospital is another commonly cited reason for opting for a hospital birth. Forty per cent of first-time mums attempting a home birth will be transferred to hospital during the course of their labour. For second-time (and beyond) mums, this rate drops to just over 10 per cent (according to 'Birth at Home' by Chamberlain G., Wraight A., Crowley P., *Practical Midwife* July–August 1999).

'From all the reading that I've done, I realise that births don't go wrong in a split second; there is enough warning to transfer in the vast majority of cases. From all the reading I've done, I have also learned how many problems arise precisely because of too much intervention, and people not trusting their bodies to do what they are designed to do perfectly well. I'm actively looking forward to a home birth. I'm also philosophical about the need for a transfer, because for 40 per cent of first-timers, it becomes necessary.' Naturelover (who subsequently had a successful home birth)

Another mother says: 'At home, the midwives refuse to take any chances. Any sign of things going wrong and they send for the ambulance. They are much more cautious and because many of them have been involved with you from early on, they know what is normal for you and what is not.' And as one mum points out: 'In the event of an emergency in hospital, they still have to get theatre ready and surgeons prepped before you can go in. If you are at home, you get transferred by ambulance, and meanwhile they can get ready for you at the hospital.'

Birth stories from the home front

'I coped by breathing through the contractions until 8.30 a.m. when I got into the pool. It was bliss! Our midwife arrived an hour later and, by this time, I was singing along to the CDs I'd selected to get me through the contractions. By lunchtime I felt I needed a bit more help and started using gas and air, which really helped with the pain. I felt totally in control at all times, was allowed to listen to my body and go with what I felt was right (both of my midwives just encouraged me, there wasn't a single instruction to push!). I even noticed that when I started feeling as if the pain was getting too much, my contractions would slow down for a few minutes to give me a breather and then start up again once I had regained my composure! Don't worry about the birth; it really is a fantastic experience!' *Betsycoe*

'During my home birth, I was so relaxed between contractions, and I'm sure that in itself made things so much easier. I didn't emerge for two days and so rested properly, unlike when I came home from hospital. I was soooo high I didn't sleep a wink all night – just gazed at my lovely wee man. Our other two children came up as normal in the morning and were thrilled to find their new baby brother in bed with us. Needless to say they were quite late for school that day but what fun they had telling their friends!' *Aero*

'I had a home birth with my fourth and it was the best experience ever; I wish I had done it with all the others. I recovered more quickly as well. The only downside was the midwives and my husband eating doughnuts and drinking coffee while I paced up and down.' *Feezy*

'I had my second baby at home 11 months ago and it was totally, utterly amazing – the most wonderful thing I've ever done, and it reduces me to incoherent gibbering every time I think about it.' *Motherinferior*

'My doula said I had a silent labour, by which we mean I just breathed through the contractions and then when I started to feel the real pressure to push I got a bit loud. The doula reminded me to breathe the baby out, and thank God she

(continued)

101   Pregnancy: the Mumsnet Guide

did, as I thought I was going to get into a panic at this stage, but she calmed me right down and I did just that – I breathed her out. Then I heard the midwife say, "Catch her," so I reached down and she swam up into my arms. It was the best feeling in the world and I'm crying typing it. She is perfect. And a girl, and ohhhh, the world is just wonderful. No stitches, no grazing, nothing, just bliss. I'm in love and so lucky and everything is great.' *Thomcat*

Maternity Leave – When Should You Take It and How Long Should You Take?

Giving up the day job, albeit temporarily, is a significant step towards motherhood. Financially and emotionally, there is much at stake. Given that you have no idea when your baby will make an appearance – only one in 20 babies is born on its due date – deciding when to stop commuting and start nesting can be a tricky dilemma, and one that there is little consensus on:

'I would stop earlier if you can because you'll never have that time again, with no baby and no job to stress about. Use the time to relax and enjoy yourself – go swimming, read novels, whatever you fancy. My sister was planning to take three weeks off before her due date, but the baby came early, so she never got any free time at all and she still feels cheated six years later.' TuttiFrutti

'Stay at work as long as possible and enjoy more weeks at home with your baby at the end of your maternity leave period. These will be the longest weeks of your life and bouncing forlornly on a gym ball in front of GMTV for days on end will only add to the torture. For both of my pregnancies, I stayed at work until the day I went into labour. I got lots of attention, a constant stream of cups of tea, gifts of biscuits and first dibs on any buffet leftovers. And in awkward client meetings my boss had a prearranged signal for me to start panting if negotiations got too difficult and we wanted to bring things to a swift conclusion!' Morningpaper

Have a strategy. If you are an employee, the first step is to find out what maternity leave you are entitled to. Start by checking out your contract, your employees' manual and consulting your HR department. Ask colleagues who have taken maternity leave before you for advice, and talk to your trade union or local Citizens' Advice Bureau. Your local job centre (or Jobcentre Plus as they are now known) might also be a useful source of information.

Working out the period when you are to start maternity leave is a bit of a head-spinning task and calls for some careful calculation. If you know a tame HR person, enlist their help in talking things through with you so that you have a clear idea of your dates and entitlement.

Statutory Maternity Leave (SML) is for 52 weeks, comprising 26 weeks of Ordinary Maternity Leave and 26 weeks of Additional Maternity Leave, plus time off for antenatal appointments. You are entitled to SML, regardless of how long you have worked for your employer, the number of hours you work and what you are paid. The earliest you can start your SML is 11 weeks before the week your baby is due. (If you are off work due to pregnancy-related issues in the four weeks before your expected birth date, your employer can make you start your maternity leave.)

But this is just the leave you are entitled to. How much of this is actually *paid* leave depends on various conditions. You may be entitled to receive Statutory Maternity Pay (SMP) for up to 39 weeks of the leave.

You should be the one to break the news to your boss, and at the appropriate time, so don't let the gossip mill beat you to it. Ideally, you should put it in writing at least 15 weeks before the beginning of the week your baby is due. Your letter should include your due date and when you want to start maternity leave, and you should enclose your maternity certificate (which you can get from your GP or midwife). It's up to you when you want your SMP to start, but it normally coincides with your Ordinary Maternity Leave period. (Most employers won't mind if you change your mind about this date later on in your pregnancy, although strictly speaking you should give 28 days' written notice.)

At the end of your maternity leave, your employer is legally required to offer you the same job with the same pay and conditions as you previously had or one at an equivalent level. If you decide to go back to work before the 52 weeks are up you'll need to give your employer 28 days' written notice of the date you intend to return to work.

'You are normally supposed to give 28 days' notice if you want to change your maternity leave start date, but your employer may be willing to overlook or reduce this in certain circumstances. I guess that will depend on whether they have your replacement sorted, etc. But don't feel guilty about going off sick if you need to – you and your baby come first.' BetsyBoop

To qualify for Statutory Maternity Pay (SMP) – i.e. any actual cold, hard cash in exchange for your selfless act of breeding – you must have been employed by your present employer for at least 26 weeks into the 15th week before your baby is due. It is paid for up to 39 weeks whether or not you intend to return to work, and is subject to tax and National Insurance. You can claim SMP only once you have stopped work; the earliest this would be is from the 11th week before your baby is born and the latest you can claim is the day after the birth. (But don't panic if you haven't got all your forms ready – you can make a retrospective claim within a reasonable period of time.)

Your employers might have their own maternity pay scheme, in which case check the details with a fine-tooth comb. Some maternity pay schemes are amazingly generous and will have you dashing to baby boutiques to deck out your little dolly like the latest Beckham babe. Other schemes are a bit of a poisoned chalice – they might seem generous but you may have to pay back some of the money if you decide not to return to work after giving birth, which could leave you with a nasty bill at a time when you don't have a lot of spare cash.

The statutory minimum for a maternity scheme will pay 90 per cent of your salary for the first six weeks, then basic-rate maternity pay for the rest of the maternity leave (33 weeks). If you qualify for SMP, your normal weekly pay must be the same or more than the basic SMP rate – otherwise the amount you receive will be the same as your normal weekly pay. This basic amount of SMP doesn't have to be repaid.

If you are not eligible for SMP, but you have been employed or self-employed for at least 26 weeks in the 66-week period ending the week before your expected week of childbirth, you can claim Maternity Allowance (MA), as long as your National Insurance contributions are up to date. This is paid when you stop work, for a maximum of 39 weeks, regardless of whether or not you intend to return to work. It is not taxable.

When you start your leave is a matter of personal choice. There is no right or wrong answer. What's right for you will depend on lots of factors: you might want to hibernate for the final weeks of your pregnancy or you might be bouncing off the walls with blooming energy and revelling in your final weeks of working life. Your decision also depends on the sort of work you do.

Bear in mind that this will be the last time for a good few years that you will be able to finish a cup of tea while it is still hot or take a pee without chatty spectators wanting to know whether you are doing a Number One or a Number Two. So whether you are at work or at home, try to indulge yourself a little bit.

As well as giving you time to adjust mentally to becoming a mum, time off pre-birth lets you make practical preparations: stock the freezer, buy baby basics, paint your nails. Sometimes your body decides when it is time to stop working: 'In both my pregnancies, I decreed that I would work till the end, but ended up leaving work both times at around 34 weeks. Your body has a way of telling you to slow down. At one of my appointments, my midwife looked me sternly in the eye and told me to finish work.' Or you might discover one morning that you are just too enormous to squeeze behind your steering wheel *and* reach the pedals at the same time.

Other women find the limbo time between the end of work and the baby's arrival more frustrating than relaxing. 'I was so bored,' says a mum who advocates sticking it out for as long as you can. 'I'm not very good being at being at home with nothing to do. When you have another few weeks off at the end of your maternity leave, you will be pleased that you did, because no one wants to go back when the time comes.' Instead of starting maternity leave early, you could take some time off as holiday or sick leave. Or approach your employer with the idea of working from home all or part of the week, or working only half days.

Whether or not you return to work is a decision that is hard to make before baby arrives, because you just don't know how you are going to feel when the time comes. On the basis of their pregnancy alone, which is usually pretty exhausting, some women decide that they want to give work up altogether, only to change their minds after a few months at home with their new bundle. Others regret their haste to return to work: 'If there is one thing I would change, it would be not to have gone back to work so quickly. I think a year off for new mothers is an absolute must. It is such a short time in your career. I wish that employers would be more understanding, and I wish I hadn't been in such a hurry to reclaim "old me" by going back to work. Old me is still here, but enhanced by being a mother.'

It's OK to admit that you haven't made your mind up yet. Motherhood is an enormous change, and it's hard to know when you will feel ready to return. Or when you'll be able to shoe-horn your thighs back into your power suits. Whatever you decide, don't sign on the dotted line too quickly.

The gap year: funny things said by soon-to-be first-time parents

'I'm going to use my maternity leave to learn Italian.' *Pagwatch*

'I will go back to work and the baby can stay in the room next to me while I am working; I can pop in every now and again to check on it.' *Sweetkitty*

'My wife wants to go back to work after three months, so I'm going to stay at home with the baby. I'm really looking forward to it. I'm going to get one of those kit cars and spend the time doing it up. It'll be fantastic to finally have the time to do that.' *Trefusis*

'Babies sleep 16 hours a day, right? So that leaves eight hours, which is what you'd do as a normal day's work anyway.' *TheUrbanNixie*

'I can't wait to get a "holiday" from work, and get the chance to do all those hobbies I never had time for.' *PotPourri*

'I will do an Open University degree while at home on maternity leave.' *FairyMum*

'My sister said, "I can't wait for baby to come; all they do is sleep for the first few months, so I'll be able to get loads done on maternity leave!" And she showed me her "Dream List" of everything she was going to achieve throughout baby's first few months of life. Nearly six years, and two more sproglets later, she has done the grand total of ONE thing off that list: master breastfeeding.' *Mananny*

'I said: "I expect I'll spend my maternity leave in the park reading magazines while the baby sleeps in the carrycot ..." (I actually did try that once, but got so stressed that the sun might be coming through the trees and burning my daughter, and trying uncomfortably to breastfeed her against a tree, that I ended up calling my husband and wailing down the phone that my life was

(continued)

officially ruined by having a baby, as I couldn't do anything any more!)' *BumperliciousNeedsToSleep*

'I'll do my two-hour Ashtanga routine every day; by the end of maternity leave I might start teaching it!' *Peacelily*

'A friend's husband said to her while she was pregnant with her first: "Brilliant! What are you going to study while you're on mat leave? You could get a new qualification!"' *Wickedwaterwitch*

'From my husband when I was eight months pregnant: "I'm really looking forward to paternity leave and having a couple of weeks off work." Followed by (about six weeks later): "It's only two days, three hours and 47 minutes till I go back to work. THANK GOD."' *Intravenouscoffee*

'I think I left work to go on maternity leave with the immortal words: "I'm off for my nine-month holiday ... bye losers!" How they laughed.' *Anonymama*

Which Classes to Sign Up For

Turning up for your first antenatal class can be as nerve-racking as your first day of school. Why did I sign up for this, you'll think, when I could have got it all from a book? But flash forwards a few weeks, and chances are you will be sharing the fleshiest of details from your private life, while panting like a warthog and perched on an upturned bucket. Post-birth, you will be with the same group (maybe not the men), squeezed around a café table, surrounded by prams, drinking coffee and comparing notes on sore nipples.

'What to expect? There'll be flip charts and biscuits and, if you're lucky, a knitted boob.

Some people will know more than you, some won't, but the whole point of being there is to learn, so don't worry. It'll be fine, and with a bit of luck you'll make some nice friends who are due around the same time.' MuminBrum

There is a host of antenatal classes to sign up for, many of which are over-subscribed. If you are interested, you would be advised to start making enquiries as soon as possible: you might want to wait until your first scan, but by then you might be too late. Classes are run by hospitals, health visitors, midwives and other qualified experts (often qualified antenatal teachers). The National Childbirth Trust (NCT) runs popular classes, but again, be sure to book up early as they are often full.

The idea behind antenatal classes is to prepare you and your partner for what lies ahead: pain relief in labour, practical tips on massage and breathing techniques, breastfeeding and how best to cope during those first weeks post-birth are just some of the topics covered, but each course will vary. One Mumsnetter rather enjoyed the handout entitled, 'What's in a nappy?' which gave descriptions and 'colour pictures of many different types of baby poo'. Oh, and expect at some point for the class to descend into anarchy when discussing how soon after birth people expect to be having sex again.

Classes might be run by the NHS and free, or be run by charities or private businesses and require a fee. Some take place one evening a week over a course of several weeks, while others are more intensive and are run over a weekend, sometimes with an overnight stay.

'There are three reasons for going to any antenatal class: 1. To make friends; 2. To prepare you for birth; 3. To prepare your partner for birth.' Springerspaniel

Signing up for an NCT (National Childbirth Trust) class has become something of a rite of passage for pregnant women. The teacher usually hosts the session in the evening, in her own home or in a local hospital or similar venue, and the groups are open to couples (although some women have to bribe reluctant partners with a beer afterwards to get them there). And sometimes you might end up wishing he had stayed at home, after all: 'My husband wanted to know how many other women would be in the birth pool with me at the same time.' If you don't have a partner, or if your partner (legitimately, or otherwise) isn't able to make it, try to take a friend, or even your mum. If you know you will have to go to classes alone, ask the antenatal teacher if they have any groups that cater just for mums-to-be, rather than couples.

NCT charge a fee which can be reduced in accordance with your financial circumstances. It can feel a bit like a meeting of Alcoholics Anonymous to start with, but the bond that some groups form can last for years. Natural births and breastfeeding are encouraged, but what is covered stems in part from what each group – and, of course, the teacher – wants to discuss. One teacher re-enacted her own C-section using Playmobil men.

Some mums feel that certain antenatal teachers focus on 'natural' (non-medicalised vaginal) birth and do not fully inform them of the broad spectrum of birth experiences:

'I was terrified when my birth ended up being about as "interventional" as possible, and there was absolutely no need for me to be. It was all fine. I didn't get a urinary tract infection from the catheter; I'm not paralysed from the epidural; my Caesarean was not the worst thing on earth. I blame the classes for building up my hopes for a "perfect" birth which, ultimately, wasn't possible, and making me think that anything else was terrible. So, if you do go, please go with an open mind. I'd hate anybody else to end up with the guilt that I had about not being able to achieve a "natural birth".' Laura032004

Hospitals and GP surgeries may offer classes, both courses and ad-hoc workshops. Local breastfeeding groups (such as the Association of Breastfeeding Mothers) may also run informal drop-ins and workshops. Swimming pools may offer classes for pregnant women (although you might feel like one in a pod of whales). Yoga schools may offer classes for pregnant women and private hypnotherapy clinics may offer courses in 'hypnobirthing' (see p. 305). Active Birth Centres, which specialise in teaching techniques to help women keep mobile during labour, offer courses; and you may have a local 'home birth' group for women who are interested in a home-birth experience. As well as all of these, you might find that there are also midwives, doulas or antenatal teachers that offer their own private classes.

While the NCT and your local hospital or GP surgery are likely to be the main course providers, you don't have to stick to just one – you can do as many courses or classes as you like.

'When I was pregnant with my son, I did both NCT classes and hospital classes. The NCT classes offered the social side of things, as we were encouraged to meet up as a group after we had had our babies, which we did. The hospital classes were much more realistic about what you will actually experience and much more down to earth in terms of discussing your options for pain relief. All in all, if I was starting with my first baby again, I would still do what I did then and attend both.' DumbledoresGirl

Some people don't feel that classes are really for them: and that's fine too. You might want to stick to books and the Internet instead. And you can always 'crash an NCT coffee morning once the baby's been born and meet friends that way' . . . 'or join in a Mumsnet meet-up on your local site.'

'I never went to any classes and felt one hundred per cent prepared both physically and emotionally for labour. I found it more useful to read books and speak to people; and I practised visualisation. Don't be pressurised by your doctors or midwives to go. When I told them I wasn't going to any, they sighed deeply and raised eyebrows, but they aren't right for everyone and certainly not at that price!' Kama

But don't underestimate the social network that classes can provide in your new life, which will be far more useful to you than the knowledge that the average couple sleeps for only 37 minutes a night and doesn't have sex again until the child is at secondary school. (N.B. These statistics may vary.) Your old social network is likely to become less relevant as time goes by – particularly if your old friends do not have young families of their own. Having someone in the same boat as you at this stage of your life can be hugely important and make a big difference to how easy the transition will be: 'The more friends you make with babies at the same time as you, the more support you'll have and the less isolated you'll feel.'

'If I was running antenatal classes it would go like this:

- Women kneel in front of men (calm down, boys).
- Men slap testicles on a stool and women place clamp around testicles.
- Women slowly tighten clamp until men go cross-eyed. Keep tight for 60 seconds. Say,

"Well done darling, you're doing really well."
Rub his back.

– Release clamp. Wait two minutes. Repeat
endlessly for 24 hours. Tell him to breathe
through it. Increase the tightness of the
clamp over this time. Don't forget to
suggest positions that might make it more
"comfortable". When he starts begging, light
a candle and suggest that he focus on this and
breathe. If at any point he suggests that he
wants to die, remind him that it's "only pain"
and "nothing he can't handle". Charge £140.'

Morningpaper

WHEN THINGS GO WRONG
Miscarriage and Loss

'I have just come home from the hospital after a miscarriage. This was the first baby for us; we tried for so long, and I just feel like my heart is going to break. I have had days where I think I'm fine, but there seem to be pregnant ladies everywhere and that just sets me off again. I have a fabulous husband who is being great, and lots of support from family, but I still feel so alone. I just can't believe it happened.' StephanieNorthampton

Facing up to the sadness of a lost pregnancy *is* heartbreaking. You might come to a slow realisation that something is wrong, or the news could come as a cruel surprise. Either way, the loss can be devastating, no matter how far along you are in your pregnancy. It can be an overwhelming, frightening and lonely time. 'I am filled with so much grief, shock, disbelief, anger and hatred,' wrote one Mumsnetter. 'How do I carry on?'

The loss of a pregnancy, or a miscarriage (sometimes called 'spontaneous abortion'), is – sadly – a very common occurrence. Statistics vary wildly, largely because it is thought that many women miscarry very early on, before they even know they are pregnant. It is possible that as many as 40–50 per cent of pregnancies result in miscarriage, although figures of around 25 per cent are more commonly cited. Most miscarriages happen in the first trimester.

Diagnosis of miscarriage

Some bleeding is common during early pregnancy and does not necessarily mean you are miscarrying (see Bleeding, p. 52, for more information about this). However, heavy bleeding, particularly with blood clots or tissue, is a symptom of miscarriage. This may be accompanied by abdominal pain and cramping.

If you start to experience any of the above, you should contact your doctor. Although some women prefer to miscarry without medical intervention, it's worth telling your GP for various reasons: so they can keep an eye on you and make sure you have miscarried fully; so that you can register that you had a miscarriage, lest, heaven forbid, you have further miscarriages and need to have the cause investigated. (Most hospitals will do this only once you have had three miscarriages.) You will possibly be referred to the Early Pregnancy Assessment Centre or Early Pregnancy Unit at your local hospital, although this may take a few days. There, they will examine your uterus with an ultrasound machine, which will examine the foetus and look for a heartbeat. (If you are at the very early stages of a pregnancy, say five to seven weeks, it is possible that the heartbeat is too small to detect, and you may be asked to return in a week or two for a further exam.) You may also have an internal examination, to check your cervix. If your cervix is open or dilated, then it is unlikely that your pregnancy will continue. Once a miscarriage has started, there is very little you can do.

When should I call my doctor?

Call your doctor or midwife at any time that you are worried about your pregnancy or want reassurance about any aspect of your own or your baby's health. They are there to look after you and won't mind answering your questions and listening to your concerns.

Call your doctor or midwife *immediately* if you:

- are bleeding a lot and are worried that you are losing too much blood (as a rough guideline, if you are soaking more than one sanitary pad in an hour)
- feel feverish or fluey – this may indicate an infection
- have severe pain on one side of your abdomen – this may indicate an ectopic pregnancy (see p. 117), which can be life-threatening
- need pain relief.

Types of miscarriage

There are several different types of miscarriage, as outlined below.

Threatened miscarriage If your cervix is closed and a scan shows a heartbeat, you may be diagnosed as having a 'threatened miscarriage'. This is a ray of hope; it means that the ball is still in the ring and your pregnancy has a chance of continuing. You may be advised to go home and rest.

Complete miscarriage A 'complete miscarriage' is where your body completely expels the foetus, placenta and tissues so that the uterus is empty and the cervix is closed. If this has happened you may need a check-up with your GP, but are unlikely to need further treatment. The pattern of this miscarriage may be a 'natural miscarriage' (see below).

Incomplete miscarriage An 'incomplete miscarriage' occurs when some tissues remain in your uterus and the cervix may still be open. There is a risk of infection, so you are likely to be offered an operation to remove the products of the pregnancy. This is called an Evacuation of Retained Products of Conception or ERPC (see p. 122 for details).

Missed miscarriage Sometimes you may not have any obvious symptoms of a miscarriage, but a scan reveals that the baby has no heartbeat and has stopped growing. This is called a 'missed miscarriage'. It occurs when an embryo dies but the placenta keeps growing, so effectively, the pregnancy continues, although the baby has died. In a missed miscarriage, the woman's body retains the placenta and the baby, so she is likely to still "feel" pregnant and pregnancy tests will still be positive. A missed miscarriage can only really be diagnosed with an ultrasound, which detects whether or not the baby's heart is beating.

'I discovered that I had a missed miscarriage at my 12-week scan. I would have been far more prepared for it had I realised that it was quite possible to be feeling all the symptoms of pregnancy and yet have actually lost the baby. As it was, it was just a huge and horrible shock

at a time when I had hoped to see a scan and share the good news.' Nauseous

When a missed miscarriage has been diagnosed, you are likely to be offered an ERPC (see p. 122).

Blighted ovum This is a type of missed miscarriage, where conception occurred and a fertilised egg implanted in your uterus, but a baby did not develop. 'I read a description once which described a blighted ovum as "an empty nursery",' writes one mum. 'The sac, placenta, etc. are all there but the baby has died at a much earlier stage and for some reason everything has stayed in place.' A miscarriage will usually follow, although it may take several weeks, so you will usually be offered the choice of medical management, i.e. a drug to bring on a 'natural' miscarriage or an ERPC (see p. 122).

Ectopic pregnancy

In normal circumstances, after being fertilised in a Fallopian tube, the egg would be shuffled along so that it could implant itself in the womb lining. An ectopic (meaning 'out of place') pregnancy occurs when a fertilised egg implants itself outside the womb; it can be in the ovary, the abdomen, the cervix or in the scar of a Caesarean section – but the vast majority (around 98 per cent) occur in a Fallopian tube.

A Fallopian tube is not designed to stretch and grow in the way that a uterus does. As the embryo grows, the Fallopian tube will burst, causing internal bleeding. This can be fatal and so requires emergency surgery. Catching it early is important.

'My first pregnancy ended with an ectopic. I didn't have the sharp pain most feel but started bleeding. I had found out I was pregnant on the Thursday, started bleeding on the Friday and by Tuesday was no longer a mum-to-be. Despite losing a tube as it had already burst I have since had healthy twin boys, now toddlers, without any IVF. Always get it checked. They are pretty prompt to respond when there's a chance of an ectopic. As soon as the blood test came back and they realised it wasn't a miscarriage I was literally ordered into hospital.' *Paula71*

(continued)

Around one in 100 pregnancies is ectopic. The causes are not really understood, but factors that increase the risk of an ectopic pregnancy include using an intra-uterine device (IUD) or the mini-pill (progesterone-only contraceptive pill), previous surgery on your abdomen or Fallopian tubes (including Caesarean sections), having had pelvic inflammatory disease (PID) and having experienced a previous ectopic pregnancy.

Symptoms can arise as early as the third week of pregnancy, but may occur as late as 12 weeks, or even later. Over half of women who have an ectopic pregnancy don't show any signs until they collapse. Symptoms include:

- one-sided pain in your abdomen
- shoulder-tip pain – a very distinctive and specific pain right on the tip of your shoulder
- pain on urination or when having a bowel movement
- dizziness
- collapse and fainting
- a feeling that something is very wrong – increased pulse rate, sickness, diarrhoea
- abnormal vaginal bleeding – a longer-than-usual period (even if only light bleeding) or a prolonged bleeding of a 'prune juice' consistency.

In cases of ectopic pregnancy, home pregnancy tests may not be accurate and may report a false negative as it may be too early in the pregnancy to show as positive. So if you are trying for a baby and experience any of these symptoms – even if your pregnancy test is negative – see your GP or, if you are very concerned, attend your A&E department immediately.

Diagnosis
If your symptoms are mild, your GP may take blood samples to test your level of pregnancy hormones and confirm that you are pregnant and also to see whether you are just having a 'normal' miscarriage; this could be an another reason for pain and bleeding. Your GP is likely to take blood samples at intervals of one or two days apart, to see how your hormone levels are changing. He or she will advise you to keep an eye on your symptoms and to go to A&E if they become severe.

If the blood tests confirm that you are pregnant, you may then be referred to the Early Pregnancy Assessment Unit (EPAU) where you will have an ultrasound scan which will hopefully determine where the pregnancy has occurred. If you are very early in your pregnancy, they may use a modern endovaginal – or transvaginal – scanning device, which is inserted in your vagina. This can give a more accurate picture of developments earlier in the pregnancy than older devices which are used on your belly. If an ectopic pregnancy is seen (i.e. a foetus and sac are found outside the uterus) then you will need to be treated.

'Looking back I did have symptoms, but I thought it was just pregnancy. I was exhausted and very breathless and had some abdominal pain. No one really took me seriously until I finally insisted that my GP check me out and he whisked me to hospital immediately where they took me straight to theatre, to stop the internal bleeding. A few more hours' delay and I would probably have died. I tell everyone now to make a note of any pregnancy symptoms and if they are at all worried, to call their GP.' *MrsMac*

If an ectopic pregnancy is suspected but cannot be located or seen on an ultrasound (for example, if there is no visible evidence of a foetus in the uterus, but your blood tests show that you are pregnant), then a diagnostic laparoscopy may be performed. This is a keyhole procedure (i.e. done via a small hole in your abdomen) where an instrument called a laparoscope is inserted and has a good look around inside. This is normally done under a general anaesthetic by a surgeon specially trained in the procedure (if the porter suggests doing it for you, you should politely decline).

Treatment
Sadly, an ectopic pregnancy cannot be moved into the uterus, and must be stopped or removed. Some hospitals may wait and see whether the pregnancy stops of its own accord (while you are monitored in hospital) but generally intervention is the course of action that most hospitals now take.

Non-surgical intervention: if your pregnancy is in the very early stages you may be given an injection of Methotrexate. This is a

(continued)

drug which interferes with the cells of the very early pregnancy and stops them from growing. In most cases, this then stops the pregnancy.

Surgical intervention: in cases where a pregnant woman has collapsed due to loss of blood (from internal bleeding) they are usually transferred straight to theatre and 'opened up'. The foetus and the Fallopian tube are removed. In cases diagnosed before this stage, a keyhole laparoscopy (or sometimes open surgery) is undertaken to remove the foetus and the products of the pregnancy. Sometimes the Fallopian tube can be repaired, but it may need to be removed.

The chance of a future pregnancy depends on the condition of the tubes left behind. It is perfectly possible to get pregnant with only one Fallopian tube. But if both tubes are damaged or have been removed, IVF may be necessary for future pregnancies. The number of Mumsnetters who have had ectopic pregnancies and gone on to have healthy babies is reason for optimism.

Approaches to miscarriage

The treatment options for miscarriage address minimising distress and preventing both infection and excessive blood loss. The treatment that you will be offered to manage a miscarriage largely depends on how your body has already progressed in expelling the pregnancy. Your doctor or consultant should inform you about your options, along with the advantages and disadvantages of each. It is quite normal to have lots of questions, and even to feel that the doctors are wrong and must have made a mistake. If you have questions that you feel have not been answered, you can always ask for a second opinion or for another person to explain your options.

Natural miscarriage

Natural miscarriage or 'expectant management', is also known as letting nature take its course. This is an option if you are not losing too much blood or running a fever (which may indicate an infection). It is usually the procedure for miscarriages in the first trimester, where the body starts expelling the pregnancy of its own accord. Only 10 per cent of first-trimester miscarriages will require an operation (ERPC – see p. 122). Some women diagnosed with a missed miscarriage may choose this option instead of an ERPC.

For some women, a natural miscarriage may be like a very heavy period: 'I was surprised at how much blood there was; that would have been useful to know.' For others, it might be more painful: 'No one mentioned that it might feel similar to labour; I felt contractions and an urge to push, which was really upsetting.'

'I miscarried at six weeks. Everyone's story is different I know, but although the bleeding was heavy, it certainly wasn't "flooding", which is what I expected to have. Yes, there were some clots and tissue, but I couldn't detect an embryo, although I'm pretty certain there was a sac (very small), and there was very little pain – no more than period-like cramps.' Charlie1000

One thing you will need is support, especially if you are sent home to wait for a natural miscarriage to take its course.

'If you're sent home to miscarry "naturally", you need industrial-strength sanitary pads and someone sympathetic with you. You can't really prepare yourself for flushing your longed-for baby down the toilet, and you don't want to have to do that alone if it comes to that. Plus, I'd stock up on ibuprofen, or get the doctor to prescribe something stronger. The last thing you need is physical as well as mental pain.' Biza

A natural miscarriage may involve bleeding for a couple of weeks. During this time, there is a risk of serious bleeding or infection, which on rare occasions can be life-threatening. There is also a risk that some tissues might remain in the uterus, which may mean having an ERPC.

'My first miscarriage – at around seven weeks – was like a very heavy period, and by the time I had a scan, all the signs of the baby had gone. When I miscarried at eight and a half weeks, I bled unimaginably heavily for several days, and had a lot of pain. After about ten days, the blood turned smelly and it turned out I had an infection, which is something to watch out for. On a positive note I was pregnant again within the month and had a healthy baby boy.' Giggi

If you miscarry naturally at home, you should report it to your doctor as a matter of record.

Evacuation of remaining products of conception (ERPC)

Formerly known as 'dilation and curettage' (or D&C), ERPC is a minor surgical procedure in which, under a general or local anaesthetic, the cervix is dilated and the uterus is scraped or suctioned out to remove any remaining pregnancy-related tissue. The decision to carry out an ERPC is based on the size of your uterus and the results of your scan, but it is more common further along in a pregnancy, and is usually recommended for an incomplete or missed miscarriage. There isn't the same waiting that comes with a natural miscarriage but, like any operation, it carries a very slight risk of infection.

One mum says: 'They were going to send me home because "everything would come away naturally", but I preferred the option of an ERPC, and my consultant agreed that I could have one the same day.'

'I was ten weeks pregnant when I realised that I had miscarried but the scan showed the baby had died at six weeks. I opted for the ERPC and it was OK. I stopped bleeding, mostly spotting, after nine days. The procedure was quick and painless. I felt a bit groggy afterwards and had light bleeding for a week. My reason for this choice was that I just couldn't face miscarrying naturally. I was very upset and thought this would be too much. It is a personal choice though.' Lcy

Medical management or 'assisted medication'

If you have been diagnosed with a missed or incomplete miscarriage, or you have just started to miscarry naturally, you may be offered the choice of taking a drug (most likely a course of tablets and pessaries over several days), which will speed up the natural process of miscarrying by causing the uterus to contract. Side effects may include abdominal pain, nausea, vomiting and diarrhoea.

'I opted for the medical route when I had a missed miscarriage (rather than a D&C) because for me the D&C just sounded too invasive. My hospital gave me a tablet and then a day later I was admitted and then given a pessary. That kicked in quite quickly. To be totally honest, it was quite painful (like really bad period pain), but as I was in the hospital they gave me drugs. I had to bleed into a bowl and a nurse would come and check it. Cloudydaze

Not all hospitals offer this option, and you may be sent home to pass the last of your pregnancy. Some women may still require an ERPC to completely clear their uterus.

'If the tablets work (they don't always), then you'll start to bleed, then there will be clots and then bits that look like liver. There might be an intact sac. Most of the bits will usually come out in the toilet. The hardest part is flushing it away. The pain can range from just period-like cramps to really quite painful. The hospital should give you painkillers and instructions about what to do, and when you should contact them or go in.'
Cmotdibbler

Why did this happen?

The cause of miscarriage is not usually identified. Naturally, this will be the only question going around in your head, but hospitals do not generally investigate whether there is an underlying cause (such as a genetic problem, blood clotting disorder or hormonal disturbance) until you have had 'recurrent miscarriages' – meaning at least three. So, in the large majority of cases, there is no answer, which may be extremely frustrating, and can leave you feeling powerless.

You may start to worry that you could have done things differently or that the miscarriage was caused by too much worrying, eating the wrong foods or exercise. It is natural to think: what did I do wrong? But it is highly unlikely that it was your fault; the embryo simply didn't develop properly.

'One of the nurses said to me that it was nature's way of telling you that things weren't right; nobody's fault. I really think that is true, so tell yourself that again and again.' AnnieLaurie

Dealing with the emotional fallout of a miscarriage

The physical signs of your pregnancy should pass after a few weeks, but it can be particularly painful to still be feeling pregnant (and carrying pregnancy weight) when your baby is no longer inside you: 'I was surprised both times that the pregnancy symptoms continued post-miscarriage for quite a while. To still have morning sickness and sore breasts when there's no baby seems so cruel and unfair.'

Eventually, the physical side of things should settle down, but the emotional side of a miscarriage may last for some time. For many women, feelings of bereavement are very strong and hard to deal with. 'I found that the emotional stuff didn't really hit full force until physical recovery was over,' writes one Mumsnetter. 'I had that awful feeling that I had nothing to show for all those weeks of pregnancy and months of trying to conceive.'

Some women take comfort from the knowledge that the experience of miscarriage is very common: 'I have always found it helpful to be reminded that miscarriages are a very common event, and that there is huge potential for things to go wrong in the very early stages of pregnancy.' There are certainly many, many women who understand the feelings of bereavement over a lost pregnancy – and you will possibly find that some of your family and friends have been through the same experience.

'Having a miscarriage is so hard because it's not the sort of thing that people talk about a lot in real life – although a couple of friends I told have also had miscarriages, but I didn't know that until I told them about mine. Just try and take it easy, get some rest and watch some rubbish on TV.' TheBlonde

Even a very early miscarriage can affect you more than you might expect: 'Don't assume that just because you have had an early miscarriage it won't affect you,' writes one Mumsnetter. 'It's still a big deal and a hard thing to cope with.' Another says, 'Be kind to yourself; allow yourself to grieve and lean on your loved ones as much as you need to.'

'I feel OK physically, and mentally I think that I am coping. But I know that there is more going on in my head than I want to admit. Fortunately, I have a very supportive boss, who told me off for coming in to work. My colleagues have also been great. I got a good piece of advice from one of them who went through a miscarriage herself years ago: to take things one day at a time. One day you might feel fine, the next you're in tears. It's a strange and unsettling time.' JanZ

There may be many things that trigger off your grief again: it may feel like 'everyone else is pregnant', and you can't walk down the high street without falling over someone else's double buggy, filling you with rage at life's unfairness. These feelings are quite normal.

Around your due date things may also be very fraught, so make allowances for yourself at this time: 'Letting go of the idea that you're having that particular baby on that date is so hard.' You might want to mark the day in some way, to acknowledge the baby that you lost.

'We planted a tree for the baby we lost. We have other children now, but we wanted to have some permanent memorial to the baby we never got to meet.' Munchpot

'I know it is such a cliché, but time is the best healer,' says one Mumsnetter. 'Let your body and mind do whatever they need to do – rest, cry, throw things, yell, get mad, curl up in a corner and tell the rest of the world to piss off, cuddle up with your man – whatever makes you feel better at the time.'

Your partner's feelings

Partners can feel sidelined following the loss of a baby, the focus obviously being on your body and what you are going through. Your partner may feel that he (or she) doesn't have as much right to grieve as you do. 'No one asks him how he is. It's always, "How is she?" writes one Mumsnetter, 'On the day of my op, his mum sent me flowers and didn't mention him. Or US.'

'My man is struggling. Although he was fantastic at the time, the more I get "better" the more depressed he seems. He really wanted this baby, probably more than me now I look back, and he feels as though his world is falling apart.'

StephanieNorthampton

A miscarriage is the loss of a partner's baby as well, and it is helpful that you both recognise this. Men are perhaps not as at ease as women when it comes to talking about their feelings with friends and family, but talking can be a good therapy, so try to talk to each other, and don't be afraid to seek counselling for either or both of you to work through issues if they are proving hard to deal with.

Alternatively, you might find that your partner doesn't seem to grieve in the way that you do: 'I felt that my husband didn't really feel the same way as I did, which was hard to cope with. He just thought it was a minor setback whereas I felt like everything was falling apart.' Some women find that their partners throw themselves into work as a way of dealing with events. Grief affects people in different ways, but it is also possible that your partner was not as emotionally involved with the pregnancy and baby as you may have been.

Things You Can Do to Help You Cope with Loss

'I'm off to get a little bit drunk and eat Brie,' declared one grieving mum. That is certainly an approach that suits some Mumsnetters, but there are other ways you might like to consider to mark this time in your life.

You may feel particularly emotional while you are waiting for the miscarriage to complete and better once it's over: 'I feel a bit of closure now I've had the op, knowing things are sorted and I can move on.'

'I have my hospital scan picture which is something to remind me of the short time my baby had with us,' says one mum. Some hospitals may issue a special certificate marking your miscarriage, which may help things to feel more tangible.

If you have the opportunity, you might want to consider making special arrangements for the remains of the pregnancy. This is more likely to be feasible if you have the miscarriage at home; if you are in hospital you can ask whether arrangements can be made, but this may only be possible with later miscarriages.

'I had my second miscarriage in the comfort of my own home with a basin. Yes, I was sad and bereft at my loss, but I kept the sac and gave it a proper burial myself, which helped enormously with the grieving process.' Spidermama

Several Mumsnetters feel that giving the remains of the pregnancy a proper 'burial' or something similar helps to confer some dignity on the baby you have lost. 'I re-potted a small olive tree this afternoon and put it in the pot,' says one Mumsnetter. 'It felt too callous to deliberately flush "it" away. The way I look at it, some teeny bit of good can come by nourishing another growing thing.'

For outside support, there are organisations that you can contact if you would like more information and support, including the Miscarriage Association (www.miscarriageassociation.org.uk).

You'll find plenty of empathy and advice from others who've suffered miscarriage on Mumsnet (www.mumsnet.com/Talk/ miscarriage) and, of course, you can also talk to your GP if you are worried about any aspect of your mental or physical wellbeing.

'I had lots of mixed feelings about the miscarriage, and needed a bit of help to get my head around them,' writes one Mumsnetter. 'Our babies will always be loved and never forgotten,' says another. 'We have found that marking certain days as a family (we already have a son) has helped us to deal with our grief. We try to mark the birth date of our baby and the anniversary of the miscarriage.'

Onwards and upwards

After a miscarriage, it is natural to start to doubt your body, and to worry that you are not able to carry a baby to term. 'I felt that there must be something wrong with my body that I couldn't hold on to this baby.' It's very hard, but try to remember that many women have miscarriages but go on to have healthy pregnancies and babies.

'I had a miscarriage many years ago and it was devastating, says a Mumsnetter, 'but now I have five children – all were uneventful pregnancies.' 'After several miscarriages I now have a gorgeous three-year-old daughter,' writes another. 'She truly does feel like a miracle!'

Your next period is likely to start around four to six weeks after the miscarriage has finished. You may be advised to wait a month or two before trying to conceive again, but there are no hard and fast rules. Some doctors suggest waiting for your next period (to rule out any signs of infection) before trying to get pregnant, but some advise that you can start trying again as soon as you both feel emotionally ready to do so: 'My husband was in the room with me when I asked how long we needed to wait before trying again and, with a slight twinkle in her eye, the doctor advised waiting until we got home.'

You may not feel ready to start trying to conceive again immediately, and that is fine too. Give yourself time to grieve, and don't rush into anything if you don't feel that you are ready: 'When I miscarried, I thought I could never go through a pregnancy again, but we've now started to try again and I'm feeling really positive about that.'

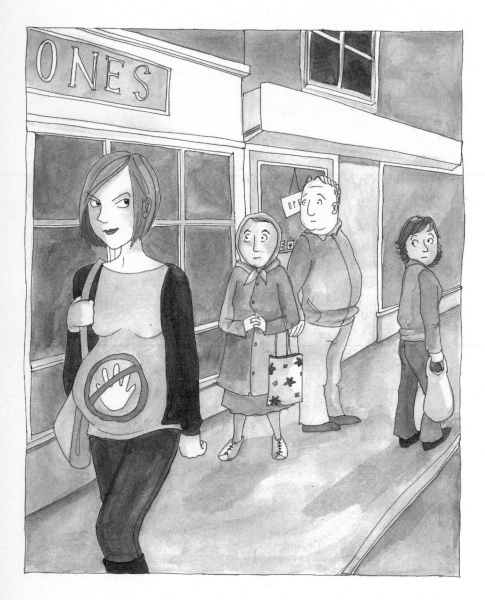

Second Trimester:

Not Ballooning But Blooming

In this chapter ...

Blooming Gorgeous

After the initial shock (and hopefully joy) of discovering that you are pregnant, added to what can be a gruelling first trimester, you are now, with a bit of luck, getting into the swing of this pregnancy lark. At last, your secret is out in the open, and you can revel in the attention and in the extra plates of biscuits proffered by kindly colleagues. Your partner is finally starting to take your pregnancy seriously, and you are both rejoicing in your new, impressive cleavage.

What's more, you may now be starting to look pregnant rather than just plain podgy. Chances are your hair has become glossy and bouncy, as though you're in a shampoo advert, and your skin has taken on a new glow. You are the poster girl for pregnant women. And the birth itself is not yet an imminent reality – hurrah!

'I was sick for the first 14 weeks of pregnancy and as a result switched to part-time work, dropped my studies and became a bit of a hermit. Now, at 15 weeks, I am feeling great! This is so strange and I'm almost in denial that I'm pregnant. I am enjoying work again and almost wish I hadn't gone part-time. I am back to cooking meals, cleaning, going out and just enjoying being me again. Is it normal to stop feeling and being sick so suddenly? I'm sure it is but I feel like I'm not pregnant now.' ChaCha

While some find the sudden absence of sickness mildly worrying, it is undoubtedly the long-straw relative to the ongoing sickness that some are destined to endure. Because, alas, the end of the first trimester doesn't always spell the start of the blooming period for an unfortunate number of us. You may still spend most of the day with your head in a bucket or asleep at your desk, dribbling on to your keyboard. Plus, aches and pains can kick in during the second trimester, sleep becomes a distant memory and indigestion and constipation continue to be a daily grind. And all this on top of piling on the blubber at a rate that would seriously impress the readers of *Heat* magazine.

Still, at least there are a million things to distract you from your off-the-scale weight gain. First, there are the milestones that will help you feel that you are heading in the right direction and that there is actually a point to all these frustrating pregnancy symptoms. Important matters such as, have you chosen a name? Are you going to find out whether you are having a boy or a girl? Have you been kicked by your baby yet? Have you invested in a cute little vest or two? Then there is all the stuff you are learning about your body: you could get a diploma with everything you've picked up about your body parts in the last three months – parts so wild and woolly that you probably didn't even know they existed. And, of course, you will have been bombarded by advice, some of it helpful and some of it profoundly forgettable – just ignore the terrifying stuff and stick with what sounds do-able, preferably things you can achieve without leaving the sofa!

For many women, as well as coping with the physical changes, now is the time when they have to make serious decisions about their pregnancy, and this is not easy: should you have an amniocentesis; would you consider a termination? Being responsible for a new life can put you under a lot of pressure. What you want is for someone else to make the decisions for you, but sadly, they can't. Remember, you are the only one who really knows what this journey feels like (despite what your mother thinks), and it is not always fun. Keep talking to your other half (if you have one) and, if you need it, seek out help from your GP or midwife.

The second trimester is the time to grasp the nettle and pull on those expandable-waist trousers, tuck into that plate of pastries and whine, 'But the baby wants it!' If your partner raises an eyebrow, just curl up with the Mothercare catalogue and a box of tissues. And if anyone rubs your belly, playfully move their wandering hands to cup your jubblies and they won't do it again!

Foetal Movements – It's Alive!

'Have you felt it move yet?' is one of those bog-standard questions that can get very boring. But feeling that first flutter really *is* nothing short of thrilling. Amazing. There actually is something in there! You may feel slightly freaked out, especially if you were a big fan of the *Alien* movies in the eighties, but rest assured that you will get used to the daily flutterings and bubblings, and will soon come to love them.

Foetal movements aren't always easy to detect. Is that a baby inside me? Or do I just have really bad wind? Some women start to feel movement from 14 weeks, but everyone is different; anywhere around 20 weeks is average if it is your first baby.

'I felt something like butterflies at sixteen weeks. The midwife said it was unusual to feel movement so early given that I was a size 18-plus (cheeky cow!) but it was definitely the baby.' JackBauer

Skinny women tend to feel more foetal activity: 'My midwife pointed out to me in the nicest possible way that I was too podgy to feel much movement second time around.' Eating a piece of fruit sometimes encourages movement because of the increase in blood sugar. Likewise a family pack of Maltesers.

Babies are generally at their busiest between 24 and 28 weeks when there is still room in your womb to move. You'll most likely notice more kicks and flutters as you approach your due date, although it would be wise to resist the urge to start a detailed tracking spreadsheet. It's not unusual for babies to change their patterns of activity, but if you are at all worried, it's worth paying your midwife a visit to put your mind at rest.

In these later weeks, eagle-eyed friends will be able to spot strong movements as your belly undulates like a carrier bag full of hamsters. Try not to feel offended if they shriek in horror: it does look odd if you haven't seen it before.

'I'm certain my baby was doing handstands the other night. I had a number of pointy-out bits. Frankly I am expecting Nadia Comaneci to exit in a few weeks' time.' Piffle

During the day, when you are busy on your feet, your baby will probably be rocked to sleep by your movements. As soon as you put your feet up, it will wake up and start jumping about and demanding attention. You'd better get used to it because this will continue for the next 20 or so years.

Soon after you notice your baby's kicking, others should be able to feel the movements too if they lay a hand on your belly. For the next few months you will probably find that no sooner do you shout, 'Ooh quick feel this, it's moving,' than your jumping bean is instantly stilled by your partner's hand. But eventually they will feel the baby moving and will share in your excitement. In the final weeks you will most likely be able to lie in bed with your belly pressed against his back and for his child to give him a good kicking.

Braxton Hicks contractions

Another joyful side effect of pregnancy are 'Braxton Hicks' contractions. These are sometimes called 'practice contractions' – they enable you to practise not swearing at your other half or begging for a gun when you are doubled over in pain. No one really knows the significance of Braxton Hicks. Some women notice them more than others, and some don't notice them at all. They may occur several times a week or even several times a day, and they are usually painless. One mother describes Braxton Hicks as 'a tightening in my belly and my bump goes rock hard'.

While Braxton Hicks are generally described as a 'tightening' sensation, you may sometimes feel your ligaments stretching, which can hurt. This can be a stitch-like pain or sharp pains, often in your lower abdomen. Rest assured: you are growing to quite impressive proportions, and a little bit of loosening and stretching is necessary to accommodate your lovely bundle of joy (and all those cakes you are scoffing). But, as always, if you *are* worried, give your midwife a ring.

One thing that you really mustn't do when it comes to Braxton Hicks – at least, it seems, in the experience of Mumsnetters – is to complain about them to your mother-in-law. 'Ooh, we didn't have those in my day, dear,' declared one mother-in-law witheringly, while another dismissed them as an unnecessary modern folly: 'I never bothered with having them: I just gave birth.'

Another thing you shouldn't do, as one Mumsnetter confessed, is to tell a mum friend that you are sure you will sail though labour because you have been coping very well with your Braxton Hicks contractions. She will probably pat you on the head and make you a cup of tea. And then leave the room and snort loudly.

What Not to Wear

In olden times, when your mother was pregnant, it was acceptable to spend your entire pregnancy in sensible flat shoes and trousers with an elasticated waist. But pregnancy is no longer an excuse to put away your skinny jeans and be a slattern for six months. If *Hello!* has taught us one thing, it is that pregnant women are not required to go into fashion purdah; it's a case of use it or lose it. Maternity wear sites and independent maternity shops are popping up all over the place, and every high-street store and mail-order company has its own on-trend maternity range.

All that choice. And yet we still complain. Sometimes it feels like it would be easier to stay indoors. Who wants to walk into a shop called Larger Than Life? Nothing ever fits quite right. It's too long, too short, too baggy or too tight. You could spend your entire pregnancy trying to find the right kit to cover your expanding bump and still look like an obese scarecrow. 'My husband suggested I just wear my son's play tent,' said one disgruntled mum.

It's the in-between stage that can be the hardest – when you feel more fat than pregnant. Your favourite jeans feel like an instrument of torture, yet it would take two of you to fill maternity clothes. How do all those celebrities do it? Well, for a start, they have a team of stylists, unlimited funds and a bump the size of a lychee.

There are a few tricks that might see you through that awkward stage as you get a feel for the shape of your tummy. 'I used to thread a thick elastic band or hair bobble through my trouser buttonhole, double it over and loop it over the button, then wear long tops to hide the gape,' advises a mum. Bump bands, which sit under a regular T-shirt but stop your belly peeking out, are an alternative (one mum recommends improvising with 'cheap large boob tubes from Primark'). But unless you are very lucky, your bump won't be the only part of your body that expands during your pregnancy; your bum and thighs will want to join in too: 'I have got away so far with a belly band on my work trousers, but this morning I couldn't shoe-horn my thighs in.'

For a while, you can often get away with buying normal clothes in a size bigger than you would normally wear: 'My best friend is a stylist and she took me down to Primark and showed me how to adapt some of the larger sizes to fit under my bump.' Elastic and drawstring waists – think Gypsy skirts rather than Saga slacks – might also give you a few months' reprieve before you need to head for the maternity section.

Alternatively, for that woman-in-the-Dulux-commercial look, borrow from your partner's wardrobe: 'Rather than spend a lot of money on maternity nightwear, I pinched my other half's old shirts – the bigger and baggier the better.'

Wearing clothes that hug your bump – showing it off rather than shrouding it – usually work better and prevent you from looking like a fat person who dresses nicely. Avoid at all costs the crop top with belly-button exposure; not only does it scream Britney, but it can be hazardous near a hot stove.

'Empire line is your friend,' advises one Mumsnetter. 'The beauty of it is that it will make you look pregnant rather than just looking like you have eaten all the pies.' And it's definitely the way forward if you are getting married sporting your bump.

Some lucky (annoying) women need very little maternity wear. But for most mums, there will come a time when they eventually outgrow even their child's play tent.

Think about how well your clothes are going to fit in a month's time, not just how you look; you want to feel comfortable as well as covered. What might look OK in front of the mirror won't always work when you start to move. 'My advice is to walk around and sit down in the changing room if there's enough space, just to make sure everything fits without falling off or gaping,' says a mum.

It will have been worth it when you get an invitation to supper and you aren't forced to wear your husband's Arsenal shirt because it's the only piece of clothing that fits. 'I remember squeezing into a pair of trousers to go out to dinner, thinking I wouldn't have to do much moving around as I only had to get as far as the restaurant table,' recalls a shame-faced mum. 'Three courses later, the button on my trousers went pinging across the restaurant.'

Bump bargains

That leap from busting out of your regular clothes to investing in a maternity wardrobe can be costly, particularly when you want to spend money on lovely, small pink and blue things instead. Try these tips for low-cost maternity dressing:

- Freecycle (www.freecycle.org) is an organisation that enables you to offload any item that you no longer want by giving it free to other local people who have a use for it. The idea is to keep reusable stuff out of landfill sites. It can be a good source of second-hand maternity wear, and remember that you don't exactly wear maternity clothes for years (no, really, we promise) so you can often get clothes in great condition. Check local listings or post your own request for what you need.
- Maternity hire shops/websites – these are particularly useful if you have formal functions or parties and want something a bit special without forking out too much cash.
- Second-hand maternity wear dress agencies (such as www. maternityexchange.co.uk).
- Local NCT 'nearly new sales' often have second-hand maternity wear for sale – contact your local branch for details.
- Mumsnet's For Sale/Wanted boards (www.mumsnet.com/ Talk/clothes_and_shoes_adults) are another good source of second-hand gear.
- Stock up in the sales.
- Friends and family: if you know anyone who has recently has a baby, chances are that they may have cast-offs that they haven't already set fire to – you can always give them back once you have finished with them.

Preghead – Are You Really Losing Your Mind?

Have you found your car keys in the fridge? Given your mobile a spin in the washing machine? Missed appointments? Lost the ability to reverse park the car? Walked into a room and wondered why? Called your boss by your partner's name? No? Maybe you have just forgotten.

There is something about pregnancy that turns your brain to mush. Not only does your growing baby leech your body's stores of nutrients and vitamins, but it also apparently eats up most of your undergraduate education as well. 'Every time I am pregnant this happens and it is a bit of a joke among my family and friends, especially since I am normally so organised,' says one mum. This prenatal idiocy is sometimes referred to as 'placenta brain' or 'pregnancy amnesia'. Forgetfulness, clumsiness, indecisiveness and a lack of concentration are all part of the package, so don't book yourself into the Alzheimer's clinic just yet: you hang up your brain with your skinny jeans and you don't get it back for at least another five years.

'I put a spoonful of butter in my coffee this morning ... bleeee! What was I doing with a spoonful of butter anyway?' Redrobin

Part of the reason could be that during pregnancy women tend to have a lot on their plate (both literally and metaphorically). It's distracting when you have so much to think about, plus you are probably not sleeping well, which can also make you fuzzy-headed. Pregnancy hormonal changes can put you in a spin, in much the same way that they do in the run-up to your period. And don't tell anyone, but studies have also found that women's brains shrink during pregnancy – not significantly, but enough for you to shave one armpit and not the other without noticing. It could take up to six months from when you give birth for your brain to regain its normal size, once your body has returned to its non-pregnant state. (OK, the latter won't actually happen, but your hormones will eventually settle down again.)

'I have recently put a firm chair in my bathroom, as I'm finding getting socks on and off a bit difficult. A couple of days ago, desperate for the toilet, I rushed into the bathroom and sighed happily as I sank on to the chair, relieved that I had made it without embarrassing myself – all the while staring at the toilet and feeling just a bit confused …' Skwiggy

One part of a woman's brain that seems to take a particular hammering is that part responsible for driving. Reversing into walls, driving down public footpaths and waiting at a green light then pulling away when it turns red all seem fairly common, as is forgetting which side of the road to drive on: 'I sat at a roundabout yesterday, smiling at people on my left and wondering why they weren't going anywhere,' admits one mum. 'Several times now I've forgotten to put the handbrake on when I park the car,' confesses another. 'I've returned to find it gently resting against someone else's car.'

'I picked up my new car and completely forgot how to drive. Didn't get it at all. My husband tried to explain it to me and I just looked at him totally bemused. The car salesman tried to explain and pointed to the pedals, but I still couldn't remember which pedal was which despite having driven for 15 years and having just driven to the garage! In the end I had to get out and let my husband drive home.' Ajm200

Bumpy Rumpy Pumpy – Is It Good For You?

When pregnant women talk about sex, it is usually in the context of whether they would prefer a boy or a girl. But should the conversation take a racier swing towards what goes on when the lights go out, you will realise that pregnancy affects people's sex lives in different ways. Maybe it has brought you and your partner closer and made you more inventive than usual; or maybe it's put both of you off sex for life. What works for you in the first trimester might be the last thing on your mind in the third. And although it is you who is going through the physical metamorphosis, it could be your other half who is most affected ...

'I am eight months pregnant and feeling really fed up. My husband hasn't wanted sex for most of my pregnancy. He assures me that he still loves and fancies me, but says he is worried about harming the baby. We had a great sex life before pregnancy and I am finding this really hard to cope with. I'm feeling quite horny. Is this the beginning of the end of our sex life?' Babygap

Sex can stop as soon as you get a big fat positive on the pregnancy stick, however much you might want it: maybe your man has come over all puritanical and feels sex with a pregnant lady is improper; or perhaps your melon-sized breasts bizarrely just aren't doing it for him; or it could be that he never had much of a thing for sea mammals. 'My hubby said it's not that he doesn't still fancy me, just that it seemed a bit wrong to be doing it while the baby was there – like it was in the same room. I have tried to convince him otherwise, but I guess once you have a certain picture in your head it's very difficult to work around. So, no nooky for me.' His zero libido can be alarming: 'I said to him, "You have needs too. Can't I just face the other way? You don't have to look at the bump." He was nearly sick at the thought. I think he is scared of doing damage.' 'Between his hang-ups and my fatigue I think it will be a while before we resume relations!' confesses another mum.

You and your partner are going through a huge period of change. You might not even know why you feel the way you do. The best you can do is to remain affectionate and talk about how you feel, rather than just shutting up shop completely. Your partner might struggle and need encouragement when it comes to sharing his side of the story, but try not to come down on him too hard. So to speak.

Sickness, achiness and tiredness make it hard for many women to get enthusiastic about sex during pregnancy. 'My sex drive has completely plummeted,' says a weary mum. 'In the first few months, I felt so knackered and, as I get bigger, the thought is becoming less appealing.' It can be hard to explain why you are feeling the way you do. 'It's like the chemicals in my brain that normally think, "Husband, you look a bit sexy, a bit of rudery would be nice," just aren't being produced and I feel like a dried-up, shrivelled old hag,' says another. Rest assured, this feeling will pass and you will blossom into a yummy mummy; albeit a knackered, short-tempered one.

It's harder if you are in pain: 'I had symphysis pubis dysfunction [SPD – see p. 78] and thought I was going to fall to bits. Sex seemed like a hilarious joke at the time – a pity as I'm quite slutty.' 'My fanjo feels really bruised,' moans one mum, 'I feel like I've had five rounds of sex with a donkey.' Sitting it out might seem like the only solution, but you will probably find other inventive ways of satisfying those cravings.

If you have previously miscarried it might make you more cautious, although there is no need to be unless you have been advised otherwise. However, one mum cautions: 'I bled for five to six weeks in the first trimester. I asked my GP about sex and he said, "Intercourse probably won't cause any problems but if you miscarry, you won't believe it wasn't the sex, and you will blame yourself." So we waited. There are lots of other things you can do, of course.' Abstinence may be recommended in some medical circumstances (for example if you have placenta praevia – see p. 250), so if you want clarification, speak to your GP.

While some women completely lose their appetite, others find their sex drive rockets, particularly in the second trimester:

'I was rampant from the minute I became pregnant and carried on being so throughout the pregnancy. I didn't feel unsexy and even my husband said it was a different kind of sexy as I was no longer worried about fat bits – I was all bump – so my skin was tighter. Poor bloke had to ask for a rest.'

You might find that your usual positions are not suited to your new pregnancy shape or you might not want your pendulous belly swinging between you like a wrecking ball. Spoons is a popular choice of sex position for pregnant Mumsnetters.

One curious thing about sex when pregnant is that the contractions following an orgasm can go on long after you have finished having sex. Experiencing this can be disconcerting when you are lying next to your snoring partner, but it won't put your pregnancy in jeopardy unless your doctor has advised you otherwise. Some pregnant women find that orgasms are uncomfortable or hurt. If you feel this way, it's probably a good idea to tell your other half to slow down tiger.

Urban myths abound when it comes to oral sex and pregnancy, but rest assured that it is quite safe to receive oral sex during pregnancy; 'in fact, I would tell your partner it is positively beneficial to the health of the baby.'

'There is no risk of air entering your body when someone is giving you oral sex, unless you are doing it wrong. You will not overinflate your baby from oral sex in pregnancy. That's not how it works. You're confusing it with blow jobs.'

FabioTheWhisperingCat

Whether you are permanently in the mood or you never want to see a naked man ever again, be reassured that things won't stay this way for ever. However you feel, you are probably well within the normal range. As long as neither of you develops a fetish for maternity clothes, of course.

HEALTH ISSUES

It's Been a Hard Day's Night: Sleep (or Lack of) During Pregnancy

Anyone who has children already will delight in telling you to stock up on sleep now as you won't get any once the baby arrives. Apart from the fact that this is rubbish advice (sadly, no one has yet worked out a technological solution to storing sleep, but we really hope they're working on it), these prophets of doom also appear to have forgotten what it's actually like to try and get eight hours' kip when you're the size of a small whale and suffering from every pregnancy ailment going. Sometimes there isn't even an explanation for why you can't sleep; it's just the cruel curse of pregnancy insomnia.

This can be a killer when you are pregnant and craving sleep. Your body is working overtime making that baby and it just needs a break, damn it, and the frustration that it isn't getting one only makes you grumpier. 'I could have slapped anyone who said, "It's Mother Nature's way of preparing you for when the baby is born",' moans one mum. 'It is terribly lonely at 3 a.m. when everyone else is dreaming. I have often had a quiet blub to myself. It's pure frustration really.'

'I am just so cross. I am shattered and look horrendous. I take three hours to go to sleep, then wake several times in the night and find it hard to fall back to sleep. Then I wake early and twitch.' Piffle

If you suffered from insomnia before pregnancy, it can be doubly aggravating now that your usual cocktail of sleeping potions and pills are forbidden. And a noisy sleeper next to you doesn't help: 'My partner's snoring makes me want to kill him; it's like he's whispering, "I'm asleep, I'm asleep," over and over.' 'I have had to

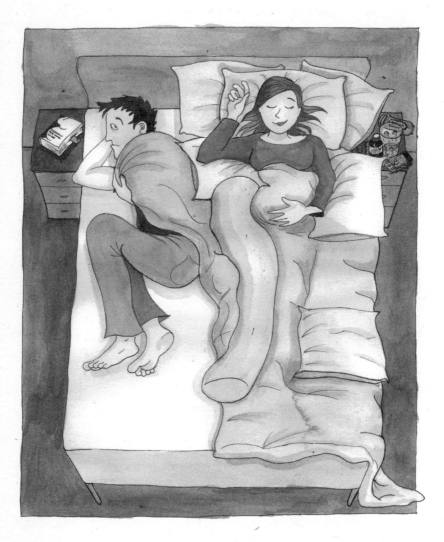

send my husband to the spare room', confesses another mum-to-be, 'because I was starting to have murderous thoughts.'

Some pregnant women get used to surviving on a few hours' sleep at night and snatched cat naps in the day. Dropping off to sleep might not be the problem, but if you wake up to go to the loo it can be hell trying to get back to sleep. Or maybe you are being woken by a wriggling baby, your mind is racing, your stomach is bubbling away with indigestion or your pelvis threatens to snap in two when you try to roll over in bed.

A warm bath and a hot milky drink or a cup of camomile tea before bed can help. If you are feeling peckish, opt for a banana or a turkey sandwich – both are rich in tryptophan, which some say may help you sleep. Persuade your other half to give you a relaxing bedtime massage – or invest in a wire scalp massager, so he can give you an Indian head massage with one hand, while holding the TV remote in the other. Aaahhh.

'Go to bed at the same time every night, get into a routine before bedtime so your body knows what's coming and face the clock away from you,' advises a sleep-savvy mum. Use pillows to make yourself as comfortable as you can. A pillow between your knees might alleviate pelvic and hip pain. Or there are enormous full-length body pillows you can buy, which some people find helpful. Some also suggest that it is better to get up and do some quiet activity, such as reading or listening to the radio, then try to go back to sleep when they feel tired again.

'Late pregnancy insomnia is a really cruel trick of nature. I had it in both my pregnancies and found it very difficult to cope with. I found a healthy dose of fresh air in the afternoon helped. With my second pregnancy, I think trying not to fight it kept me sane. I bought some really good books and when I woke up, instead of tossing and turning I went downstairs and read. Sometimes, I slept better on the sofa than I did in bed. I also think if you can avoid taking a nap during the day, you will sleep better at night. If your toddler still has a nap, put your feet up for a bit, but try not to go to sleep.' Bugsy

You may be very well read by the end of your pregnancy. And familiar with your partner's snoring patterns. You could try wearing earplugs or listening to the radio with earphones. And to settle a racing mind, you could try making lists in your head – like going through the alphabet, for example, thinking of girls' names beginning with 'A' then 'B' ...

Relaxation techniques can help to calm a racing mind, whereas lying in bed feeling cross will make things worse: 'It's important not to get too agitated about not sleeping, because it just makes you more awake.' 'If you have worries or stresses that are keeping you awake, it really helps to keep a diary,' says one mum. 'I used to write them all down just before bedtime. It allowed my brain to stop thinking about them.'

Although you can try various things, there is no magic answer to pregnancy insomnia. But don't forget, you are not the only angry fatty creeping around in the early hours – there are many other pregnant women out there who understand your frustration; just check out the pregnancy Talk boards (www. mumsnet.com/Talk/pregnancy) on Mumsnet at 2.30 a.m. if you need convincing. And if it all gets too much, you can always consider a career change: 'I'm thinking about taking up burgling!'

Pregnancy dreams

When you actually do fall asleep, you might find that your dreamtime is so hectic that you wake up feeling even more exhausted and stressed than you did when you went to bed. Many pregnant women report having extremely vivid dreams throughout pregnancy, which can be quite traumatic.

Some women find that they are plagued by pregnancy nightmares, often about bad things happening to the baby. 'For the last few nights I've woken up screaming out loud,' writes one mum-to-be. 'My husband didn't notice but the dog was very worried.' Other dreams may be more symbolic: burglars or kidnappers invading your house are very common (amateur psychologists may chalk up some obvious explanations about those), and driving in a car with no brakes is another frequently reported night-time adventure (you can imagine Freud chuckling to himself). Some leave even less room for misinterpretation:

'I dreamt I had turned into a dairy cow and my assets were reaching my knees. After I'd finished, all that was left were two bits of empty, awful-looking sausage skins. Now I'm worried that this is really going to happen …' DelGirl

It also seems quite common to have dreams in which your partner has been very naughty, perhaps running another family which he has previously failed to mention. These can put you in a very bad mood with him when you wake up:

'I had a dream that the anaesthetic for the birth knocked me out for three weeks, and by the time I came round, my husband had called the baby Shelby. I pulled up a cane from the sweet peas and chased him round the house with it shrieking: "F**king SHELBY? What the F*CK were you thinking?"' Ninedragons

Birth dreams are quite common, and giving birth to animals is normal (we are still on dreams here, so don't panic): hamsters, guinea pigs, litters of kittens and even a moth ('I was trying to catch it with a jam jar … '). 'I dreamt the baby had been born, but it was a ferret,' reports one stressed mum-to-be; 'I had hold of this ferret with my norks out and kept trying to latch it on …'

'I dreamt that I went to my 20-week scan, and the doctor congratulated me on the size of my baby's trunk and ears. He kept on about how great they were then showed me the picture and I was carrying an elephant.' Lissie

The other type of dream that can plague the pregnant lady is the erotic dream, sometimes complete with orgasm. 'I took my filthy dreams as compensation for 21 weeks of morning sickness,' concludes one happy mum, and another agrees: 'Erotic dreams? Oh dear god yes! Gang bangs, girl on girl, everything. And every night too!' 'I dreamt that Doctor Who had got me pregnant!' confesses one lucky lady, although you might pull a shorter straw: 'I had a rather rude dream about Boris Johnson.'

'In my dreams I have had sex with most of the men in my office. And I work in a VERY big office.' Missnatalie

From shagging ex-boyfriends to murdering your mother, there is no repressed fantasy that is immune to the technicolour dreams in pregnancy. But exhausting though they may be, they won't last for ever. 'I had the most realistic dreams I'd ever had in my life when I was pregnant, but unfortunately they passed as the pregnancy progressed,' recalls one mum. 'It was a shame, as I was quite enjoying the show!'

Sleeping positions

The general advice is that you should, if you can, get into the habit of sleeping on your left-hand side from the end of the first trimester. This apparently makes it easier for the heart to pump blood to all the places that need it, as well as helping your kidneys to expel waste products and fluids from your body more efficiently, which should, in turn, help to ease any swelling in your ankles, feet and hands (nice). By comparison, lying on your back puts pressure on your intestines and the inferior vena cava (the vein that transports blood from your lower body to your heart), with the result that you might feel dizzy, faint and generally uncomfortable.

So far, so gloomy. But the good news is that unless your GP has advised you otherwise, sleeping on your back for part of the night is very unlikely to cause you, or your baby any harm, so don't sellotape a marble to your back just yet: 'It soon becomes too uncomfortable to sleep on your back, which is your body's way of telling you not to – but there's no need to worry until then,' reassures one pregnancy veteran.

Weight – How Much Should You Put On? (And Does It Ever Come Off?)

You are a woman – so unless you have been living in an exclusive Brethren commune on Exmoor for the last 20 years, you probably have some idea that our society places great value on the less cumbersome lady. But stepping on the bathroom scales takes on a whole new significance when you become pregnant. What if you break them? How are you supposed to view the digits through your blur of tears? And why is your maternity bra full of pastry crumbs?

It is inevitable that you are going to pile on the pounds, and, at some point, you will be busting out of your jeans, and possibly even getting wedged behind the car steering wheel. But what you eat – and how much – is no longer just about having a pert bottom and Rosemary Conley's thighs. You have your baby's wellbeing to think about. You are now a baby carrier, and, on top of that, you have the equivalent of a marathon ahead of you. Pregnancy requires stamina, and a healthy and varied diet is an obvious step in the right direction. Point made, now pass the chocolate HobNobs.

Some books will tell you that pregnant women gain on average between 10 and 12.5 kilograms (or 1½–2 stone); this is over the course of the entire pregnancy, by the way, not just during the first month. It won't seem like that if you have been scrutinising the yummy celeb mummies in the glossies. But everybody is different – not everyone has a personal dietician or a trainer or a friendly surgeon to whip the baby out at eight months and sew everything back neatly and the right way up (allegedly, of course).

Your pre-pregnancy size can also be a factor in how you gain weight. If you were overweight before conception, you might drop pounds, at least in the early stages. 'I'm 21 weeks and haven't gained any weight, although I have an extremely big bump,' says one bemused mum. 'I suspect it was because I started out overweight. I was already eating for two before I became pregnant. My appetite has decreased quite a lot since then.' A combination of giving up alcohol and morning sickness can also make a difference to the ominous numbers on the bathroom scales.

'As I was overweight at the beginning of my pregnancies, I was careful to eat well so as not to gain too much. But I lost two stone in the first trimester of each pregnancy due to awful sickness. I had put it on again by the end. I had two healthy children, and finished the same weight as I had started. Some of the weight gained in pregnancy is extra blood, fluid, the placenta, the baby itself, the uterus, an increase in breast size – that isn't noticeable until further along. If all is well with the baby, then don't worry.' Lulumama

Doctors no longer expect you to eat for two, although sometimes you may feel like you'd like to. But these days, midwives and doctors are not as worried about weight gain as they were in the past, and you probably won't be weighed regularly if your pregnancy is progressing normally. If you are weighed and you'd rather not know the bad news, a kindly midwife won't mind a jot if you explain that you'd prefer if she didn't tell you. She will just write it down with a cheery and reassuring smile and a knowing look instead of gasping in horror and declaring that you now weigh slightly more than a Routemaster.

'I'm paranoid about not gaining too much weight,' is a common concern. 'I was pretty happy with myself before becoming pregnant – not really a careful eater, not a dieter. But between the Internet, books, the midwife and my mother, I am so conscious now of having to lose baby weight after birth that it's stressing me out.' It can be particularly hard if you have lost a large amount of weight prior to conception. 'I'm petrified I'm going to end up an absolute heifer again,' wails a newly slimmed-down mum. But now is not the time to diet or to cut out specific food groups – unless we're talking Mars bars. Talk things through with your midwife or doctor if you are concerned about your weight either way.

'My tip is: don't weigh yourself. At 37 weeks, I have put on more than three stone. For someone who is a neat size eight, it has all been a bit of a shock. But I think as long as you are balancing healthy food with the occasional treat, you will be fine. I believe that if you are craving something, you obviously need it. I can strongly recommend a daily walk, a swim or some antenatal yoga. I reckon people who do some exercise spring back into shape quicker.' Alfie72

Pregnancy weight is not just about looking glam in your Isabella Oliver maternity coat. Backache, high blood pressure, breathlessness, indigestion and oedema can all get worse the heavier you are. And too much weight also increases your risk of gestational diabetes (see p. 255). It also becomes even harder to move around – especially at night, when you might want to call in a crane and a winch.

Overweight women are also more at risk of birth complications. 'I'll be so embarrassed if I have a section and the doctor has to cut through three inches of doughnuts before he reaches anything,' confesses one mum. If your bump is feeling 90 per cent cake and 10 per cent baby, it can be easy to give up and indulge for the remainder of your pregnancy, but getting the weight off can be a slog with a new baby. There is a saying that what takes nine months to put on, takes nine months to take off.

Whatever your size and shape, brace yourself for inappropriate comments: 'I'm starting to develop a complex,' says one mum. 'People are very blunt: "Are you sure it's not twins?" I'm not going mad with what I am eating, but I'm starting to feel a bit down about this.' You may find that most of the daft comments come from people who haven't had children yet, or for whom it was so long ago that they have forgotten how pregnant women look at 20 weeks. Ignore them. Or perhaps give their bellies a cheeky pat before trilling: 'Well, at least I've got an excuse!'

Mumsnetiquette: Tummy touching – how do I tell people to bog off (politely)?

Some people don't mind a little bit of fondling by strangers, but others find it rather repellent.

If you feel this way, try some of the responses below to fend off straying hands (and if you are regularly approached by people trying to cop a feel, be reassured that – 'At least you know you look nice and approachable!'):

'Excuse me, that's my colon you're rubbing.' *TheDoctorsWife46*

'I'm not pregnant.' *Princess*

'When's yours due?' *Honeybunny*

'I AM NOT A LUCKY BUDDHA!' *Pingviner*

'Ouch. That really hurts.' *MoonRiver*

'Anywhere else you would like to rub? Or have you had enough?' *custardtart*

'Do you mind not doing that? It gives me bad wind.' *uptheduff*

'Careful, it's catching.' *pearlgem*

'Have you lost something?' *toodlepip*

Of course, if none of the above does the job, you could always try a slightly different approach:

'I loved strangers grabbing my bump, especially men, because I never ever failed to reach over and start fondling their bollocks when they did so – which ALMOST made it worth being pregnant. They only ever did it the once. But I worked with about 500 men so got LOTS of handfuls of bollocks, I can tell you.' *Morningpaper*

Bleeding Gums and (Bleeding) Heartburn

According to an old wives' tale, pregnant women who suffer from heartburn give birth to babies with lots of hair. As if feeling gassy and bloated isn't enough to deal with, now you are faced with the prospect of bearing an ape. But take heart. It's just another (made-up) thing to wind you up. 'I was expecting a baby gorilla but my daughter was balder than a coot and stayed that way for 12 months,' reports a relieved mum.

Pregnancy can be a gastric nightmare. You might feel like you are feeding a totally different body. You probably haven't paid a great deal of attention to your oesophagus until now, but the food pipe that carries food from your mouth to your stomach can play some nasty tricks: as pregnancy hormones relax the valve connecting your stomach and oesophagus, it allows stomach acid to come sneaking back up into your oesophagus towards your mouth. The resulting burning feeling in the back of your throat and pain in your chest area are known as heartburn. But don't panic – it has nothing to do with your heart and it doesn't affect your baby.

'People never warn you about the sheer hell of heartburn during pregnancy. Absolute agony. Can't understand how people live with it in "normal" life.' Dondletella

You might feel breathless, or like a very large elephant is sitting on your chest: 'My heartburn was so bad, I was convinced I was actually having a heart attack on several occasions,' recalls one mum. Another says, 'I used to see the adverts and wonder what was meant by heartburn.' But she is wiser now: 'The bigger I get the more I know. I am waking up five times a night on average in need of a swig of Gaviscon. I have grown to love the stuff and am developing a serious addiction.'

Symptoms are usually worse in this trimester, as your growing baby presses against your stomach, pushing acid back up the oesophagus. Things may improve, however, as the pregnancy progresses and the baby drops down.

Over time, you will work out which foods settle best in your stomach: you could try keeping a food diary to identify trigger foods. Avoid anything spicy, fatty, fried or rich. Some Mumsnetters say cutting out wheat, caffeine and alcohol makes a difference. Pastry, pickles, bacon and cheese are also on the Mumsnet blacklist. As one mother puts it: 'Basically, you are left with really boring, bland foods.'

Try eating little and often, rather than having three big meals a day. Drinks that come recommended are: milk, peppermint and fennel tea, soda water, ginger beer, ginger cordial and warm water with a squeeze of lemon. Eating yoghurt, ice cream, rice pudding and bananas helped some. And, 'It sounds daft, but nibbling a few almonds (shelled but with their brown skin on) when the heartburn came on really helped me.' Others swear by liquorice, digestive biscuits, aniseed and chewing gum, or even 'hot chocolate with melted marshmallows. Honestly, it really works!'

'Love Hearts, Refreshers, and Giant Fizzers worked for me. Packets of them. Rot your teeth but leave your tummy calm.' Suzywong

In addition to watching what you eat, don't bend over as that just squashes your tummy, and avoid wearing anything tight. Sleeping propped up against pillows can help or the sofa might even be an option if you want to try sleeping upright. It will also give your partner a night's peace, but only do so if it suits *you*; after all, you are the incubator. Acupuncture, osteopathy and reflexology can also offer relief. Homeopathic remedies include Arsenicum and Nux Vomica – but always consult your GP before taking any alternative or complementary medicines.

The most common approach to dealing with the hell of heartburn, however, is to turn to an antacid or other over-the-counter remedy. Your GP can prescribe Gaviscon, so at least you don't have to pay for it. It doesn't work for everyone but there are alternatives and your GP should be able to advise you. 'Zantac is the only thing that worked for me,' wrote one mum. 'I nearly wrote to the manufacturers to thank them!'

'I had a string of GPs who told me to go away and drink Gaviscon, but I couldn't keep it down. In the end, I saw a female GP who had taken Ranitidine herself for heartburn when she was pregnant, and said it would sort me out. She wasn't wrong.' Bakedpotatohoho

Heartburn during pregnancy can be horrific, but the best cure is to give birth – that *will* happen eventually and, when it does, the heartburn will disappear instantly, as if by magic. In the meantime, if you really want to scare fellow commuters, pop your Gaviscon in a hip flask or brown paper bag and swig regularly.

Mumsnetiquette: What can I do about my bleeding gums?

Brushing your teeth during pregnancy can leave the bathroom sink looking like the opening scene from *Saving Private Ryan*. Your gums swell up in pregnancy, partly because the amount of blood pumping around your body has shot up, and because pregnancy hormones have softened them, causing them to bleed at the slightest graze – a condition known as gingivitis. You need to keep your mouth spotless or a build-up of plaque will result in painful inflammation, which, left untreated, could end up with you

(continued)

losing a tooth. Add to that the research that links gum disease to premature labour and low birth-weight babies and you begin to see why dental care is free on the NHS during pregnancy and for one year after the birth. So make sure that you take care of your pearly whites – after all, Pregnant Dracula is *not* a good look. Here are some tips:

'It's thought that pregnancy hormones can make your gums more sensitive to even tiny amounts of plaque on your teeth. Gingivitis is very common among pregnant women, and assuming you have a clean, healthy mouth, it usually disappears as soon as the baby is born. In the meantime, keep your teeth as clean as possible; brush your gums as well as your teeth and floss every day. If you are not used to cleaning your gums, they will get worse before they get better. Getting them cleaned by a dentist or hygienist is a good idea – there might be hard tartar on your teeth which won't come off with your ordinary toothbrush. Get some Corsodyl (chlorhexidine gluconate) mouthwash from the chemist and swill it round twice a day after brushing. You should see an improvement after a week.' *Jasper* (a dentist!)

'I knew it was a symptom of pregnancy, but wasn't quite prepared for a mouthful of blood every now and then when just having a conversation with someone. If your gums are swollen, try rinsing your mouth with salt water a couple of times a day.' *Puppie*

'If you have problems with sore or bleeding gums while pregnant, a baby's toothbrush is great for gentle, thorough cleaning.' *Vivie*

'A sour taste can be from bleeding gums or a build-up of bacteria in the gum area. Unfortunately, during pregnancy, it can really get bad because you are more prone to gum bleeding and the little bugs think it's a buffet and hang out there. You need to scrape your tongue and brush more. I use mouthwash and floss a lot.' *Whomovedmychocolate*

Constipation

Constipation is a common, slightly embarrassing side effect of pregnancy. It makes you feel bloated and incredibly uncomfortable, and leaves you wondering how on earth your body is managing to accommodate everything you have eaten – oh boy – without giving way at the seams. The urge to grab a pencil and start scraping it out may be strong, but you must resist. It's also important not to strain when you are on the loo because it can cause, or aggravate, piles (see p. 75).

Constipation can be disconcerting, especially with all those doctors and midwives prodding your tummy at every opportunity; and you will start to worry about what, in fact, you might end up giving birth to.

For starters (and don't worry, that's not a food reference), your growing baby is putting pressure on the bowel, making everything take that much longer to process. Pregnancy hormones have relaxed the muscles in the wall of the intestine so everything is moving along at a snail's pace. As your poo trudges through your colon, more water than usual is absorbed and the stools harden, making it more of a struggle to push them out. With everything that is going on, you might also be more tense than normal, causing the wall of your intestine to contract and – you guessed it – slow down bowel movements. Some women find that certain foods, such as wheat and milk, make constipation worse.

Another reason you might be clogged up is if you are taking either iron tablets or iron-rich pregnancy supplements. To aid absorption, take these one hour before a high-fibre meal with a vitamin-C-rich drink. You could talk to your doctor about switching to another type of supplement or dietary change instead. 'I couldn't take iron pills, but managed to get my iron levels up several points by taking the liquid herbal supplement Floradix Floravital – it seemed to help with the constipation too!'

The good news is that constipation doesn't affect your baby and there are plenty of tips – not all pleasant – that might help to get your bowel movements back on track. Let's start with one of the more enticing suggestions: 'My midwife told me to eat a small amount of very good dark chocolate.'

But besides this, the main thing you can do to avoid or relieve constipation is to eat lots of fibre, keep up your water intake and heave yourself off the sofa to engage in some moderate exercise. High-fibre foods include fruit, vegetables, wholegrain bread and cereals like porridge and All Bran. Try adding a tablespoon of linseed or flaxseed to your cereal or stir it up in a glass of warm water or juice.

'I found that fresh apricots – not dried, as that gives me a lot of gas and wind – are a startlingly effective way to get things moving. But you have to eat five or six. Do it before you go to bed, then hopefully you'll be ready to go in the morning.'

Wilbur

Some mums recommend a bedtime glass of prune juice, or a one-hit wallop of 'one pint orange juice blended with a bag of pitted prunes'. Drink plenty of water throughout the day or herbal teas, to keep your stools soft. 'Drink hot water,' one mum advises. 'Take a cup to the loo with you. It sounds odd, but it worked for me.'

Gentle exercise such as walking, swimming or yoga will aid digestion and improve circulation.

Lots of Mumsnetters swear by over-the-counter remedies, but you should check with your GP before taking this route, and always try to change your diet and exercise first. 'I ate mountains of fruit and veg, but that didn't work. Lactulose was the only thing that softened my stools when I was pregnant. You can buy it over the counter or get it free on prescription.'

Olive oil also comes highly recommended: 'Lots of it, on pasta and salads, and dip brown bread in it.' But not castor oil, as this can have nasty side effects. And definitely not Castrol oil, even though you might be the size of a Boeing 747.

Rough and ready: dietary sources of fibre

When it comes to fruit and vegetables, don't peel them if possible, because most of the fibre is in the skin. As far as wheat and rice are concerned, most of the fibre is in the grain, so the more processed it is, the more fibre will have been removed. So always choose wholesome wholegrains over the feeble white stuff. Good choices include:

- fresh and dried fruits
- vegetables (including potatoes in their skins)
- nuts and seeds
- wholemeal, granary and seedy breads
- wholegrain breakfast cereals (check packets for dietary information)
- wholemeal pasta and brown rice
- pulses and lentils.

Pregnancy Skin – What's Going On?

Pregnancy can be so unfair. Some women bloom; their hair shines and their skin looks airbrushed. The rest of us suffer like teenagers with bad skin and greasy locks. 'My usually perfect skin is flaky,' weeps one distraught mum-to-be.

Along with greasy hair and patchy skin, your tummy is as tight as a drum and can be very itchy. At times, you might feel as though you're carrying an ant hill, not a baby. Could that explain the faint line that has appeared as if out of nowhere, stretching from the top of your pubic bone to your belly button – the ants are on the march ...

The linea nigra – or 'black line' – is a dark line that goes from your navel to your pubic bone. This tattoo is one of the more mysterious side effects of pregnancy. Not everyone gets one, and some women get it in one pregnancy, and not in another. But all women, pregnant or not, have a 'white line', which pregnancy hormones turn into a 'black' one, only it tends to be more noticeable on women with darker skin. 'My line was a centimetre wide and almost black,' says a mum. 'My niece thought it was the place that the doctor unzipped to get the baby out.'

'I have had two pregnancies and have never had a noticeable linea nigra. But I do remember going for a hospital check-up in the winter, where the consultant had a student with him and asked him what the line on my tummy was called. He got it right – but I didn't have the heart to tell him it was the imprint of the seam on my tights!' Batey

Another weird side effect is chloasma – the 'mask of pregnancy' – consisting of blotchy brown or yellowish patches that some women get on their face. It is caused by pregnancy hormones stimulating the melanin cells in the skin to produce more pigment. 'I look like I have a black eye, or I've smudged mascara down my face days ago and left it there. It's a bit depressing, and I didn't have it there the first time I was pregnant.' Another fed up mum says: 'I have a very large, dark mark on my top lip, which looks exactly like I've got a great fat moustache.' Chloasma can't be prevented completely but you can reduce the darkness of the patches by avoiding the sun or using sunscreen: exposure to the sun will stimulate the production of melanin and make the patches more intense. Chloasma doesn't always go away straight after giving birth so you may have to invest in some Touche Eclat to cover up.

Another glamorous pregnancy accessory are skin tags, which can pop up anywhere – on your neck, along your knicker line, under your breasts or under your arms are all common sites. Skin tags are small flaps of skin that are harmless, but can be annoying. 'I keep thinking it's something I've given birth to, it's so big,' says one mum. They don't always disappear after the birth, and although you can get them burned or cut off, doctors will usually remove them only if they are in places where they are causing a problem or chafing, not just for cosmetic reasons. You can always ask your GP for advice. (Look away now if you are squeamish, but one mum was advised by her doctor to go home and lasso hers with a piece of thread: 'I've found you don't have to tie it particularly tight, it just takes longer to fall off. When it does fall off, there's no wound – just a small mark that fades pretty quickly.' It might be best to leave trying this until after the baby is born though, just in case you do open up a gaping wound in the removal process and you have to be pumped full of antibiotics.)

Pregnant women are also susceptible to a skin rash called 'polymorphic eruption of pregnancy' or PUPPP (pruritic urticarial papules and plaques of pregnancy). PUPPP is the most common pregnancy skin rash; it manifests in itchy red bumps over your abdomen and thighs, and a gradual slowing down of offers of dates by attractive men. It starts around your belly button, often setting up camp in abdominal stretch marks before spreading to the rest of the body, but never the face.

PUPPP is harmless, but the itching can drive you crazy. Let your doctor take a look, as you may be prescribed an antihistamine or steroidal cream. Calamine lotion, E45 cream, Sudocrem, Aveeno cream or a warm bath with sodium bicarbonate might also offer some relief. 'I used to keep loads of wet flannels in the fridge as they helped to relieve it for a short while,' says a mum, who kept her E45 cream and aloe gel in there too. The good news is that it generally disappears post pregnancy, and is unlikely to return in a subsequent one.

'I had PUPPP with my first pregnancy. It came on around week 36 – severe, itchy lumps all over my thighs, abdomen and back which looked like a nettle-sting rash. The only comfort I found from it was calamine lotion or splitting open aloe vera plants and getting my partner to spread them all over the area. It looks really attractive – white and green stripy skin.' Loubiehigh

While itchy skin during pregnancy is common and usually harmless, it could also be a symptom of the liver condition obstetric cholestasis that can occur during the second or third trimester. It is, therefore, important to get itching checked out, because this condition can be dangerous for mum and baby.

'At 33 weeks, I started to get itchy skin, which is quite common in late pregnancy due to stretching skin and hormones. However, I had persistent itching all over, particularly on my hands and feet. I told my midwife and she sent me for a blood test. It turns out that I have a common pregnancy condition called obstetric cholestasis. This is when your liver doesn't process bile chemicals properly and it can potentially make your blood toxic for mum and baby. The itching is caused by chemicals being deposited back into the blood. No one knows what causes it or why it happens. It is likely that I am going to have to be induced at 37 weeks, as the risks may be more significant if I carry to full term. Once the baby is born, the mum's liver usually returns to normal and the baby is not affected. I would advise that you tell your midwife if you get any itching so that OC can be ruled out.' Gemtubbs

Itching from OC is most often worst on the palms of your hands and soles of your feet. You won't get a rash, but there is a small chance you will get mild jaundice. You are more likely to get it if you are carrying multiples or if you have had it in a previous pregnancy. If you are at all worried, see your GP.

Backache Blues

Back pain is a particularly grim type of pain, simply because you can't really *do* much without involving your back in some way.

You are loaded up with baby like an old pack horse and your poor old back is crucial in helping to carry that extra weight. However, pregnancy hormones loosen up your ligaments and muscles, which can leave you vulnerable to back pain. This is compounded by your posture which can often suffer as you try to accommodate your growing bump (or stick it out proudly as you waddle through the streets like a fecund Mr Greedy).

In some cases, the strain of extra pressure and inflammation on the sciatic nerve can result in pain that spreads through your buttocks and thighs: this is called sciatica. Sciatica is quite literally a pain in the bum. It can also happen if the baby sits on or gnaws through the sciatic nerve (actually, this doesn't happen, but it can *feel* like it).

Backache can be agony, so don't be afraid to ask for help from friends and family. You need as much help as you can get, particularly if you have other children to look after.

Some people find that warmth can provide relief from back pain: applying a hot-water bottle or similar to parts that are aching can be soothing, as can warm baths. 'The best thing I found for immediate relief is a lavender wheat cushion,' advises a mum. 'It can be heated in the microwave or oven and was fantastic throughout my pregnancy and labour. I would sleep in the foetal position with it wedged into the back of my big knickers.' You can also try alternating warm things with cold things (like a pack of frozen peas), which some people find helpful in relieving muscle spasms.

Gentle exercise can help: swimming and antenatal yoga are good (but make sure you tell your instructor about any problems you are having). Sadly, your pregnant state precludes you from taking any really useful painkillers. Folks will suggest the occasional paracetamol after the first trimester, but take it from those who know – for full-on pregnancy backache, it's not going to make any difference.

Your GP or midwife should be able to refer you to a physiotherapist who will assess your pain and give you advice on exercises or practical tips that you can use to relieve the pain. 'I found the physiotherapist very knowledgeable,' writes one mum. 'She showed me how to do simple things like climbing in and out of bed a certain way, which reduced the strain on my muscles and ligaments.' A physiotherapist will also assess whether an elasticated pregnancy support belt or a 'belly bra' (just as sexy as it sounds) could offer you some relief, and may even be able to lend you one for the duration of your pregnancy.

'I had dreadful backache during my pregnancy and for six weeks after the birth. I went to see a physiotherapist and the relief was immense. The physio was excellent and she showed me some very specific exercises to do to get relief from the pain.' Bugsy

One mum was camping when she hit on the right solution for her: 'I was in pain from nine weeks until about 16 weeks when I discovered that sleeping on a hard floor is much better for my back than a soft bed.'

For any kind of back or pelvic pain you can also try complementary or alternative therapies such as acupuncture or osteopathy.

'I had tried everything for my pregnancy back pain (I had an inflamed sacrum, which is just as scary and horrid as it sounds) and was spending a part of every day in tears because everything I did made it hurt. My osteopath did some gentle manipulation and basic acupuncture and although it got a bit worse for about a day before it got better, the relief when the pain stopped was just wonderful. I could have kissed her.' Zoots

Pelvic girdle pain

Another type of back pain that affects pregnant women is pelvic girdle pain or PGP.

First the science. Your pelvic girdle (pelvis) is made up of your two 'hip' bones (called ilia), which are joined to a bone called the sacrum at the back. They are connected at the front by a joint called the symphysis pubis, while at the back they are connected by joints called sacro-iliac joints. All of these joints are normally stuck together very nicely by good, firm ligaments. But in pregnancy, your hormones make all of this 'looser' in preparation for the birth. For some women, this loosening seems to place too much stress on certain parts of the pelvis, resulting in feelings of pain around the pelvic area: 'I feel like my pelvis is about to split open and my hips dislocate from their sockets!'

Although it is called PGP (also known as symphysis pubic dysfunction or SPD), the pain can extend to more joints than just the symphysis pubis.

'I'm 30 weeks pregnant and in a lot of pain. It feels like I've been kicked hard in the groin and the muscles running from the pubic area to the top of my inner thighs feel really sore. I also have an aching pain right at the bottom of my bump. I'm having trouble with everyday things such as getting in and out of the car, walking up the stairs and getting dressed. The worst, though, is when I'm lying in bed and I try to roll over; it's agony.' Brighteyes

Most women who suffer from PGP will feel the pain when standing from a sitting position, when getting up after sitting or lying for a long time, and it may be painful just to part their legs (although a physiotherapist will be able to advise you on other positions that you can adopt should you wish to engage in any activities requiring leg parting). PGP can be so debilitating that some women end up on crutches or in a wheelchair during pregnancy. For others, the discomfort is mild.

'I had SPD and I thought I was falling to bits,' says one mum. Another says: 'It's a terrible thing to live with. Mine didn't subside for a long time after my son's birth. I had physio and that helped.

I was taught exercises to strengthen my tummy and pelvic floor muscles.'

A physiotherapist is the best person to see if you suspect you are suffering from PGP, ideally a women's health physiotherapist. They will assess you and work out which bits are hurting and/or falling off. They will drill home the message, 'Keep your legs together' (to which you, of course, will respond: 'It's too late for that!'), and they may recommend an elasticated pregnancy support belt which 'holds it all together' and gives instant relief for lots of women. They may perform some manipulation techniques or teach you some self-manipulation and basic exercises which will give you a bit more support. You will be advised to avoid twisting movements, and to think about keeping your body as symmetrical as possible, to avoid stressing the pelvis (for example, by carrying two small bags of muffins in each hand, instead of one enormous bag in one hand).

Back pain and labour

When your secretary is pushing you around the office on a wheelie chair because your back is too painful for you to walk, you might start to worry whether you are going to be in any fit state to labour when the time comes. Try not to worry: unless they have serious or very severe back or pelvic problems, most women find that they are able to give birth without any problems. As one mum says: 'PGP is miserable, but I found labour quite distracting!'

Talk to your midwife about your options, make sure your condition is clearly written on your notes and that your partner is ready to explain the situation to your caregivers if you are too busy squealing like a pig to provide any coherent self-advocacy.

The general advice to avoid lying on your back applies, particularly if you have PGP: upright or kneeling positions are preferable. A birthing ball might be a comfortable option and labouring in water might be helpful in supporting your weight. 'Avoid stirrups at all costs!' advises one Mumsnetter – but you probably don't need to be told that. Delivery on all fours, on your side or in water could all work well if you are suffering from PGP, but birth is an unpredictable event, so don't worry too much at this stage about managing your back or pelvic pain during labour. Talk things through with your midwife and physiotherapist, but, for now, focus on making yourself comfortable during your pregnancy and on keeping up with any exercises you've been asked to do.

The good news is that most pregnancy-related PGP and back pain should go away after the birth. It could be immediate or it might take a few months, but your body should gradually get back to normal. So be optimistic and try to concentrate on the days when you'll be back to your old self, bounding up the stairs with nothing more to worry about than the (high) likelihood of wetting yourself.

'I had a home birth with PGP and it was great. The only thing I would say is that I was on crutches for the first 24 hours after the baby was born – the symptoms didn't disappear immediately; in fact, they were much, much worse. But by day three I was skipping around the house.' Peabody

Thrush – A Fungi to Be With (Not)

During pregnancy, it is not unusual to feel that you have turned into some weird, wobbly blob that oozes and spurts gloop. In a sexy, fertility-goddess sort of way, of course. An increase in vaginal discharge is quite normal, but if it is thick, white and creamy (cottage-cheesy) and accompanied by itching, it could be thrush.

Thrush (also called candida, vulvo-vaginal candidiasis, or vaginal candidosis or monilia) is a common vaginal infection characterised by itchiness and sometimes burning in the infected areas. It is caused by a yeast fungus, most often Candida albicans, which generally lives quite harmlessly on the skin and in the mouth, gut and vagina. Ordinarily, it is kept in check by friendly bacteria, but when the normal conditions go a bit haywire (thanks to those pregnancy hormones again – although antibiotics can also aggravate things) then the yeast can increase, causing the following grim signs and symptoms:

- itching, soreness and irritation around the vulva
- vaginal discharge (odourless: usually cottage-cheese like, but can also be watery and contain pus)
- pain or discomfort during penetrative sex
- possibly pain or discomfort while urinating
- vulvo-vaginal inflammation: redness, soreness, swelling or even cracked skin of vagina and vulva (and sometimes sores in the surrounding area, which may indicate other infections too).

If you suspect that you have thrush, go to your doctor to get checked out. They will generally diagnose it based on a description of your symptoms, but they might want to take a swab if you have recurrent bouts and/or to rule out other infections: 'I went to the GP as my thrush wouldn't go away, and it turned out it wasn't thrush at all, but Group B Strep, which can be very harmful if the baby catches it while passing through the birth canal,' explains a mum.

Thrush won't affect your pregnancy, other than make you fidget excessively, but because it can be passed on to the baby as it travels through your vagina during birth, it's important that your GP or midwife knows if you are still getting symptoms close to your due date. They are then prepared to treat the baby, if necessary.

A cream is typically the first line of defence, and should be applied as your doctor recommends (usually rubbed into the vagina and surrounding skin with your finger, twice or three times a day). You may also be prescribed an antifungal pessary. You will be advised to be very gentle applying this, to use your finger rather than the plastic applicator and not insert it too far up towards your cervix (you don't want to bumble away too roughly up there with a plastic stick). The pessaries tend to be jolly messy, and it will look like you have shoved a handful of chalk up your glory hole for a few days. (Oral tablets to treat thrush aren't generally allowed during pregnancy, although you might be prescribed them at other times.)

Thrush thrives in warm and damp conditions, so you should wear loose cotton pants (no thongs) and avoid tight clothes – stick to hold-ups or stockings instead of tights or just wear a big, airy kaftan and go commando. Always wipe front to back when you go to the loo. Don't use bubble bath or soap, as these can irritate your vagina further and, if possible, avoid baths (unless you want to try adding a drop of tea tree or salt to the bath for therapeutic reasons) and just have showers instead (or a swim in the sea if you're hard enough!). Wash towels and underwear 'as hot as you dare' – ideally at 60°.

If you get recurrent thrush, you might be advised to treat your partner as well if you are still having intercourse: 'Make sure your man uses the cream too. Otherwise, you might be clearing yours up and then getting it back every time he has his wicked way.'

Some people swear that dietary changes helped to get rid of their thrush – in particular, avoiding foods with sugar and yeast in them – but you need to make sure that you are still getting a balanced diet, so speak to your midwife if you are considering this route. Others swear by alternative remedies: 'I had a couple of bouts of thrush before my midwife put me on to a wonderful acupuncturist who has gently and successfully put my body back into balance.'

There are also lots of traditional home remedies for thrush, the most common of which is to fight it with natural bio yoghurt. The yoghurt should be nice and cool, which will provide relief from the itching, and the live bacteria are supposed to help to fight off the thrush. But remember you need *live* yoghurt here, not a Müller Corner. 'Nothing is as good as plain live yoghurt whacked up in there, smear a bit around the outside and layer knickers with some toilet paper.' Although one mum warns: 'You don't half get funny looks from the men in the family when you walk upstairs with a pot of yoghurt and a syringe.' Another traditional home remedy is a clove of garlic delicately positioned in your special place – also handy if you are being stalked by vampires.

'Here's what you do – I did it after advice from my fab midwives. Peel a clove of garlic, splash a few drops of tea tree oil on to it, thread a piece of cotton through it for easy retrieval and put it up your fanjo overnight. Voila, goodbye thrush.

Garlic has antifungal properties as does tea tree, which is also antibacterial. You need to make sure the thrush doesn't come back by starving it of yeasty food (bread, wine) and sugar. Also dried fruit should be avoided. You may well crave these things, but be strong and don't feed the thrush. This really worked for me and it was a blessed relief.' Spidermama

> Whether this is a good plan or not should perhaps be left to your midwife to decide, although as one mum points out, it does beg the question: 'I'm happy to stick a clove of garlic up my fanjo, but where should my husband put his?'

TESTS AND SCANS

Antenatal Appointments – Perfecting Peeing in Jars

The moment you are pregnant, all the exciting red-letter days in your diary are instantly distilled into those containing your antenatal appointments. The business of being pregnant can be all-consuming, so you will probably quite look forward to regular one-on-one sessions, where you and your baby are the focus of attention. Unfortunately, however, your appointments might be a bit of a disappointment. The pattern is usually the same: you rush like crazy to get there on time, with a list of questions as long as an umbilical cord and your precious vial of wee upright in your handbag. Finally, just as you are about to get your hands on the copy of *Heat* magazine that has been doing the rounds in the waiting room, your name is called. In all your excitement you forget completely about your questions, and, before you can say 'hyperemesis gravidarum', you are back in the waiting room, none the wiser.

'My first proper appointment was horrendous,' says one mum. 'I felt that the midwife wanted me out of there sharpish.'

'Antenatal care is important, if only for reassurance. Having said this, my appointments were also a source of major stress for me when I was pregnant. I went to one when various people had told me I looked small for my dates, and I was worried whether the baby was all right, only to be told by a locum doctor that he couldn't hear the baby's heartbeat, but that he was "sure that everything was OK" – just what a concerned pregnant woman wants to hear. Then, towards the end of the pregnancy, the midwife kept telling me that the baby was breech. I got very stressed about how I was going to cope with a C-section, until my sympathetic GP sent me up to the hospital to discuss turning the baby. They did a scan and we found out that she was head-down after all.' Azzie

Antenatal appointments are a necessary part of pregnancy. They are a way of keeping a check on any potential problems that may arise for you and your baby. If everything is straightforward, most pregnant women will be seen once every four weeks after week 12, every two weeks after week 32, then weekly until the baby finally arrives. Where you go for your appointments will depend on your area; it could be your hospital, GP surgery, a health centre or even your home.

By now, you should already have had your booking-in appointment, discussed your health and family medical history and most likely had your blood pressure and urine tested. Once you start your second-trimester appointments, as well as blood pressure and urine tests, you will probably have your tummy felt and your fundal height checked with a tape measure (to assess foetal growth and development) in centimetres from the top of the pubic bone to the top of the uterus. According to the text books it should match the foetus's gestational age in weeks within 1 to 3cm, e.g., a pregnant woman's uterus at 22 weeks should measure 19–25cm. Your midwife will also check your baby's heartbeat, which can be a source of joy or stress, depending on whether or not they do actually manage to locate it:

'When it works and you hear their little heart going like galloping horses it's amazing. But try not to get too upset if they can't find it; it doesn't mean it's not there.' Biza

You may be given a plastic folder with your notes inside to look after. Should you look at them and be concerned about something that has been written, make sure you ask your midwife or doctor to clarify. The idea is that you carry these around with you in case you need to go to hospital in an emergency. As with everything during pregnancy, your notes will grow, and by nine months, you will need a handbag the size of a bin liner to accommodate them.

If you feel that you aren't being listened to, or that your questions and concerns are not properly addressed, don't be afraid to speak up for yourself or even request a different caregiver:

'Antenatal care can be hit and miss. I have a choice of two hospitals and the care at each couldn't be more different. If you are unhappy, it might be worth exploring alternatives, and possibly changing GPs or hospital as I did to get the care and birth I wanted. If you truly feel the care you are getting is inadequate speak up. My midwife tried to cancel my 37-week home visit, but once I explained that I wanted the appointment to be kept and the reasons I couldn't go to her, she came out. Don't think you can't ask for what you want. Sometimes we just need to be a little bit more assertive.' Foxybrown

Don't be surprised if you come away from an antenatal appointment feeling dissatisfied. 'I cried after one, as I just couldn't believe that I was in and out in four minutes without hearing the heartbeat,' says one disappointed mum. When it's your first baby, it's all new and exciting and you expect to be treated like you're special. But a quick visit is usually a sign that there are no problems. And some people prefer a hands-off approach: 'It was a bit disconcerting at first, but now that I am 20 weeks, I'm quite glad of the lack of interference,' says one mum.

Your other half will probably want to be there for the scans but whether they accompany you to all the antenatal appointments is another matter. 'I've always found them pretty routine and boring, so I wouldn't put him through it,' advises one mum. And if he is the feeble type then you are probably better off alone: 'My husband fainted while the midwife was doing my bloods; she left me sitting there with the needle in my arm while she picked him up off the floor.'

Always take a snack and something to read in case you are in for the long haul. And don't forget your notes and your jam jar of wee.

Twenty-Week Scan

For most women, this is the scan they get really excited about, as it's the first time they will see something that vaguely resembles a baby.

'My 20-week scan was great. I got to see lots of detail and it made me all teary. On the serious side, it flagged up a problem with my son's kidneys which, left untreated, could have been life-threatening.' fastasleep

As well as – possibly – revealing your baby's sex (depending on the position they're in!), the scan will check the following:

- The head will be measured to check for any obvious brain or developmental problems, and to make sure there is a nice big head growing there to do the job of ripping you asunder a few months down the line.
- Baby's heart will be checked to make sure it is working properly.
- Baby's hands and feet will be checked.
- The spine and abdomen will be checked, as well as kidneys and bladder.
- The stomach will be checked – you can sometimes see a little black mass of stomach contents, which is swallowed amniotic fluid (don't worry, the baby is supposed to do this).
- The placenta, umbilical cord and amniotic fluid will all be measured and checked to make sure they are working and developing correctly.

'I had a 20-week scan and would do so again. Sometimes 'problems' that are brought to your attention can be corrected before, or after, your baby is born. And it gives you a chance to prepare yourself for any issues that may arise on its arrival.' shhhh

Various other things are measured to check that they are all growing well and in proportion. It is not uncommon for discrepancies to be picked up at this stage, but they do not necessarily mean that there is anything wrong with your baby. 'The scan showed a shortish thigh bone and a large head, and we were called back for more scans,' recalls one mother. 'But in the end I just had a perfect daughter who has short legs and a big head – much like myself.' If any measurements are outside the normal range, you will be called back for further scans a week or two later.

'One of the best days of my life was the 20-week scan when we found out everything was fine (there had been concerns). We also found out we were having a girl after two boys.' Chocolateface

Invasive Tests

Few pregnancies are completely trouble-free, but being faced with the option of whether or not to go ahead with an invasive test can be particularly harrowing. Depending on the stage of your pregnancy, you might be offered CVS (11–13 weeks, see p. 86) or an amniocentesis (from 15 weeks) if you are considered 'high risk' after other screening has been done (see p. 86). Or you may just decide that no matter how low your risk, you want to know for sure that your child is free from some of the more common chromosomal abnormalities. Whatever your reason for heading down this route, it is one of the toughest decisions that you will have to make during your pregnancy.

The tests are called 'invasive' because they are just that – they literally 'invade' your body with a long, fine needle. The results are more than 99 per cent accurate but for every hundred women who have CVS approximately two will miscarry, with the rate slightly lower for amnio at one in 100. This means that around 320 healthy pregnancies of babies without Down's syndrome or other chromosomal abnormalities are lost each year in Britain because of invasive tests.

What happens when you have an amniocentesis?

Under local anaesthetic, a fine needle is inserted through your abdomen, using ultrasound to guide it, to extract fluid from your baby's amniotic sac. This is tested for Down's and other chromosomal disorders. 'I was a nervous wreck,' admits one mum. 'I viewed myself as a racehorse with three big hurdles to get over: the test itself, the risk of miscarriage and then getting the result.' Another mother says: 'I didn't find my amnio at all painful and I'm a massive wimp. Just don't look at the needle – it's rather large.'

Afterwards, you will probably feel some cramping pains. There may also be some bleeding and amniotic fluid leaking from your vagina; if so, contact your doctor or midwife immediately. Take it easy for the next couple of days, don't lift anything heavy or do anything too strenuous.

Cases of infection are rare, but may lead to miscarriage. 'I had already had two miscarriages so was taking no chances,' says a mother who had an amnio. 'I went home and lay on the settee for two days and did absolutely nothing. The midwife knew I was really scared about it and came round the morning after to let me hear my daughter's heartbeat, which was very reassuring.'

Around 8 in every 100 amniocentesis tests fail to obtain enough fluid (usually due to the position of the baby), so the needle has to be inserted again. If a second attempt is not successful, you will probably be asked to return on another day.

Agreeing to something that will increase the risk of miscarriage is a hard step to take, but one that many people do choose. It can be a frightening time. Your mind is probably racing with various scary scenarios, made worse because you are feeling under pressure to make a quick decision. Ask your doctor if you want to be referred for counselling to talk things through further.

For some people, the risk of miscarriage is enough to put them off taking the test. 'My sister-in-law had CVS and miscarried a few days later,' says one Mumsnetter. 'She bitterly regrets it, and it's completely put me off, especially as the results came back clear.'

Others feel that the need to know is important for them and their family:

'I teach children with severe learning difficulties and love my job. I have five students with Down's syndrome in my class, so I am very well aware of all the implications of having a child with special needs. Personally, I didn't want a screening test that would give me a 1 in 50 or 1 in 50,000 likelihood of having a child with a chromosomal abnormality – after all, I could still be that one. I wanted a diagnostic test that would tell me "Yes" or "No".' I understood all the risks and I honestly don't know what I would have done if the results had not been normal. The amnio itself is not pleasant, and waiting for the results seems to take for ever, but once I got the all-clear I was able to relax and enjoy the rest of the pregnancy. I must stress, again, that I did what was right for me and my husband, and you must do what is right for you.' Christie

Waiting for the results can take anything from three days to three weeks. Getting to know the sex of your baby early is a bonus for some, but make sure that you tell medical staff if you don't want to know. Don't be surprised if you get some vaginal bleeding afterwards, but inform your doctor. If you were to miscarry due to the test, this would happen within the five days that follow.

'Here's a good-news story, to give you some hope. We were given a 1 in 13 chance of Down's syndrome, and a risk of a heart defect. I was convinced that it would be bad news. We had to wait a week for the CVS test as I was bleeding internally and another week for results. They were the longest two weeks of my life. Our CVS results came back clear. We then had two heart scans at 15 weeks and 23 weeks and both came back clear. I was dreading my 20-week scan, as I was convinced there must have been a reason for the high measurement but all seemed fine, and our daughter is perfectly healthy.' Porridgebrain

The first non-invasive, prenatal blood test to detect Down's is now on the horizon; it looks for genetic markers that show whether your baby has the chromosomal disorder. Currently on trial, it has been shown to diagnose 90 per cent of Down's cases, while also identifying 97 per cent of foetuses that do not have the condition. It could be offered to every pregnant woman, not just those at high risk.

'I didn't have anything other than basic scans and blood tests done when I was pregnant. My daughter was born with Down's syndrome. I'm so pleased I didn't know before and have never, not for one second, regretted not being scanned or tested. I'm pregnant again and I'm not having tests this time round either. Knowing how wonderful my daughter is, and loving her as passionately as I do, there's even less reason to have the tests this time round. But it's not the sort of thing you can advise anyone on; it's far too personal. Each person has to do what they feel is right.' Thomcat

Finding Out the Sex – Now You See It, Now You Don't!

Even for those who have decided that they're not going to find out the sex of their child, there must be moments of weakness. After all, how much do you like surprises? Could you cart a large, wrapped gift around with you for nine months and not take a single peek? Most hospitals give you the opportunity to find out whether you are going to have a boy or a girl when you have your second scan at around 20 weeks. But some hospitals have a policy of not telling (in case they get it wrong and you try to sue them for all that money you wasted painting the nursery with Farrow & Ball's Calamine Pink). If you do want to know and your hospital won't tell, you can opt to pay privately for a scan.

Bear in mind that scans aren't always 100 per cent accurate. You can be told that you are definitely having a boy, no question, for absolute certain. You can buy blue everything, decorate the nursery with sailboat wallpaper, pick out a name, even tell a few friends. And then have a beautiful baby girl. Of course, this would serve you right for pandering to outmoded gender stereotypes. But pregnancy hormones can distort a baby's genitals in the womb (making labia puffier, for example) or sometimes your baby is just sitting with his legs crossed and being coy.

There are lots of good arguments for finding out though. Why should the doctor know and not you? And on a practical level it makes sense, if it is going to make a difference to the colour of your cot bedding or the baby clothes that you buy: 'We found out that we were having a boy, we picked a name and had a lovely time shopping for him.'

'It's a totally personal decision. We found out both times and I loved knowing. I felt like I knew my sons before they were born.' Piglit

If you have other children, it can be easier for them to adjust to the new arrival when they can start imagining a little brother or sister and fantasising about all the fun they will have together. If you're feeling brave and could live with a child called Iggle Piggle, Bob or Miss Hoolie, you can even let them help with suggesting names.

Others feel that the birthing suite will offer quite enough surprises already:

'I am 26 weeks and have been told that I am having a girl; I am so pleased I found out. The moment when the sonographer turned to me and my husband and said, "You are having a little baby girl," was probably one of the best moments of my life. I felt like fireworks had gone off as this little thing inside of me suddenly became a real person.' Newby29

But some parents would rather not spoil the surprise: 'I didn't want to know the sex at the scan; it feels a bit like opening your presents before Christmas,' says one Mumsnetter. 'Finding out the sex at the birth is one of the last true surprises in life!' argues another.

'We chose not to find out the sex. It's so much more romantic (even after a long and painful labour) when your partner tells you, "We have a

little boy/girl", than a sonographer announcing, "Well, it's probably a boy/girl", while you lie in a semi-dark hospital room halfway through your pregnancy. We specifically told the midwife at the birth that we wanted my husband to announce the sex of the baby, which was a truly unforgettable moment for him.' Murcimari

For a lot of parents, finding out the sex of their baby can be an emotionally complicated issue. You may have a fixed idea that you would prefer a boy or a girl, which might make you want to know in advance, so that you can 'come to terms' with your feelings, although as one mum says: 'I reckon if you have strong feelings about a preference, you shouldn't find out, because it won't matter once they are born. Why set yourself up for 20 weeks of upset, worry and confusion?'

'I'm not sure that finding out the sex was best for me. I so wanted a girl and when I found out, I could only feel disappointment in the boy that I hadn't yet met, whereas when he was born, at least I had the cuddly baby and it was much easier to love him.' Chipmonkey

On the other hand, if you are desperate for a girl/boy and unsure how you will bond with a boy/girl, finding out now will give you 20 weeks to get used to the idea, rather than having to deal with it in the delivery room in front of an audience of hospital staff. Feeling sad and disappointed – 'devastated' even – when you learn that it isn't the girl/boy you had wished for isn't uncommon. But it's not something that is always easy to talk about. Don't be afraid to give voice to your feelings though, because they are quite normal. And they also usually pass, often halfway through labour when, frankly, you won't care whether you give birth to a boy, girl or small dog, as long as it's healthy and your body doesn't actually explode.

THINKING AHEAD

Doulas, Independent Midwives, Maternity Nurses and Night Nannies – Are You Allowed One of Each?

Until you have been pregnant, given birth and looked after a newborn, it is hard to know what sort of help you are going to require, both in terms of medical attention and emotional support. You might already feel overwhelmed with worries about how you will cope. Family members often live far away, and they're not always as helpful as you might have hoped (or they're just too annoying to have around for any length of time); friends usually have their own busy lives to conduct.

Most pregnant women want more than just a hand to hold, although that would be nice too. What you really want is someone who knows about pregnancy and childbirth, who will fight your corner when it comes to getting you the best medical attention, and give you confidence as a mum. In a perfect world, you would get all the guidance and reassurance you are going to require from your attentive midwife and caring family, but that is not always the case.

Unfortunately, expensive extra help is not available to everyone. For pregnant women who feel let down by the NHS – and who can afford to go private – there is help out there in the form of independent midwives and doulas. For others, the time to fork out might be post-birth, with the services of a postnatal doula, maternity nurse or (hurrah!) cleaner – for the time when you are stuck at home, maybe post-C-section, with sore boobs and a newborn to feed, a house to keep clean, piles of laundry (not to mention piles) and months of the graveyard shift stretching ahead of you.

Surviving the first few months is crucial if you don't want to get overwhelmed by this mummy lark, so it's important to get the best start that you can. But finding the right 'fairy godmother' to suit you takes time – and they do tend to get booked up, so start cleaning out the fireplace now and praying that one will appear.

Of course, not everyone wants an extra person involved – 'it's such an intimate time' – and the idea of a stranger taking over seems wrong. Plus, many couples cope well on their own, and some even enjoy it! But if you think you might be in the market for some paid extra help, read on.

Independent midwife

An independent midwife is fully qualified and will usually visit you at home for your antenatal and postnatal care; they will be there for the birth and will visit for up to a month afterwards. They are freelance and work alone, and what you are paying for is continuity of care, which is often lacking in the NHS, where midwives tend to work in teams. With an independent midwife you have the opportunity to build up a relationship of trust with one person who is going to guide you through your pregnancy and, in many cases, deliver your baby if you are having a home birth. 'I'm pretty sure that I'm going to plump for an independent midwife to get some personal attention, otherwise I think I'll freak out,' says one first-time mum-to-be.

Most independent midwives specialise in home births and some may be experienced in particular areas, such as twin or breech births. The majority of hospitals will allow an independent midwife to accompany you in the event that you are transferred from home, and even into theatre if that becomes necessary. If you have chosen to have a hospital birth, your independent midwife is likely to play more of an advocate's or a doula's (see below) role, rather than be involved in any medical capacity, unless she has a contract with them.

'I employed an independent midwife, even though I planned to have a hospital birth. She was fantastic. Well-connected independent midwives can make things happen in hospital. So many of my friends reported spending much of the time on their own, not being able to get epidurals, not being allowed enough time to deliver naturally, not getting the help they needed breastfeeding or being encouraged to use the bottle if the baby wasn't gaining the "required" amount of weight, etc. My midwife was a total buffer for me from all of that nonsense – she was really diplomatic. You shouldn't need to employ an extra person like this in principle, but unfortunately, in so many cases, you do.' Genidef

If you feel that you are not getting the support that you need from the NHS, the general consensus from Mumsnetters who have employed independent midwives seems to be: 'If you can afford it, do it.' There are circumstances in which the fee can be altered to fit your budget: some independent midwives are sympathetic and will try to come up with a payment plan, and may even reduce their rate. But be mindful that they can't take on many clients each year, so you are asking a lot if you start to haggle. 'I paid a lot less as my income was very low, but it was still an eighth of my annual take-home pay and worth every penny,' says a grateful mother.

'My friend recently gave birth to her fourth son. She had an independent midwife and wishes she had done it with all of them. She said it was fantastic, and it was her only birth with no medical intervention. However, I had two great births and didn't feel compromised not having the same midwife with me throughout.' LilyLoo

Doula

A doula and Mumsnetter describes her role as: 'What you would want your ideal mother to be. She's your support through pregnancy, labour and beyond. She doesn't come between you and your partner; she supports you both. She doesn't do anything clinical or medical. She is a constant presence through your labour and birth.'

The word 'doula' comes from ancient Greek, meaning 'handmaiden'. There are two types of doula: a birth doula, who gets to know you during pregnancy and offers antenatal support, but is primarily there for the birth; and a postnatal or baby doula, who helps after the birth, supports you through breastfeeding, shows you how to look after your baby and possibly helps by keeping the house in order or cooking meals.

'The doula I had was the single best thing I did during pregnancy. I called her when I started having contractions three days before my daughter arrived and she chatted happily on the phone to me, texted regularly and came over to take me for a walk in the park to try and get the little one moving. On the day, she arrived at 8 a.m., helped my husband put up the pool in the kitchen and then ran around doing all the things he would have had to do – getting water, timing contractions – so that I could just lie with my head on his lap and have him stroke my forehead. Research I've read shows that couples who use a doula rate the experience of childbirth much better than those who don't. Also, you are less likely to have a Caesarean or any other kind of intervention, labour is usually shorter and relations between the couple are less stressed after the event.' Worktostaysane

Doulas do tend to get booked up, so give yourself time to find someone you feel comfortable with (see p. 439 for useful websites). Trainee doulas may offer cheaper rates than more experienced ones.

'My doula was brilliant,' says one relieved mum. 'I was scared to death of labour and I knew that neither my husband nor I knew enough to fully understand the delivery process when our time came. She knew exactly what I wanted and helped to communicate our needs successfully to the midwife team. It was also lovely to have a friendly face there at shift changes.' Another mum who had a doula says: 'I felt completely in control and she made sure that my husband was "looked after" as well. I'm sure without her I would have gone in earlier; I was 12 days late and five centimetres dilated when I arrived at the hospital. I was fortunate enough to have no pain relief; I'm sure this was due to her fantastic back massage and encouragement that I could do it.'

'I've got a postnatal doula, who is lovely and will do anything from housework to taking my toddler off to the park or soft play. She's less expensive than a maternity nurse and leaves me more time to bond with my baby, get feeding established, etc. I wish I'd done it first time around.' Liath

Maternity nurse or night nanny

Not everyone has the funds to hire a specially trained maternity nurse (or the room to put them up, if you want one to live in, Mary Poppins style). But some mothers consider them a necessity. As well as changing nappies, doing laundry, bathing and getting your baby into a routine (if you are a fan), a maternity nurse will also help with the night feeds, either doing it herself if your baby is bottle-fed or by bringing your baby to you to be breastfed. Some people would feel uncomfortable delegating this to a stranger ('getting up in the night is part of the bonding process') but for others it is a life-saver. We all cope differently when it comes to looking after a newborn and, whatever way you choose to do it, this stage won't last for ever – although it might feel like it at the time. The good thing is that it's never too late to hire a maternity nurse, but your choice will be more limited if you wait until after your baby is born.

'Most of the maternity nurses I know are incredibly energetic people who can't bear to sit around and who spend the 30 minutes when you are feeding at 3 a.m. catching up on a bit of ironing,' reports one mother. 'If they have previously been nannies, that works well because they are usually good with siblings and know how to get on in a family context, but I would say that experience counts for everything and, obviously, a willingness to get stuck in.'

But not everybody has good things to say: 'I would prefer a doula who looks after you and any siblings, who will help with the shopping and housework, as well as help with the baby. A maternity nurse only looks after the baby, so, in theory, you could end up looking after her, making cups of tea and tidying up, while she cuddles your baby. On the other hand, doulas don't do the overnight stuff that maternity nurses do.'

'My big tip is don't waste your money. I had a maternity nurse who had an impressive CV and qualifications; she was an ex-special-care nurse and had worked for a string of celebrities. She was a lazy madam who watched me mop the floor two weeks after a C-section – the cat had brought in a dead mouse and she had just left it there. I assume it was beyond her to clean it up. This is just one of many stories I could post, and the woman in question was the most expensive mistake I have ever made.' Twinkle3869

The real life-saver for some is a night nanny, who is only there for the evenings. 'She arrives at 9 p.m. and goes straight up to bed, in the same room as the baby,' says a mum. 'She either gives him a bottle of expressed milk or brings him to me for feeds, does all the nappy changing, winding and settling down. She writes a diary of what happened at what time during the night, then leaves at 7 a.m. I'm planning on using her until my son can go from 11 p.m. to 6 a.m. without waking, or until we run out of money.'

The best way to find a maternity nurse or night nanny is to look up local agencies or, best of all, see if you can get a personal recommendation. But however you find one, always make sure that you check out their qualifications and references thoroughly: anyone can call themselves a 'maternity nurse', so if she only has an HND in horticulture, you might want to reconsider. Bear in mind also that maternity nurses and night nannies may want to adhere to strict routines, with the aim of 'getting baby to sleep through'. If that isn't your top priority, or if you're not over-keen on strict routines, you need to make that clear and find someone whose approach tunes in with yours.

For anyone who doesn't have the funds to consider these alternatives and wishes they did, there is plenty of satisfaction to be found (albeit retrospectively) in having spent those tender moonlight moments with your baby and knowing that you did it single-handedly. 'I loved waking up with my daughter and breastfeeding her throughout the night,' writes one mum. 'And when I felt frustrated or tired, I remembered all the other millions of mums around the world who were up with their babies and doing the same thing. It made me feel part of some sort of worldwide community of mums, all doing the night-shift with their lovely newborns.'

Umbilical Cord Blood Banking

One additional and not particularly cheap extra offered to parents is the facility to bank their baby's umbilical cord blood. This is the baby's blood that remains in the placenta and umbilical cord after the birth, and which contains stem cells, transplants of which can be used in treating various blood, immune and metabolic diseases. They are easy to collect and are immediately available for use, or can be frozen and stored for years.

The Royal College of Obstetricians and Gynaecologists warns

parents that storing cord-stem blood is unlikely to be of much use to families with no history of blood disease: 'The RCOG remains unconvinced about the benefit of storing cord blood with a private bank for families who have no known medical reason to do so.' (The RCOG does, however, support public cord-blood banking and donation to the NHS cord-blood bank – see below.)

'Has anyone ever used the cord blood they stored? It sounds like a rip-off to me, taking advantage of poor pregnant paranoid mums. Mind you, if you have money to burn ...' Triceratops

Cord-blood collection may not be advisable in certain circumstances, for example if your baby is premature, you have a multiple pregnancy, the cord needs to be cut early to deliver the baby (e.g. if it is around the baby's neck), you have an emergency Caesarean or you are prescribed certain medication.

The procedure

If you are using a private cord-blood bank (see below) you will need to check in advance that your hospital will support you. Not all hospitals are happy to help, or even allow you to bring someone in to collect the sample and, as the extraction of stem cells should ideally be done by a trained health professional, you need your hospital on board. Prior to the birth, your chosen company will send you a sterile collection kit which your midwife can use to collect a blood sample from the umbilical cord once you and the baby are well and happy. The cells are collected after the placenta has been delivered, using a special needle connected to a sterile bag. UK regulations require that a small blood sample is taken from the mother either immediately before the baby is born or just after the birth to check for viruses or infection. The sample is then sent by courier to the relevant laboratory where your baby's stem cells will be separated from the blood, frozen and stored for future use.

There are two types of cord-blood bank: private and public. Private banks are usually run as businesses, and store your baby's cord blood for the sole use of you and your family should it be needed in the future. Public banks (like blood banks) are usually run by the NHS or a charitable organisation and the cord blood they store can be used by any patient who may need it.

If you don't use a private bank and your child develops an illness in the future that may have been treatable using cord blood, there are still, of course, other options for their treatment, such as cord blood from public banks and bone-marrow transplants (including those from a sibling).

There are also organisations, such as the Virgin Health Bank (part of the Branson empire), which are private blood banks but which also donate some of each 'deposit' to public cord-blood banks. For a fee, parents can have half of the blood collected put aside for their family, while the other half goes to the National Blood Service for anyone to access.

Some hospitals will give you the option of donating cord blood to a public bank (such as the NHS cord-blood bank). Like blood donation, it is voluntary and you don't pay anything to do it. A public bank stores cord blood for use by anyone in the world who might need it.

'My hospital collects the cord blood if you give them permission. It's a donation, like giving blood, so it's not stored for you, but for anyone who needs it. The way I see it, I can't afford to store it myself, so if it can help someone with leukaemia, for example, then I'm happy. It would only be disposed of otherwise.' Princesspowersparkle

For families with known genetic problems, stem-cell collection is usually done by the NHS. If a child in your family already has leukaemia or a blood disorder, your caregiver may be able to arrange for cord blood to be donated and stored in the NHS cord-blood bank, but reserved for the future use of your family. You should discuss this possibility with the team in charge of the care of the person who is ill.

Naming Names – Avoiding the Pitfalls of Everyone's Favourite Topic

'Have you thought of any names yet?' An innocuous enough question – yet one that can unleash no end of controversy. Discussing baby names is a tempting but, ultimately, dangerous game, involving comments like: 'I knew someone at school with that name and she was a right bitch,' or 'Oooh yes there are five Finlays in my son's nursery class – it's quite common now isn't it?' It's easy to find yourself wondering why you entered this conversation in the first place. Although it can be useful if you were thinking of calling him Bob Junior, but hadn't considered the hazardous initials ...

'It is easy to object to a name, but a lot harder to object to a baby with that name.' Hedgehog1979

Picking out a name is probably one of the first choices you and your partner will make together as parents – and quite possibly the first baby-related issue that you'll argue about. His ideas will sound to you like a wind-up, while he will laugh out loud at yours. Or, worse still, tell you that he'd assumed you would be carrying on his family name: 'My husband's dad died when he was young and there was pressure to include his name in my son's, but I refused on principle,' says a disgruntled mum. 'I think it's unfair to include one side and not the other. And it was a really bad name.'

For some couples, it's an easy decision. They know their baby's name even before it is has been conceived. But for most couples it is an agonising struggle. Draw up a (joint) list, and don't discount any suggestions for now. Keep adding to it, then start to cut it back as you head towards the end of your pregnancy. Even if you haven't decided on *the* one, at least have a shortlist ready by the time your waters break. If you really can't agree, and are planning to have more children, you could take it in turns choosing.

Once you think you've come up with something, you'll also need to consider whether you like the shortened version of it because that is the one that friends are likely to use. You don't want to be the crazy mother barking, 'It's Sam*antha*!' every time you introduce your child to someone.

It's also crucial to make sure that the name works with your surname. 'I was at parentcraft classes with a couple who wanted to call their daughter Iona,' recalls one mum, 'until it was pointed out that it wouldn't go well with their surname, which was Squirrel. Iona Squirrel?'

You might also want to think about what your child's initials will be: 'My sister-in-law is ASH and, funnily enough, she is the only smoker in the entire family.'

The big debate on Mumsnet is whether you should give your child a poncey name or play safe with something from the Top 100 list (www.statistics.gov.uk). 'I always breathe a sigh of relief when I meet children with nice, normal names rather than being called Englebert or Waterlily,' says a mum. Another mother admits that her son was going to be called Tiger until her husband persuaded her otherwise: 'The hormones took over!'

'Think about what your child's name will sound like when calling it loudly across a park: "Cardamon, stop hitting Flavian!"; "Cyrus, put down the brick!" If it makes you cringe or worry what other people think, then maybe have a rethink.' PetraDish

Cool names don't stay cool for long. And a cool name doesn't make a cool child. If you shift uncomfortably at the thought of a priest hovering over an ancient font declaring, 'I baptise this child Espresso', you should probably go back to the drawing board (or just go for a funky humanist naming day instead).

Surnames can also be a challenge. You may have taken your husband's surname if you are married, but crossing out your family name for the next generation can be painful. Some opt to give their maiden name as a middle name. If you are not married, or are married but have not taken your husband's surname, then you have a bit of thinking to do. You might want to hyphenate your surnames to make a double-barrelled mouthful, or just tack it on the end à la Hillary Rodham Clinton.

'My children have both our surnames: his first, then mine. Non-hyphenated (on account of their potential children). Unfortunately this means they have not one, but two surnames, one Bengali, one Swedish, neither easy to spell, preceded by Jewish first names. I am already saving for their therapy bills.' Motherinferior

If you have children from previous relationships with your surname, then you might want all the siblings to have the same surname. Or you might want to give each child its father's surname to make it easier for the CSA to cross-reference them all for the purpose of invoicing.

'I am very, very proud to have given our daughter my surname as well as my partner's. It is my name – something I can and have passed on to her to do with as she pleases. It is nothing to do with convention at all, just what felt right for us all as a family.' Batters

Or you might just feel that stamping the children with your surname is only a fair swap after the horrors of pregnancy and childbirth:

'My first two children both have my surname which my other half wasn't very happy with, but after nine months of pregnancy (which I hate), and childbirth (ditto), I tend to feel I have been the one to suffer most for the offspring and won't concede anything. I can't honestly see why I have to go through all that trauma for the child to have his name not mine …' Fennel

Either way, these days there seems to be little or no expectation that children will bear the father's surname, and people who have chosen various approaches rarely report any confusion or even raised eyebrows. The only people who are really likely to have any feelings about the matter are relatives, who, regardless of how many times you spell it out to them, will none the less for ever write an incoherent hash of the wrong thing on every single birthday card and letter, in the same way that they call you 'Mrs' followed by his initial and surname. Grrr.

WHEN THINGS GO WRONG
Coping with Loss

All miscarriages are cruel, but late miscarriages – between weeks 14 and 24 – are particularly brutal. Around a quarter of all miscarriages happen in the second trimester when, having carried your baby for so long, to be parted from it can be a heartbreaking wrench.

While it is more unusual to miscarry at this stage, you are more likely to find out what went wrong. Possible factors include: chromosome and genetic problems; an infection; a womb that is partly divided in two – bicornuate uterus; an issue with the placenta (see Placenta Praevia, p. 250); or an 'incompetent' or 'weak' cervix, where the cervix opens too early (this causes a quarter of late miscarriages, and is more likely to happen if you have had surgery for a previous miscarriage or abortion).

'I have an incompetent cervix – I found out by going into very early labour and losing a baby. They can do something to help with this though. In my next pregnancy I was scanned to see if my cervix was shortening, and they put in a stitch (suture). I went on to have two perfectly naughty children with cervical sutures.' DimpledThighs

Signs that you might be having a miscarriage include cramping and a pinkish vaginal discharge. These can often mean nothing, but it is always best to check with your doctor. A 'spontaneous miscarriage' starts naturally – your waters might break and most women feel something like labour pains. A 'silent miscarriage' is one in which a baby dies in the womb; something you might not discover until you have a scan.

At this stage of pregnancy, if you discover that your baby has died in the womb, or you start to miscarry naturally, you will probably be induced, which means you will be given hormones (in pessary, tablet or injection form) which will start labour. 'I was four and a half months pregnant when I found out during a scan that the baby had died,' says one Mumsnetter. 'I was induced. Despite it being traumatic, it was the best way to do it for me. I was able to leave the hospital 12 hours later and go home. They gave me very good pain relief.'

Afterwards, you may be offered the chance to hold your baby if this is something you want to do. 'After all that you have been through, it's not a terrifying moment at all,' says a mum who wondered how she would cope seeing her baby. 'Spend time with them. Bring a shawl in case they are too small and fragile to dress. Name them.' Some parents say that they were grateful for the opportunity to take photographs of their baby while they could.

Afterwards, you will probably feel tired and you may bleed for several weeks. Your breasts will produce milk, which can be upsetting, but there are hormones you can take to slow down production. You might lose your pregnancy shape quickly or continue to attract comments about your bump from people who don't know. Either way, what you are going through is an enormous emotional hurdle.

Most hospitals will offer a burial or cremation service, which might be shared with other parents who have suffered a similar experience. You can also make your own arrangements.

'The cremation gave me closure,' says one mum. 'It helped to see the coffin.'

You might want to make up a box of mementoes to keep with a hand- or footprint, scan pictures, photographs, condolence cards and letters. One mother bought two identical teddies; one to put in her son's coffin, the other to keep on a shelf in the bedroom for her other children to cuddle whenever they felt the need. Some plant a memorial to remember their baby: 'We bought a rowan tree to plant in our garden in memory of our daughter,' says one mum. 'The most important thing is not sweeping everything under the carpet and pretending the baby never existed, which is what some members of our family wanted to do.'

Mumsnetters who have had late miscarriages recommend seeing a bereavement midwife or specialist grief counsellor: 'Sometimes, you get so pent up with it all that even your partner doesn't understand. It was fantastic for helping me let the feelings out, as trying to make sense of it all was sending me insane in all sorts of ways.'

The cause of miscarriage is discovered in over half of all those that occur after 13 weeks; it can be a source of comfort and can also be helpful if you are considering a future pregnancy. 'Finding out that my baby was genetically perfect helped me get further treatment and testing to discover why it kept happening to me,' says one mum. 'The only downside was the waiting, which took six months. I couldn't move on during that time and even leaving the house was impossible some days. But I'm glad I did the testing.'

Many Mumsnetters recommend Sands (Stillbirth and Neonatal Death charity), www.uk-sands.org, whose forums and helpline assist people whose pregnancies end from 14 weeks onwards.

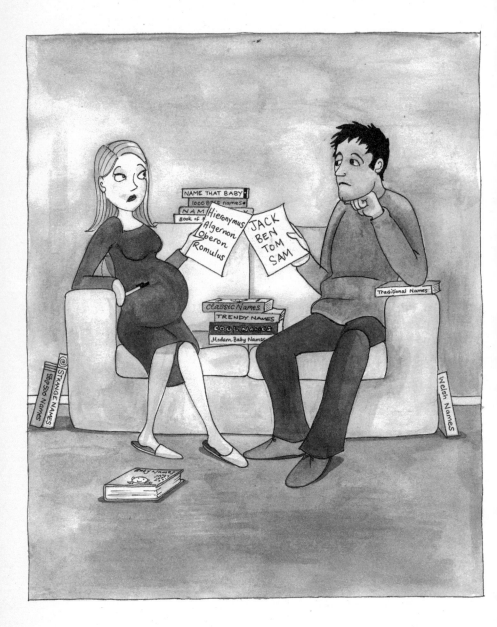

Third Trimester:

OK, Fat Ladies – It's Nearly Time to Start Singing

In this chapter ...

Nearly There

'Something weird and wonderful happ[...]
to me as the birth of my daughter got [...]
Up until then, I had been petrified; I'm such a
physical coward and a total quitter in general.
But I stopped worrying about the birth because
I got so fed up with being pregnant. The thought
of not carrying the baby inside me began to
seem really deeply enticing. I got quite gung-
ho: "Bring it on!" In those final weeks you get
really huge and uncomfy and therefore keen to
crack on with it.' Bakedpotatoe

At last, some light at the end of the birth canal. The idea that
you are going to get a baby, after all this time, effort and serious
additional poundage, might finally be sinking in. Alternatively,
you might just feel like you are sinking. It is mind-blowing how
far and wide that once neat little bump can expand in your
third trimester. Heck, one of these days someone on a bus might
even give up their seat for you. Or they might just try to climb
aboard.

What do you do with yourself during these last weeks and
days? It's hard to concentrate on nice lunches and shopping trips
when you are obsessed with the elephant in the room. No, not
you, dear: the birth itself. This is a subject lurking on the edge
of your consciousness that you are none too keen to focus on.
You will have discussed your options with health professionals
in theoretical terms. Maybe even written out a birth plan
plotting out your ideal delivery. But there's one question you
are not even sure you want to ask: how freakin' painful is it
going to be?

If you do ask, everyone will tell you something different. The
helpful woman in the corner shop says it is as easy as shelling
peas; your best mate describes it as like having your shell ripped

off. It's so mind-boggling and terrifying at the same time, you might as well have signed yourself up for open-heart surgery. Except that they don't make you do that fully conscious.

'I think the key to childbirth is not to worry about what anyone else thinks about your "performance". I remember getting a lot of praise for giving birth vaginally to one of my children without any pain relief, but it wasn't really a difficult birth. I was lucky. I think birth is a lot about luck and people make it into a performance instead.' FairyMum

> First-time childbirth is very hard to predict; for some, it is a nightmare, and for others, it is a more positive experience. Adrenalin can be a wonderful distraction. And controlled drugs aren't that bad either. The only thing that you can do at this stage is to steer towards the type of birth you want, while keeping an open mind, because anything could happen: 'Try to focus on having a baby, not having a "birth experience",' advises one wise mum.

'Birth is not a consumer choice, no amount of preparation will provide you with a magic formula to give you the "birth of your dreams". Don't put yourself under unnecessary pressure or set yourself up for disappointment. But at the same time, try to fight your inner Eeyore: "Ah, birth. It's miserable whichever way you look at it. A choice of pain during, or pain after. An option of whether you'd like the scar tissue where the sun shines or where the sun don't shine."' jaype

For some, giving birth can be an incredibly exhilarating experience. 'That sensation of the baby's body coming out after its head and shoulders is close to orgasmic,' raves one mum who liked it so much she went on to have more. This is not a view shared by many, it has to be said, but even so another mum swooned: 'I would do it again just for that feeling of, Oh my god, it's over, and my baby is here. Oh and the gas and air isn't bad either. Enjoy that part.'

'Sometimes I feel reluctant to share my birth stories because I was so lucky and relaxed. But I met a girl the other day saying she is trying to get pregnant and the only thing putting her off is an absolute terror of giving birth. She was in tears at one point because she said it had made so much difference to hear a positive birth story. I would do it again in an instant. However painful the experience, it *will* end! And you will meet your little one.'

MrsNormanMaine

It's natural to have doubts about life beyond the birth, too: Will my vagina be around my knees? Will I turn into my mother? Do I actually like children? But it's a little late to start interviewing potential surrogates. You're on the home straight. You want that gold medal, don't you? Or at least a gold necklace from Tiffany's? Now is the perfect time to drop a big hint ...

Birth Plans – 'Dear Santa ...'

Birth plans are a bit like essays. The swotty types set to work on them as soon as they discover that they are pregnant, writing dissertations complete with bullet points, cross-references and footnotes. The slackers are more lax and might eventually scribble something down on the back of a coaster from their local or crib a few ideas from a friend. One succint Mumsnetter wrote on hers: 'Have baby. Have tea and toast.' And some women simply never get round to handing in anything at all, hoping they will be able to wing it on the day.

'I didn't have a birth plan with my daughter, figuring that I'd go with the flow and trust the professionals. I was positive and open-minded, but pretty soon felt powerless and confused by what was happening. So for my second child, I will have a birth plan. I will specify that I don't want unnecessary intervention, want to avoid Syntocinon at all costs, do not want my waters broken manually, do not want internal examinations, want to remain mobile, want to be encouraged to try water birth, do not want to lie down, do not want time limits imposed on me, will consider an epidural as a last resort, but don't want pethidine, and if the baby is in distress and my options become limited would rather a Caesarean than a prolonged, ineffective, exhausting, natural delivery. Oh, and I would like the midwives to be aware this time that I have SPD. That's about it I think.' Happynappies

A birth plan is not a legal or professional document: it is just a wish list of your own personal preferences, which your caregivers should read and refer to when choices are made. You don't have to write a birth plan (lots of people don't bother, particularly for second births), but if you feel that you want your preferences put down on paper, then your birth plan is the way to do it. Usually, there is a space in your maternity notes for you to write a plan, or you may want to write it on a separate piece of paper and staple it to your notes.

Keep it simple – no more than one side of A4. When you've written it, discuss it with your midwife (some time in the third trimester – not when you are still staring at your positive pregnancy test). Whatever you include in your birth plan, try not to sound like the head girl from St Dunces and include the phrase 'if at all possible' as much as you can. Being patronising won't go down well with the midwives and remember – they are the ones with the needles and thread.

Don't just focus on the birth; think about the bit before and afterwards. Who do you want to be there? Do you want music? Low lighting? What are your thoughts on pain relief? Do you want to be active, or do you just want to be presented with a menu of the drugs du jour? Do you want to breastfeed? Do you want an injection to expel the placenta or wait for it to happen by itself? Do you want to apologise to your partner for all those obscenities you will be volleying at him in writing or just verbally?

'No one will have the time to read an essay if it is a mad rush, so I'd try to make sure that they know your top priorities. I was adamant about breastfeeding and having no drugs. You need flexibility but that doesn't mean you don't have a few things that you really want to have done in a certain way. Have those things clearly displayed so there is no misunderstanding.' Lua

Of course, it can be a bit irritating if you have a carefully crafted plan that no one bothers reading: 'The midwife looked at mine and said, "That's nice", then ignored it!' recalls one disappointed mum. And some babies arrive so quickly there is no time to discuss the finer details. In the whirlwind of a fast labour, it is easy to forget to even take your plan out of your hospital bag. Others lose their nerve at the last minute and chicken out of handing it over when faced with a midwife with six other women to see and a half-eaten ham sandwich to finish. But don't be shy. It's your birth, so be assertive; hand over your work and make sure the midwife reads it. And – more importantly – make sure that you discuss your feelings with your birth partner, so that he/she can be an advocate when you can't do anything but moo. Also, remember to warn them that your plans might have to change. One Mumsnetter asked for pain relief only to have her husband interrupt: 'No. We agreed it would be a natural birth.' No doubt they laughed about it later ...

Bear in mind that the road to hell is paved with good birth plans, and giving birth rarely goes to plan. 'I wrote that I was to have no pain relief and would do everything naturally,' says a mum. 'About an hour after arriving at the hospital, I had an epidural.' Another mum whose plan went to pot suggests: 'Write a birth plan, put it in an envelope and stick it at the back of a drawer. When your baby is six months old, read it and have a right laugh.'

I had visions of a water birth and even made tapes of the music I'd listen to. In the actual event, I didn't fancy getting into the bath let alone the birthing pool. I ended up watching car chases and Nigella in bed while on pethidine. It was fine, just not what I'd imagined.' wild

Even if your midwife never gets round to reading your birth plan, writing one can help you to consider different scenarios. 'What's an episiotomy?' is not something you want to be asking mid-labour, neither do you want to be leafing through your dog-eared copy of Sheila Kitzinger while your ten-minute slot with the anaesthetist is slipping by. Putting a plan together will help you to collect your thoughts, and at least you will have an idea of what you would like to happen (just as long as you also know that it might not work out that way).

'My birth plan started with a TENS machine, included gas and air and epidural and any other drugs deemed necessary, flirted with a water birth and ended with a Caesarean option. I ended up having almost everything on there including the emergency C-section. Not everyone's idea of an ideal birth but at least it was on the plan and I'd considered it, so it wasn't so much of a shock or disappointment.' Biza

Your birth plan is about imagining your ideal birth, much like the fantasies you had about marrying Prince Charming when you were younger. The more open-minded you are, hopefully the less put out you will be if all does not go to plan and the man holding your hand is an overweight and less amusing version of Jack Dee.

Birth plan – what should I write?

Like all good stories, your birth plan needs a beginning, a middle and an end. Whether it's just a few ideas, or a full-length exposition of your hopes and fears, here's our handy crib sheet to help you formulate your own birth plan.

Beginning – labour
- Write a sentence or two summarising your approach to the birth, for example: 'I would like to have a birth with no drugs'; 'I do not want an epidural'; or 'I would like a Caesarean' (obviously you would need to mention this particular one before you are in the labour suite).
- Who do you want to be with you? Your partner? Your mum? The helpful lady in the corner shop? And do you mind students witnessing part of your birth or labour?
- Monitoring: do you want, or would you mind continual foetal monitoring or would you prefer occasional monitoring with a Doppler (a hand-held sensor) or similar?

(continued)

- Location: of course home births need to be discussed well in advance, but do you want to try to labour in water?
- Pain relief: do you feel strongly about certain types of pain relief? Do you want to see if they have a mobile epidural? Do you want gas and air? Have you had problems in the past with any of the drugs used? Do you want to carry on with just a TENS machine for help for as long as possible?
- Speeding things up: would you like to avoid artificial rupture of the membranes? Or a Pitocin drip?

Middle – birth
- Birthing positions: what birthing positions do you think you might prefer? What would you like to avoid?
- Do you want an episiotomy or would you rather avoid one? Would you rather avoid tearing?

End – immediately after the birth
- Would you like the baby to be delivered straight on to you, or would you prefer the baby to be cleaned up first?
- Do you want the baby to be wrapped separately, or would you prefer skin-to-skin contact?
- Who do you want to cut the cord? Do you have any preferences about when the cord is cut? Are you donating cord blood?
- Do you have strong feelings about the delivery of the placenta? Would you be happy for a managed third stage (an injection to hurry it up), or do you want to try for natural delivery?
- Feeding: if you are breastfeeding your baby, would you like the midwives to help you with this?
- Stitches: what pain relief would you like if you need stitches?

Too Posh to Push – Should You Have an Elective Caesarean and How Do You Go About It?

A Caesarean section is an operation by which a baby is born via a surgical incision through the abdomen skin, muscles and walls of the womb. An 'emergency Caesarean' occurs after labour has started, when complications prevent labour from progressing. An 'elective Caesarean' is when the operation is planned before labour starts.

'My elective section was a lovely experience. My husband had immediate skin-to-skin contact with our daughter and sat next to me the whole time. The medical team were absolutely wonderful. It was nothing like an emergency one. There's no panic for you or the doctors and you will not be exhausted from labour. Everyone is happy and excited. If I were to have another child I'd choose an elective again.' LilRedWG

The World Health Organisation has a target of no more than 10 to 15 per cent of deliveries to be by Caesarean section in Western countries, but in the UK, around 20 to 25 per cent of births take place this way. Caesarean sections may avoid some of the risks associated with vaginal birth – such as perineal tearing and a long, stressful labour – but they are not without risks of their own. As far as the mother is concerned there's increased risk of emergency hysterectomy, increased risk of infection, bladder injury and a risk of uterine rupture in future pregnancies. For the baby there's an increased risk of breathing problems. Although extremely rare, maternal mortality is also higher for women having a Caesarean section than it is in vaginal births.

There are several medical reasons why an elective Caesarean can be the recommended route (see below). However, there are also women who want to choose a Caesarean for reasons of their own, even though doing so gets a bad rap. In the popular imagination, elective Caesareans are the preserve of WAGs and bankers' wives who want to minimise the pain of giving birth and keep their five-star pelvic floors intact – and perhaps have a little tummy tuck while everything's being chopped open. But in reality, there are many reasons that women might want to choose to deliver by Caesarean section.

Delivering a baby via your abdomen is not the soft option, but for some women it is the least terrifying scenario at a time when there is so much uncertainty. At the very least, you get to know when, where and how your baby will be born. Instead of whimpering on your knees for days on end, it should all be over before you have had time to reapply your mascara. It saves you from the trauma of a last-minute emergency Caesarean, and you won't have to worry about your bits being ripped to shreds. 'There is no easy way of giving birth,' points out one mum: 'My main bugbear is those who only see the fluffy romance of a vaginal birth and refuse to accept or discuss the things that can go wrong with your fanjo/waterworks/pooworks as a result of a vaginal birth.'

'I requested a C-section as I regarded the birthing process as unimportant to me. My priorities were breastfeeding and parenting. I didn't want a nasty labour to cloud that. As it turned out, the C-section was a wonderful experience and the obstetrician agreed afterwards that there was no way I could have had a straightforward delivery. My son was positioned badly and required a ventouse even with a C-section. Way too much focus is on childbirth in antenatal classes, and too little attention is given to the really big issue of parenting.' Highlander

Lots of women feel a great deal of fear around childbirth – and that is quite normal. It is a big roll of the dice and you really have very little control over the outcome. So a planned section may feel like one way of gaining a bit of control. But the risks – particularly the long recovery period – are not inconsiderable. So, before making any decisions, it is worth asking your doctor or midwife if there is someone, such as a counsellor, with whom you can discuss your fears and concerns. There are also private counsellors and doulas who specialise in discussing and working through birth fears, who might help you to make an informed choice.

If you decide early on in your pregnancy that you want a Caesarean, unless you go privately your first hurdle will be persuading your doctor and midwife to your way of thinking. A Caesarean will cost the NHS considerably more than if you give birth naturally, so elective Caesareans are not undertaken lightly. Doctors' views vary on whether women should be able to have a Caesarean on request if they are otherwise healthy. Some consider it to be a safe alternative based on personal choice, while others believe such a risky operation should be avoided at all costs.

Securing a Caesarean should be straightforward if you have a specific medical reason such as pre-eclampsia (see p. 242), if your baby is unusually large, you are expecting multiples, your baby is breech, or the placenta is obstructing the entrance to your womb. Or you may have more personal reasons, such as bad tearing from a previous birth, or a previous emergency section and either don't want to risk another or don't fancy taking the small risk of uterine rupture that comes with a VBAC (vaginal birth after Caesarean).

'In some circles you have failed as a mother if you have had a C-section. Only this morning I got the response: "Why did you have a second child if you had to have it by C-section?"' Ladymuck

Opting for an elective is still generally regarded and referred to as 'unnatural', so prepare yourself for people to be disappointed for you, even though it was your decision. In new-mum classes, there is often an unspoken hierarchy of 'birth experiences' and a planned Caesarean usually appears somewhere near the bottom. 'When I started to tell people that I was considering having an elective Caesarean, I was amazed to find that quite a lot of people thought I was being very selfish,' says one pro C-section mum. 'It seems I might have been a bit naive to think people might accept it as my decision.'

It is worth bearing in mind that full recovery after a Caesarean usually takes far longer than for vaginal deliveries.

'A section is not necessarily an easy option in terms of recovery. It is major, invasive operation and you should be realistic about that.' MrsMattie

Some women do go on to regret their choice: 'It was one of the worst decisions I have made,' says a mother who had an elective. 'I really wish my consultant hadn't made it so easy for me.' Of course, only you will know what is best for you and your baby. (And, quite frankly, yah boo sucks to everyone else.)

Elective Caesarean: pros and cons

Pros
- You can schedule it in – no ghastly endurance of the 'Am I, aren't I ... ?' stress of the final few weeks, and no having friends/family on stand-by to look after other children if your waters break in the middle of the night.
- Your perineum will remain intact (although bear in mind that most tears heal nicely in time).
- You will avoid the risk of a long drawn-out labour.
- You will avoid the risk of emergency Caesarean if your labour has begun but is not progressing as it should.
- It may be less stressful for the birth partner watching you in pain through a long labour.
- You may have an existing health complaint that you have been advised might be exacerbated by labour or a vaginal delivery.

Cons
- Generally, higher health risks for mother and baby.
- Longer recovery time than a vaginal birth – lots of women are up and about immediately after a vaginal delivery, but it will be some time before you are up on your feet without pain after a section. It can be hard to sit up properly which can make life difficult when you are trying to manage a newborn. If you can't bear being looked after or are the sort of person who feels the need to hoover twice a day, this will be very tough. You will need a lot of help at home.

- Your hospital stay will be longer. You will need at least two or three days in hospital after a Caesarean and it's no fun on a ward – it's hellishly noisy and the food is, frankly, grim; this can be frustrating and stressful when you want to be settling in at home with your newborn and partner.
- Some people can't drive for about six weeks on doctors' orders (check with your car insurers for their conditions, too). This is a pain if you want to get out and visit friends or ferry older children around, particularly if you don't have a partner off work for this time.
- Breastfeeding can be tougher: you won't be able to pick up your baby so easily after surgery. And some women report that they felt pressurised into bottle-feeding by ward staff who were worried about their milk not coming in quickly enough or the baby not latching properly.
- A section is more expensive to the NHS: a Caesarean costs about £1000 more to the NHS than a vaginal delivery. This might not worry you too much unless you are an NHS manager, of course.
- Increased risks to your future pregnancies: a Caesarean section will result in a higher risk to future pregnancies for placenta problems such as placenta praevia (see p. 250) and placenta accrete; higher risk of uterine rupture and emergency hysterectomy for future deliveries.
- The scar – not only does it hurt for quite some time afterwards (and some folks complain of itching and tenderness for months, if not years) but you will probably also end up with a lovely 'lip', like a spare tyre or mini muffin top hanging over the top of it, which no amount of diet or exercise will shift. Nice.

Buy Buy, Baby: Equipment – What You Really Need

Becoming pregnant is a bit like wandering through a market in Marrakesh. You are overheated, sweating like a pig and you can't turn a corner without someone trying to sell you something. It is easy to become caught up in this madness but, for the sake of your bank balance and sanity, it's probably best that you keep a rational distance.

'We decided that after the final scan and the baby being given a clean bill of health we should actually start buying stuff for her. So we went to Toys R Us to play with prams and ended up coming home with a cot blanket and two little body suits.' RGPargy

The most important thing to understand is that you don't have to buy everything now. Although the imminent birth of your beloved baby really should be marked by a national holiday, chances are that Mothercare will be open as usual. Even with a baby in tow and a brain scrambled from lack of sleep, you will still be able to shop after you've given birth, although you might need a little sit-down first, of course. The exciting prospect of shopping might even get you out of your dressing gown and through the front door. If not, there is also online shopping or the option of sending your partner out to forage.

'You only need the bare basics,' advises one mum. 'You'll discover the other things you need and get them as required.' And the less you buy now, the more room you will have to move, because baby equipment can quickly swallow up floor space.

Bare essentials – what pretty much everyone needs

Infant car seat They won't let you drive away from the hospital without one, and you will not want to be waddling home on the Number 17 with your vagina hanging around your knees. A car seat should be bought new or borrowed from someone you know, because a car accident can weaken or damage a car seat, and you need to know it is safe. Check out the reviews on Mumsnet to give you some idea of the type you might want. Then double check that the car seat will fit safely in your car (ideally the shop should physically fit it and check this before you commit to purchasing).

Once you've made the purchase, make sure that your partner knows how to fit the damned thing properly, and remove it as well.

Cot Your baby will most likely be up and down all night needing feeds and nappy changes, so there is rather a lot of activity involved in nocturnal parenting. According to advice from FSID (the Foundation for the Study of Infant Deaths) babies should sleep in the same bedroom as an adult for at least the first six months of their lives. Most parents put a cot next to the mother's side of the bed, but the precise arrangement will depend on how much room you have. Cots come in all sorts of sizes and if your room is small you may be tempted to start small, but bear in mind that while your baby might look a bit lost in a giant cot now, it won't be long before he is a strapping lad, scaling those bars and rocking the cot like a teenager looking for an ASBO. 'A cot with adjustable mattress heights is useful,' advises one mum 'so you can raise the base to stop you breaking your back when lifting your newborn in and out.' Cots (like Moses baskets – see p. 225) are a good bet to get hold of second hand, as folks are keen to get them out of the house when they're no longer needed, but do invest in a fresh mattress.

If you like the idea of co-sleeping, then a bedside cot is the thing to look out for – it attaches to your bed so you are on the same level as your baby, but gives you a bit more room. You can easily drag baby across for a cuddle or push her out of the way a bit to give yourself more room when she is in a deep sleep.

And while you're choosing a cot, invest in some appropriate night-time lighting too:

'A dimmer switch or dim light in the room that the baby is sleeping is essential. It's nigh-on impossible to put a sleeping baby to bed in pitch darkness, but if you turn on the lights it's suddenly brighter than Blackpool illuminations. If the baby is still in your room with you, you can just swap your bedside light for a 12-watt bulb – much easier on the eyes for those middle-of-the-night feeds.' Nailpolish

Sling Slings and baby-carriers are no longer the preserve of hippy mothers who studied anthropology at uni. They are a great way to carry your baby around for the first few weeks, and pretty much essential for any baby who is crabby or loves being held (i.e. most babies). Studies have shown slings to be beneficial to tiny babies, who love being close to another body for both physical and emotional comfort. With a bit of practice, you should be able to get into town and do your shopping with baby snug and happy, bobbing around on your chest.

'I wish someone had shown me a really good sling two years ago, rather than me being seduced into buying an expensive pram that was bloody awful and which my daughter yelled in.' Mimia

Slings are also great for dads, because every woman loves the sight of a man with a baby in a sling, and he can revel in the admiring gaze of any woman of childbearing age who happens to pass. 'I keep thinking I am being eyed up by pretty ladies,' confesses one new dad. 'Then after I've given them my most charming smile, I remember I've got my son strapped to my chest.'

It can be hard finding a sling to suit you, and learning the various ways of wearing them, so check out the Mumsnet reviews or ask friends for advice and try a few on if you can.

Tons of vest and babygros 'You can never have too many,' advises one mum. 'They get covered in sick and poo every five minutes.' Don't buy all "newborn" sizes though, cute though they are – some newborn sizes might not fit larger or longer babies even from day one. You will probably be given lots of lovely baby outfits, but sleepsuits are a more sensible purchase because you will need to change the baby frequently and they are so much easier to get on and off than denim jeans and matching cowboy shirt combos. If in doubt, attempt to dress your pet cat in the outfit you are considering, and then decide whether it represents a good investment or not.

'DO NOT buy the baby sleepsuits which have buttons on the back. Newborns don't really like having their face squashed into the carpet for five minutes while you swear and fiddle with tiny poppers.' Stephanie 1974

Hat Newborn babies are usually dressed in little hats. This is partly so they look extra-specially cute, but also so they don't lose too much heat through their heads when they are fresh from the warm of your womb. It's not such a good idea to let your baby sleep indoors in a hat though in case they overheat. So make sure it's a hat you can get on and off easily, as there is NOTHING more annoying than arriving home with a sleeping baby and anticipating a bit of kip for you, then waking them up while trying to take their hat off.

Swaddle blanket Lots of babies love being swaddled because after being squished up in your belly for months, their flailing limbs can be terrifying to them. A fine-knit blanket will do the job, or you can buy specially designed 'swaddle blankets' which have Velcro at crucial points. If you're using a blanket, a midwife will be able to teach you the required origami as soon as the baby is born.

Muslin cloths These are great for wiping up sick and dribble, and for draping over guests' shoulders to save their nice visiting outfits from being ruined by your regurgitated breast milk. It's only polite.

Scratch mitts or an emery board Maybe not essential to all, but some babies slide out with long nails and can easily scratch their little faces with their uncontrollable flapping around. This is what scratch mitts are for, so it's worth having a couple of pairs just in case (although you can just use socks instead). Alternatively, you might be able to lightly file their nails with an emery board so they are shorter and smoother, though this will involve an element of luck as well as good judgement. 'You can also bite their nails off for them; probably not recommended in every baby manual, but it worked for us,' says one mum.

Bath support Baby baths are a terrible idea: you have a perfectly good bathtub already which comes with the convenience of handily located taps and a useful hole that drains into the sewage system, instead of on to your bathroom floor. But without a decent bath prop, bathing a newborn is a bit like bathing a large oiled toad, and you will need both hands to keep him from slipping, which results in you desperately swilling him around in the water trying to shake the poo off his legs. What you need is a moulded bath support, which holds your newborn in place in the bath and leaves your hands free to wash him properly.

Bottles and steriliser If you are planning to bottle-feed, you will need to stock up on the necessary equipment in advance. If you are planning to breastfeed, you will find the equipment stuffed down your top already.

Expressing equipment If you want to be able to leave your baby with breast milk so you can go out or go to work, or you'd like your partner to take a share of the night feeds and don't want to use formula, you're going to have to get your head round one of the odder pieces of baby equipment – a breast pump, which in most cases looks like an instrument of torture, particularly for those whose breasts are already protesting about the amount of suction they're getting. Your main choice is whether to go electric or manual. Electric pumps are usually much speedier and more effective at extracting the milk. But on the downside they can be noisy and you have less control over the strength of the suction, so they're not always ideal for sore nipples. They don't come cheap either, so are more suitable for those who think expressing will be part of their regular routine.

'I had a dual electric breast pump which meant I could express from both breasts at once which was really efficient. It meant that my partner could do the last feed each night when I was exhausted, and I could get an early night, knowing I'd be up a few hours later.' BigBertha

Obviously, if you go down this route, you will also need a bottle to feed the expressed milk to the baby and some means of sterilising this. The usual advice about not introducing this bottle too soon applies, but if it's important to you to be able to give your child expressed breast milk from a bottle at some stage, introduce it once breastfeeding is established, so the baby doesn't reject the bottle later on.

Changing gear

Glamorous new nappy bag: 'Any excuse for a new bag!' jokes one mum. But be warned: make sure it looks good for either sex to carry, unless you want to be the one lugging the nappies around for the next two years. Rucksack-style changing bags in a dark colour are less likely to humiliate your partner than something with flowers and diamante bits. A changing bag should have lots of room for stashes of nappies and spare clothes. Some also have a fold-out bit that can be used as a portable changing mat, which is useful for laying on top of discarded needles and bodily fluids on the baby changing tables in public toilets.

Nappies: even if you are a hardcore eco-warrior, disposables are easiest for the first few days when you are still feeling a bit shell-shocked. Oh, and the baby emits a horrifying sort of black sticky ectoplasm from its bottom for the first day or so, exactly like the no-nails glue 'Sticks Like Shit' purveyed by builders' merchants. Now you know where they got the name from.

Baby wipes or cotton wool balls: to remove ectoplasm from all surfaces, including baby. Some people don't like the fact that baby wipes contain a lot of fragrances and chemicals, and can sting some people's skin ('I wiped my own bum with these once and had to sit in a bucket of cold water for an hour afterwards,' one mum complains). Although as another mum points out: 'You can always run them under a warm tap to take out any chemicals if you want to.' Their woven surface doesn't disintegrate like toilet tissue, so they are better for wiping sticky stuff. (Some people use flannels and warm tap water instead: dirty ones are bunged in a traditional lidded nappy bin for later washing at a high temperature: 'If you use washable nappies, make your own wipes from cheap face flannels or tea towels cut into eight and wash them with the nappies.')

Barrier/nappy cream (Sudocrem or similar): this is the stuff that you can slap on babies' bottoms if they are a bit sore and acts as a barrier to the ectoplasm and urine, which can trigger nappy rash. You should have some in case you need it.

Changing mat: sticky poo gets everywhere and baby will let it all out as soon as you whip off that nappy, so invest in a waterproof changing mat (or two – if you live in a house with several floors). You can buy changing stations which are pieces of furniture with a changing mat on top. These are better for your back than constantly changing the baby on the floor and they also have handy drawers for changing paraphernalia and clothes. Using one can be tricky though if you have a wriggly baby as you need to keep one hand on them so they don't crash to the floor while you scrabble around trying to wipe poo off your sleeve.

Wish list – what you'd like to have if you could swap your maisonette for a mansion

Prams A pram – not essential? We can hear you spluttering already. Prams are like cars – you can spend months trawling through posh showrooms and sighing over lovely brochures and then take a deep breath and commit yourselves to an expensive hire-purchase agreement for the next few years. Or you can just look at your budget and find a nice homely old banger that gets you from A to B with your shopping in the back.

'Prams are becoming more ridiculous as time goes on. A pram needs to be somewhere for baby to sleep and have walks in laid flat. No need for one that makes you tea!' NAB3

The fact is, while lots of ladies love their on-trend Farkaboo Starship Baby Manoeuvre Solution, lots of others can manage with a sling and a buggy or with a simple, cheap pram.

'The best advice I ever got on Mumsnet was to borrow a pram where the baby could lie flat, and then buy a lightweight reclinable buggy from six months. It's not easy to contemplate second-hand stuff for your precious firstborn, but it saved me a fortune and was definitely the right thing to do.' Munchpot

Whether an all-singing pram is essential for you depends on your lifestyle, your budget, whether you live in the town or the country, whether you use a car or a bus and whether your baby likes travelling in a pram (unfortunately you can't really plan for that one). And, of course, how highly you rate maintaining your street cred.

'Maybe if you have decent pavements or hardly walk anywhere you can get away with a buggy. Living and working in a rural area, I need a decent all-terrain pram, with a carrycot. Five and a half years of *constant* use later, mine is still going strong. FromGirders

Travel systems

Travel systems usually feature a pram chassis on to which you can clip either a carrycot or an integrated car seat. This gives you the choice of lifting your baby out of the car and on to the pram chassis without all the faff of taking the baby out of their car seat each time and having separate gadgets for each part of the journey. The carrycot can sometimes be used instead of a Moses basket, though some aren't recommended for overnight use so check this in advance. Travel systems are particularly useful if you need to carry your car seat for any particular distance (for example, if you can't park near your house). However, babies do need to lie flat so shouldn't be kept in their car seats for long periods.

'It's always better to get a good car seat that fits your car correctly than compromise on safety in getting a cheaper travel system.' LadyVictoriaOfCake

Travel systems are useful while the baby is small, although remember that you will need to buy a new car seat in about a year when your baby reaches the right size and weight for a second-stage car seat, so it won't last for ever. Quite a few travel systems can be used as a regular pram once the car seat is too small. Or once your child has outgrown the car seat you can easily transfer to a cheap lightweight buggy.

Strollers – the great debate: forward- or backward-facing?

Most prams and buggies on the market face forward: the assumption being that the passenger wants to see out into the world, and, as one mum admits, 'It feels like there is so much social pressure to be forward facing.' However, studies have shown that babies are not actually that interested in watching car exhausts and the backs of people's legs on Basingstoke High Street. They much prefer – and benefit from – the stimulation of watching their parents.

Backward-facing prams enable a lot more interaction between the pusher and the pushee, and this is thought to be a benefit to the baby's development. 'I think it's great for their language development to be Mummy-facing, as you can have a proper natter to them,' declares one mum, although another confesses, 'I have walked into a few bollards while talking to him.'

Lots of pram seats can be set up on the chassis to face either way, although showrooms tend to display them only facing forward. So when you are looking to buy a backward-facing pram, you will probably need to do quite a bit of research to find the model that best suits your needs.

'My six-month-old son is still Mummy-facing, with no plans to change yet. I thought this was the "norm" until friends commented on why I did it that way! However, I frequently get stopped by older ladies in the street who tell me how nice it is to see a baby facing the person they love most in the world.' *busywizzy*

Baby monitor Most people will end up getting a baby monitor at some stage, so that they can keep an ear out for their baby in the evenings – particularly in the winter when you are likely to have your doors closed. You can get all sorts of baby monitors, from basic listening devices and breathing and heart-rate monitors to infrared night-vision wireless CCTV – what suits you will depend on the layout of your home, your levels of parenting paranoia and your innate geekiness.

'My husband set up a webcam as a baby monitor. He can see our daughter napping during the day while he is at work!' Chiiicken

'We've never had a baby monitor because we've lived in terraced houses where you're never very far away – and both babies were noisy!' writes one mum. 'Why not wait till baby arrives and then buy one if you feel you need it? To begin with, your little one probably won't be out of your sight anyway.' Some come with a two-way communication system where you can hear the baby and speak soothingly back to them. Do be careful around monitors though – you don't want to become one of those clichés in which the hosts discuss their dinner guests' failings in the baby's bedroom only to come back downstairs to stony silence in the kitchen.

Baby monitors are needed for:

1. Deaf dads. If you've sloped off to catch up on sleep and left your partner in charge, he may need a little help to hear the little one – it's all those years of selective hearing.
2. Winter nights when you are downstairs watching TV and don't want all the doors between you and the baby kept open.
3. When you go to someone else's house and put the baby to sleep where you can't hear her – especially if there's a raucous dinner party going on.
4. Summer nights if you have a garden and want to spend time in it after the baby goes down.

Moses basket Moses baskets are totally unnecessary, but they do look awfully pretty and make you feel like you've got a proper baby on the way. 'You can just use the cot from day one,' points out – well, just about everyone. But a Moses basket is often a little treat that we buy ourselves because it's charming and, of course, looks very nice in photographs.

'Moses basket accessories exist just to take your mind off the fact that you've paid £50 for a wicker basket.' ConnorTraceptive

Baby toiletry box Plastic two-tier boxes for baby 'stuff' haven't changed much since you were a baby, and that's because they are rather useful for gathering all your baby clutter (shampoos, flannels, creams and unguents) into one place. And once your baby has graduated from nappies, they are jolly useful for storing paints and craft stuff.

Baby gyms There are lots of 'suitable for newborn' toys available on the market, but most are rather useless because the only toy a baby really wants is Mummy or Daddy's face – and, for the first few months, most babies will scream their heads off if they aren't playing with *that*. However, a baby gym – basically a brightly coloured play mat with a mobile arching over the top – is great for 'baby entertainment'. You can chart your baby's progress as they move on from screaming with terror at the very idea of being put down, to contemplating the mobile with a modicum of interest, to starting to kick the heck out of it and, if you're unlucky enough to have a musical mobile, setting off the irritating tunes.

Baby sleeping bags Warm 'bags' that you can zip your baby into are very popular, and the right tog will provide the ideal temperate for your baby to sleep in his cot without worrying about the need for any sheets and blankets. Lots of babies seem to sleep better in sleeping bags, and they can't be kicked off like sheets can. A definite essential for some parents, as they become part of the night-time routine: 'After a few months just putting him into the sleeping bag seemed to calm him down and prepare him for sleep.'

Cot-beds Cot-beds are cots that turn into small beds, so you can get more use out of them than regular cots. 'A cot-bed works for some, but they are expensive,' warns one mum. 'A reasonably priced cot followed by a single bed would do both jobs just as well.' One advantage of a cot-bed is that it will last longer. 'However, if you have a second child within a couple of years you'll probably move your first child into a normal bed and use the cot-bed for the new baby, so there won't be any real cost savings.' Cot-beds tend to be smaller than regular-sized single beds, so if you are very short on space, this might sway your decision.

What not to buy (things a second child will never see)

Top-and-tail bowl Not for preparing vegetables, but for giving your baby a sort of bed bath. It's basically a bowl with three compartments, two large ones for filling with water and a smaller one for balls of cotton wool. The theory is that you wash your baby's face with the 'top' end by dipping the cotton wool into the warm water on the 'top' compartment and then wash his 'tail' with the warm water in the other compartment. (Note: do mention to your GP if your baby actually does have a tail!) Really it should be called an 'eyes and arse bowl', but regardless of its name, this bizarre piece of equipment and its accompanying ritual appear to have been invented purely to sell you one more co-ordinated plastic item for your nursery. If you want to bathe your baby this way, use an 'old margarine tub' or 'a cleaned-out summer-pudding bowl'. Or just swill him around in a sink or bath.

Matching nursery furniture and wallpaper No one will blame you for wanting to create the perfect nursery for your perfect precious newborn, but it's by no means essential and can end up being costly when you have to keep updating it.

'Don't bother with the matching nursery furniture and wallpaper. Just buy an ordinary chest of drawers, wardrobe, bedside table, etc., paint the walls in whatever colour you fancy and buy accessories to make it look nice for a baby, then change accessories as your child grows up.' Nailpolish

> **Bath thermometer** Unless you regularly emerge from your own bath needing skin grafts, you can probably judge when a bath is too hot for a baby.

Baby toiletries Lots of babies seem to break out with eczema as soon as you wave the baby shampoo over them, so most parents stick to warm water for the first few months, or a mild liquid baby soap at most.

'We didn't use any toiletries whatsoever on our son until he was a year old, just water. We now use an all-in-one mild soap/shampoo.'

Foundintranslation

Yummy Mummy: what do I need for ME?

Maternity pads Maternity pads are big, thick sanitary towels designed for mopping up the flow of blood that occurs post-birth (lochia). As one mum cheerfully puts it: 'I bled like a sacrificed bison for six weeks!' Maternity pads will remind you of the enormous monstrosities that your mother gave you when you had your first period: 'There is something strangely comforting about maternity pads: just like those schoolday sanitary towels that we used while reading Judy Blume and *Sweet Valley High*!' While you could use sanitary towels, maternity towels are really made for the industrial amounts of waste you will produce for the first few days; they also tend to be softer than normal sanitary towels, which can catch on stitches (oooh!) because of their slightly webbed surface. The extra padding in maternity pads will also provide you with a bit of cushioned support, which feels reassuring and more comfortable after a vaginal birth, when everything feels like it is turning inside out.

'Think how many pads you could possibly need for nine months of missed periods suddenly all turning up at once in your knickers. And then double it. Then send your husband out to Boots to buy them and add another six packs on top.'

toomuchmonthatendofthemoney

Cotton knickers in a larger size than normal Although some people might recommend paper pants, they are not very comfortable or easy to get on, and cheap cotton knickers are about the same price. 'For my first baby I went and bought paper knickers,' recalls one mum. 'BIG mistake. They rubbed and made my legs sore and didn't hold the pads properly in place. Second time around, out came the granny pants!' Buy a size or two larger than normal (at least) because they will be stuffed with a maternity pad, and you will want to be as comfortable as possible, particularly if you have had a C-section.

'Buy packs of cheapo pants that you can throw away. Despite the pads, you will still leak and you don't want to ruin your lucky pants.' Claricebeansmum

Breastfeeding bras You are probably already living in ugly maternity bras, so will be familiar with the cheerless ladies who measure your ever-changing bosom and regularly hand you a new pack of joyless floppy white bras. Nursing or breastfeeding bras tend to be a similar sort of thing, with the added excitement of a clip-down flap that turns your matronly bra into a matronly peephole bra to expose your nipple for feeding. Get a couple of basic ones at the end of your pregnancy, but you may as well wait until after the baby is born before you invest in the expensive leopard-print ones, because your bra size will undoubtedly have changed again by the time your baby is born.

Breast pads Breast (or nursing) pads are for absorbing the milk which will leak from your breasts – probably for the duration of the time you are breastfeeding, although it normally lessens over time. The amount of leakage varies from one woman to the next, but most women need breast pads to save the annoyance of streaky shirts every time they hear a baby cry. You can buy disposable breast pads, which, like disposable sanitary towels, you just use for a few hours and then bung out. Or you can buy more environmentally friendly reusable silk or cotton breast pads, which you throw in the washing basket at the end of the day. In the long run, the latter work out much cheaper. And unlike disposable nappies where you need a separate hot wash, you can put breast pads in with any old wash.

'It's like the Trevi bloody fountain inside my bra.'

reluctantincubator

'Always buy the best disposable breast pads, not the cheapest,' advises one mum. 'They will work better, are less likely to irritate and less likely to show through clothing.' Brands do seem to vary quite a lot – some, for example, are more formed, which will prevent the 'fried-egg look'. But different pads will suit different baps – so try lots to find the right ones for you.

eBay Baby: how to do it on the cheap

Your granny will no doubt be sniggering at you and your Mothercare store card and will gleefully inform you that she raised ten babies in a chest of drawers. And for once, she might have a point. The only things you really need to buy new are (for reasons given earlier) mattresses for Moses baskets or cots and car seats (because you need to be 100 per cent sure that the seat has not been damaged). Otherwise, eBay is your oyster, so beg, borrow and buy second-hand where you can, and don't max out that store card unnecessarily.

'If you do have a Moses basket, don't buy special sheets for it – put the mattress inside a pillowcase instead. If you have any spare single flat sheets, cut them in half and hem the raw edges to make cot sheets. Single flat sheets can often be cheaper than cot sheets – and you get two for the price of one! Also, avoid pink or blue newborn and 0–3 months clothes – then you can use them again if you have another baby of the opposite sex. Buy only white bodysuits for the same reason.' *Gemmasmummy*

'I wish I hadn't wasted money on cot blankets. I should have just got a sleeping bag plus one or two cellular blankets. You don't need cot bumpers.' *Amber1*

'Don't bother to buy one of those poncey changing tables. They look fab, but you can only use them for about four or five months

before they become dangerous. Complete waste of money.'
Caligula

'Don't bother with a baby bath; they take ages to fill and are
heavy. If you don't want to bend down to the bath, use a
washing-up bowl.' *martianbishop*

'They grow out of clothes so unbelievably quickly that it really is
worth accepting every single offer of hand-me-downs you get.'
Wickedwaterwitch

'Car-boot sales!' *hillary*

'Go to your local NCT second-hand sale.' *Cappuccino*

'Freecycle is a great place for acquiring baby equipment,
like stair gates, baby gym, etc.' *PandaG*

'Join all the baby clubs from manufacturers, supermarkets –
they will send you money-off coupons.' *TheBlonde*

'Don't bother buying books by baby gurus and other such
"experts". They'll only addle your brain.' *CorrieDale*

Of course, buying things for the new baby is all part of the
excitement of pregnancy and anticipating the change in your
life. Having a cot in a pink nursery or a neatly pressed rail of baby
clothes in your wardrobe will make you feel all emotional and
blubby inside. But the overriding message from Mumsnetters is
don't get carried away and think you need to transform your home
into a nursery showroom.

**'One person's essential kit is another's waste of
money. Best to buy as little as possible before
they're born, then look at how you're actually**

doing things day-to-day, and what you need to make that work.' welliemum

Discover what type of mum (and dad) you are first. And don't forget to save some pennies for a nice new outfit for you after the birth, so that you don't have to live in those ghastly maternity dungarees for ever.

'Spend any money you do have on things to make life a bit easier *after* the birth – the odd takeaway, babysitter while you have your hair cut or whatever really helps!' PandaG

Mumsnetiquette: Should I have a baby shower? (Or would a cold bath be more fun?)

Do baby showers make you 'Oooh' and 'Ahhh' or is it more of an 'Eugh'? Some people think it is a nice tradition, others think it is a vile American consumerist import that should be rejected at all costs.

For the sugar-coated Charlottes among us, it's the pinnacle of pregnancy. 'I just want the presents and the cake and all my friends looking at me adoringly,' declares a mum. The Samanthas, on the other hand, would rather stick nappy pins in their eyes. What sort of a party is it when you can't get drunk and leave with a man? 'In both my pregnancies I looked like a poached egg on legs and was alternately weeping, giggling insanely and cramming food into my face,' recalls one Mumsnetter. 'I can't think of anything that would thrill me less than an alcohol-free, women-only party to celebrate my alarming transition into Mr Stay Puft, the Marshmallow Man from Ghostbusters.'

When it comes to decorating the venue, think homely Martha Stewart rather than naughty Nigella: 'I decorated the house with washing lines of beautiful baby clothes from car-boot sales and put up a few helium balloons in blue, white and pink,' gushes a baby-shower pro. 'I fed everybody with dainty sandwiches, tea in china cups and saucers, and made tonnes of cakes and scones with clotted cream. We also had a bit of pink champagne.' Bless.

'If your friends ask what you want as a gift go for home-cooked food for the freezer. For my third child my friends threw me a surprise baby shower and each presented me with a frozen meal that would feed six. It was the best pregnancy present ever.' *Biza*

What to Pack for Your Hospital Mini-Break

'The boot of my car is currently full! There's a bag for:

- labour (nightie, light dressing gown, some toiletries, juice cartons, custard creams (for the sugar!), bed socks)
- the ward (big pants, two sets pyjamas, more toiletries, magazine, towel, slippers, outfit for going home)
- the little one (a few nappies, couple of babygros, snowsuits for going home, wee cuddly toy)
- in case of C-section and longer stay (two extra sets pyjamas, more big pants, extra toiletries, book).

I'm an events organiser...' Suis

Essentials

- Your Maternity Notes
- Money for the car park, telephone and television
- A list of phone numbers of people you will need to call to make the big announcement – you don't want to wait until after the birth to discover that your partner doesn't actually know his own mother's phone number
- Camera
- Pain relief: TENS machine and birthing ball ('You can always use it as a punch bag'); most hospitals should have birthing balls, so ask in advance
- Something to tie your hair up with if you have long hair; it can be irritating hanging in your face
- Something to labour in (which should be something you can bung away afterwards: a large, old T-shirt is ideal)
- Drinks for you: small cartons of juice, bottle of mineral water, bendy straws so you can suck at any angle
- Snacks for you: muesli bars, biscuits, glucose sweets
- Food for your birth partner: you don't want them sneaking out to buy fish and chips and missing all the action
- Toiletries: toothbrush, a mild body wash/shampoo
- Hairbrush
- Something to wear afterwards: massive, old T-shirts are fine, or 'a dark-coloured, front-opening nightie – not pyjamas – with short sleeves that you won't mind throwing away afterwards; they are more comfortable and convenient'
- Lots of pants: 'Big granny pants – not paper pants which cut right into the incision site if you have had a Caesarean; buy plenty of cheap ones so you can bin them afterwards'
- Flip-flops or dark-coloured slippers (because you might bleed on them; sorry if that's tmi) – flip-flops are particularly good for the showers, which can be a bit grim (sorry – again!)
- Maternity pads – not just sanitary towels but brick-thick maternity pads
- Breast pads (although if you are only in for a couple of days, you might not leak too much as your milk might not 'come in' while you are there)
- Spare batteries for everything (camera, TENS machine)
- Something to wear home – make sure it's baggy; very baggy.

'We took champagne, but nothing to drink it out of. The Orderly found us some specimen bottles.' fisil

Desirables

- A handbag-sized travel fan: 'Labour and postnatal wards are hot, even in winter'
- Antibacterial hand gel and wipes: 'Hospitals are not always as clean as you would hope'
- Cordial: 'Water is freely available, but it can get a bit dull'
- Something to suck: 'After many hours sucking on gas and air, my mouth was the driest thing ever and no amount of juice could do the trick'
- Ipod
- Massage oil – for your partner to use on your lower back while you are having your contractions
- A pillow: 'It makes the labour suite feel more like home and is comfier than the hospital ones; take one that is colourful so you don't leave it behind'
- Eye mask and earplugs: 'If you are in long early labour, you can block all the usual ward crud out and concentrate; these will also help you to sleep after the birth if the ward is noisy, but still allow you to hear your baby'
- A water spray or flannel: 'So your partner can soak it in cold water and slap it on your face; it's bliss to feel the water dribbling down your face and neck'
- Socks: 'My feet were freezing during labour'
- Lip balm, moisturiser and hand cream: 'It's amazing how your skin dries out in hospital'
- A bit of slap: 'Make-up for those first photos'
- Dried fruit: 'Constipation is bad enough without having just given birth'
- A big tube of Anusol: 'Piles after labour can be a killer'
- Peppermint tea bags: 'You may end up with a Caesarean and trapped wind is painful combined with a fresh scar'
- Gaviscon: 'If you suffered from indigestion while pregnant then I'd recommend packing some Gaviscon, or whatever works, for

you in your hospital bag, just in case you're one of the unlucky few for whom indigestion doesn't disappear straight after the birth'
- Magazines or a book: 'A really simple book to read because you can't sleep, but your brain is fried –*The House at Pooh Corner* worked for me!'
- Clothes: 'Something comfortable to wear other than pyjamas, like a tracksuit, for when visitors turn up – like your boss'
- A sarong: 'Good to wear with T-shirts (it was fab, especially as I had a section) – comfy and a bit more glam than a big nightie; if you have one in a dark colour with a busy enough pattern it can hide anything (we're talking blood here, no one ever says quite how much blood there is after the birth)'
- Dressing gown: 'A lightweight dressing gown'
- Chocolate: 'You're in hospital, you've just had a baby and dropped 5kg anyway'
- Pen and notepad: 'To make lists for your partner to bring things in and to write down questions you want to ask.'

'Get your birth partner to repack your hospital bag so they know where everything is. They will be the one finding things for you.' LenniEd

Baby bits and bobs

It is a good idea to keep this stuff separate, either in one section of the bag, or in a small carrier bag inside your bag (that way, you won't have to rifle through a hundred maternity pads every time you need a new nappy):

- Three vests
- Three babygros
- A pair of scratch mittens or emery board
- A hat
- A blanket
- Twelve nappies
- Cotton wool balls
- Six muslins

- Feeding gear if not using breasts (if you are bottle-feeding, ask your hospital what they will provide, or what you need to bring, as this varies between hospitals).

'I packed everything that it told me to in the Mothercare catalogue. I still haven't used that baby oil and my son is five!' belgianmama

And ... what *not* to pack for your hospital mini-break

- Thongs
- A Wonderbra
- High heels
- A negligée
- Your best moccasins
- Condoms.

Flying – A Good Idea or a Flight of Fancy?

'I have been nagging my partner for ages about a pre-baby holiday. So after hours trying to find dates that work for both of us we have just booked a week in Portugal and are set to fly in my 29th week. I am now freaking out about the possible risk of premature labour and harm to the baby. I am feeling guilty about it already and I'm beginning to regret the decision.' EmmyJo

Sounds like someone is in need of a break. As long as you have consulted your doctor and there's no medical reason why you shouldn't fly, the end of the second trimester/beginning of the third is the perfect time for you to make the most of a last nappy-free trip. It will probably do you good to get away. OK, so you feel a little on the heavy side now, but imagine what it is like to board a plane with a baby that flails, wails, feeds, throws up, drops toys, pees and poos – and requires more kit and kaboodle than Victoria Beckham on an overnight stay.

The concern in the third trimester is that you could give birth early on the plane which wouldn't be fun for anyone and would get in the way of the in-flight drinks trolley. If it is a multiple pregnancy or you have previously had an early labour, it is recommended that you don't fly beyond week 24. Otherwise, it's usually up to 28 weeks for a long-haul flight or 36 weeks for a short-haul, but different airlines have different policies.

After 24 weeks, you may be required to provide a letter from your GP or midwife stating that it is OK for you to fly (you could get one anyway, as a precaution). 'I almost went without a letter thinking that I could get away with looking fat,' admits one mum. 'But I'm glad I got one in the end because I felt really rough on the plane home and was legitimately able to ask the cabin crew for extra help without feeling embarrassed.'

It's important that your travel insurance is up to date and valid for pregnancy, bearing in mind that you may need to cancel your trip at the last minute should a medical concern arise. Some insurers might want to see a letter or other formal document stating your expected due date.

'I've just returned from holiday and was able to book seats with extra leg room. Make sure you go to the gate early and ask them to let you pre-board. It was great not having to stand around in the queue on the plane while everyone puts their bags in the overhead locker. When you get to the airport find out if the flight is busy; if it isn't, ask to be put in a middle row with no other passengers so that you can lie down when the seat belt sign isn't on. I was able to do this both ways and it was bliss.' gr1973

Depending on your size, you might be handed an extra length of seat belt to strap underneath your bump. Don't be offended

– you've got a good excuse. As long as they don't actually advise you to enter the toilet cubicle backwards, you are well within the boundaries of a normal pregnant shape.

'I flew to Turkey when seven months pregnant with our son – it was our last holiday before children. The bloke at the check-in desk in Turkey was funny. He leaned over the desk towards me with his hand sort of shielding his mouth and, whispering, he said: "You are pregnant, yes?" He took my midwife's letter from me, while glancing around to check if anyone was looking – I think he suspected I was smuggling stuff in under my frock.' LadyOfTheFlowers

Deep-Vein Thrombosis (DVT)

Deep-vein thrombosis is the formation of a blood clot in the leg – usually in the calf or thigh. One risk factor is inactivity during long flights ('economy-flight syndrome') and another is pregnancy – so naturally, if you are flying when pregnant, this is the sort of thing that will make your mother suck her teeth and perhaps turn slightly grey.

In order to reduce your risk, it is a good idea to get up and stretch your legs at least twice an hour. You will probably need to make frequent trips to the loo anyway so try to book an aisle seat. Kick off your shoes, slip on some flight socks (elastic compression stockings that help the blood flow, available at most chemists and airports) and rotate your ankles while seated. You want to keep your circulation pumping. Also, drink plenty of water to keep hydrated. Have a stash of your favourite snack to hand, as airline food ain't even what it used to be. On board, your feet are likely to swell, so travel in shoes that you will be able to fit into again once the plane has landed.

Few pregnant women get the urge to holiday off the beaten track, but if you do:

1. Avoid places where there is malaria – pregnant women are more susceptible, and you can't wolf down the requisite hardcore anti-malarial drugs.
2. Check with your GP – or the Medical Advisory Service for Travellers Abroad (www.masta.org). They should be able to tell you which vaccinations and drugs are suitable for travel during pregnancy.
3. Avoid anywhere too hot, too high, too remote, too uncivilised or too far from a mini-bar.
4. Beware of small planes with unpressurised cabins – another no-no – not because you are too heavy but due to lack of oxygen.
5. Steer clear of mosquito repellents that contain DEET, drink bottled water instead of tap, and always carry your medical notes.

Oh, yes, and relax – enjoy yourself. It might be a while before you have another trip like this.

Alternatively, if boarding a plane sounds like too much effort right now, follow this mum's simple but effective plan: 'I wanted some peace and quiet at home for a week, so I sent my husband away.'

HEALTH ISSUES

High Blood Pressure and Pre-Eclampsia

There is nothing more likely to send your blood pressure rocketing than someone in a white coat telling you that it is starting to creep up and you should relax. Most pregnant women find their blood pressure increases slightly at around week 20, although it is usually nothing to worry about. However, if the increase is significant, there are steps you can take to bring it under control before it develops into something more serious. Of course, by the time your child is a toy-throwing toddler, your blood pressure will be permanently high, but that's another story.

What is blood pressure?

Your blood pressure is measured by your midwife at each antenatal appointment using the tight strappy thing that progressively squishes your arm and makes you want to beg for mercy. If you are prone to very low blood pressure and drama, you might feel a bit faint and feeble during this exam.

Blood pressure is measured in 'millimetres of mercury', for example, 140/90 mmHg, usually written as one number above another number ('140 over 90'). When your heart beats, it pumps blood around your body, and as the blood circulates, it pushes against the sides of the blood vessels. The measurement of the strength of this pushing is your blood pressure. The first (top) number is known as systolic blood pressure and is the highest level your blood pressure reaches when your heart is beating. The second (bottom) number is your diastolic blood pressure, and is the lowest strength your blood pressure reaches as your heart relaxes in between heartbeats. A good blood pressure reading is 120/80 or less.

(continued)

Note: some women enter pregnancy with a tendency towards high blood pressure (or hypertension). If you were on blood-pressure medication before you got pregnant, consult your doctor immediately as some of these drugs shouldn't be taken during pregnancy.

Gestational hypertension

Gestational hypertension (pregnancy-induced high blood pressure) is the term used for high blood pressure that develops after 20 weeks of pregnancy. It is usually defined as blood pressure over 140 (systolic) or 90 (diastolic). Any expectant mum with high blood pressure will be carefully monitored with blood pressure checks and urine tests (those sample bottles again) to check whether it will develop into pre-eclampsia or other complications, which can harm both mum and baby.

Pre-eclampsia

This is a serious condition involving grave risks for both mum and baby. It can affect the placenta, kidneys, liver, brain and other organs. You have to be pregnant or have just delivered your baby to have pre-eclampsia. The cause is not known, though it is thought that it may stem from problems with the placenta. Left untreated, pre-eclampsia can be fatal for both mum and baby.

Pre-eclampsia affects 5 to 8 per cent of pregnancies. For one in 100 it will develop into something more serious. It can occur suddenly and needs to be dealt with swiftly.

During the early stages it can be symptomless. You may feel fine and might be surprised to hear that something's up. It is often only discovered at routine check-ups when your blood pressure and urine are tested which is why antenatal checks, dull though they can sometimes be, are so important.

'I felt fine all through my first pregnancy. Had a routine check at 34 weeks and was rushed in to hospital by ambulance. My midwife couldn't get my blood pressure it was so high and I had a high result for protein in urine. Three hours later I had an emergency C-section and a baby weighing just short of 4 lb. I spent three days in a high-dependency unit and was said to have been an hour away from full-blown eclampsia and seizures. Thankfully it all worked out well in the end!' klolav

Symptoms to look out for include nausea, headaches, swollen hands, feet and face (known as oedema), and strange things happening to your vision. 'I was told to watch out for "fairies" floating in front of my eyes,' says a mother who felt that was a nice change from her usual pink elephants.

Pre-eclampsia is progressive and cannot be 'cured'. The main treatment of pre-eclampsia is the delivery of the baby (and the placenta, which is thought to cause the trouble). If it is early on in the pregnancy, this will obviously put the baby at risk, but continuing the pregnancy can carry risks for both mum and baby. In severe cases, a woman might be admitted to hospital so that she can be carefully monitored to make sure that the problem does not get out of the control and that the baby is growing properly. Sometimes, blood-pressure medication and anti-convulsants may be administered to prevent symptoms from worsening.

'I had pre-eclampsia with my son. He was born at 29 weeks and spent ten weeks in the Special Care Baby Unit. My blood pressure came down during the C-section though and I had no problems afterwards.' abgirl

You may be kept in hospital for a few days after the birth so that you can be monitored and to keep an eye on you in case you develop eclampsia (see p. 246). If you have suffered from pre-eclampsia with one pregnancy, then your risk of having it again is higher, so you will probably be carefully observed as each pregnancy develops.

'I had pre-eclampsia that developed very suddenly and severely. My son was delivered prematurely at 30 weeks – thankfully, all is well with him (he's very nearly two). I had a bleed on my spleen and my blood pressure took some time to stabilise. I was on medications for three months, but all was well after that. I'm now due number two and all is good so far – I'm on daily aspirin and being watched like a hawk, seeing my consultant every two weeks and having my blood pressure measured twice a week. I am feeling positive.' madmumNika

Symptoms of pre-eclampsia

You are more likely to suffer from pre-eclampsia if it is your first pregnancy; you have had a child previously and had pre-eclampsia; you have hypertension or diabetes; you are in your teens or over 40; you have a high body mass index (BMi); it is a multiple pregnancy; your mother or sister had pre-eclampsia; or it has been ten years since your last baby. To find out more, visit Action on Pre-Eclampsia at www.apec.org.uk.

Often, there are no symptoms at all – high blood pressure is called the silent killer for a reason, so make sure you attend your antenatal appointments, particularly in the third trimester. However, you may experience the following:

- hypertension (high blood pressure)
- swelling or oedema (water retention – particularly in hands and face)

- proteinuria (protein in your urine)
- sudden weight gain – if you are crying over a spreadsheet of your weight gain every week, you might notice a sudden gain of more than two pounds a week or six pounds a month; while cakes are a likely culprit, this can also be a symptom of pre-eclampsia, so be aware
- headaches (dull, throbbing migraine-like headaches)
- nausea or vomiting (if onset is sudden)
- changes in vision (flashing lights, auras, blurred vision)
- racing pulse, mental confusion, heightened anxiety, trouble catching your breath
- stomach or right shoulder pain (epigastric pain, possibly under the right-side ribs: similar sensation to heartburn)
- lower-back pain (while back pain is common, it can indicate liver problems)
- hyperreflexia (e.g. if your reflexes are checked, your leg kicks very hard – you are unlikely to notice this yourself unless you have an awful lot of time on your hands)

(List of symptoms from www.preeclampsia.org)

HELLP

A variant of pre-eclampsia is HELLP (Haemolysis, Elevated Liver enzymes and Low Platelet count), which is a group of similar symptoms, particularly right-side pain below the ribs and vomiting and headaches. HELLP syndrome occurs in approximately 3 per cent of pregnant women with pre-eclampsia or eclampsia. 'I had pre-eclampsia in my last pregnancy and was forced to go into hospital every time I had a headache and pain under my ribs,' says a mum who ended up staying in hospital for six weeks. 'HELLP can be very dangerous and it's hard to control, so always be safe and call.'

'At the time I was ill, I don't think I appreciated how sick I was. One thing that really helped me was to get an appointment with my specialist at the hospital to talk about my fears and my prognosis and to clear up any questions I had. I would recommend doing this if you are worried. I'd always sailed through life in good health and getting HELLP really knocked me for six.'

BeachedWhale

Eclampsia

Eclampsia is a severe disorder of pregnancy resulting in eclamptic convulsions (seizures). It occurs in around one in 2000 pregnancies. Eclampsia can result in a coma or a stroke: for this reason it can be fatal for both mum and baby and is treated immediately, usually by the delivery of the baby and the administering of drugs.

'I skipped pre-eclampsia and went straight for the eclamptic seizure while in the third stage of labour. All was going well at the birthing centre, head visible, then the contractions stopped. While the midwife was calling the hospital to have them set up the drip to get them restarted I had an eclamptic seizure, fell off the birthing stool and woke up with a crowd around me in theatre and no idea I'd been pregnant! It all ended well though and our daughter is now a gorgeous, cuddly seven-month-old. Salleroo

Summary

It is easy to become obsessed with your blood pressure and the battle to keep it down. And of course, being told that the most important thing you need to do is 'Relax, Relax, Relax!' is enough to drive anyone to the brink of a breakdown. The main things you can do to ensure good health throughout pregnancy are to follow a good, healthy diet (avoid salt) and get exercise where you can – just a walk in the fresh air is better than nothing.

But don't worry too much if the exercise and healthy-diet regime doesn't quite work out all the time. Lots of us spend our pregnancies sobbing with our heads in a bucket, occasionally sucking on a Haribo and watching awful television. Just do what you can to stay healthy and make sure you go and see a medical professional if you have any concerns.

Group B Streptococcus

You don't have to be pregnant (or even a woman) to carry Group B streptococcus. It is not a sexually transmitted disease: it is one of a host of many strains of bacteria that live inside about 30 per cent of us and usually go about their bacterial business very quietly without causing any trouble.

It is estimated that around a quarter of pregnant women in the UK carry GBS in their vagina and rectum, and during labour and delivery, their babies will come into contact with these bacteria. Most babies born to mothers with GBS are unaffected. But, for some, the consequences are serious: every year, around 700 babies in the UK will develop GBS infection. Of these, about one in ten will die and some will be left with long-term problems.

There are two types of GBS disease in newborns: early- and late-onset. Eighty per cent of GBS disease is early-onset, and occurs in the first six days of life. It is usually diagnosed at birth, and is characterised by the sudden breathing problems that are symptomatic of blood poisoning. Late-onset disease (usually GBS meningitis) can occur after the baby is six days old and any time up to three months (but development after one month is rare). After three months of age, GBS infection is extremely rare.

'When no other risk factors are present, about 1 in every 500 babies born to mothers with a positive test is likely to develop early-onset GBS infection.' NHS Choices information

The NHS does not test for GBS routinely because, given the relatively low risk that most cases carry, a positive test may result in unnecessary stress, and would increase the use of routine antibiotics during labour, which in itself carries risks. However, if you've already had a baby who has suffered from early-onset GBS infection, you may be offered testing and treatment. Sometimes, GBS is picked up in tests that are performed for other reasons. The test usually takes the form of swab samples taken from the vagina and rectum (or both). Some tests are more sensitive than others: the most accurate are available only in private hospitals and clinics.

'I know it is a rare occurrence, but I knew someone who had lost their baby because of GBS, so I wanted to be tested. My GP refused (though I've since heard that some GPs will do the test, so it's worth at least asking), so I went privately. I sent off for a kit, did the swabs myself, sent them back and they phoned with the result. It didn't cost much – about the same as a meal out – was very easy to do and when my results came back negative it was just one less thing to worry about.' Bebee

'I sent off for a private testing kit and the result was positive. Although it was a shock to know I was a carrier of GBS, it meant that I was able to read up on it, discuss my options with my midwife and incorporate it into my birth plan. The birth and my lovely baby boy were fine in the end, I'm glad to say, but I'm still pleased I had the test.' Champagnesupernova

The treatment in high-risk cases is to administer antibiotics during labour. These cannot be given before labour begins, because it is possible that the infection will return. Antibiotic treatment is not recommended for elective or planned Caesareans.

'I had GBS, and although I was very worried about it at the time, I had antibiotics via an IV drip and it honestly didn't make any difference to my labour.' TuttiFrutti

If you have previously delivered a baby who has suffered from a GBS infection, you will be considered high-risk and will probably be offered antibiotics during labour.

'I had GBS in my first pregnancy and it wasn't picked up until after my son was born. He was critically ill and spent two weeks in special care needing help to breathe. It was terrifying. The hospital decided to give me IV antibiotics with my second baby during labour. After seeing my son so ill I would definitely say have them. At the end of the day, a healthy baby is all any mother wants.' Rowangirl

If you carried GBS during a previous pregnancy, but your baby did *not* develop a GBS infection, then antibiotic treatment during labour is not usually recommended. If GBS has been detected during your pregnancy, either through urine testing or vaginal or rectal swabs, then your midwife or consultant will discuss the possibility of treatment during labour. The case for taking antibiotics is stronger if any of the following additional factors come into play: if you have a high temperature in labour; if you go into labour before 37 weeks; or if your waters break more than 18 hours before you give birth. In these cases, your healthcare professional should discuss with you the option of antibiotic treatment during labour (you should put the book down and listen at this point).

Most babies born to mothers who carry GBS are born healthy and will not need any special care or treatment. Newborn babies may be 'colonised' with GBS without having a GBS infection. If it is suspected that a baby has a GBS infection, blood samples may be tested.

If you have GBS you may be advised to stay in hospital after the delivery for a 24–48-hour observation period, although not everyone does: 'I was happy that my baby was OK, so went home 14 hours after her birth. My swabs came back that my daughter was positive with GBS, but she didn't show any signs of illness so the doctors weren't worried.'

Placenta Praevia

Placenta praevia (or low-lying placenta) may be a cause of bleeding in the third trimester. The problem with a low-lying placenta is that it can lie over all or part of the cervix, preventing the baby from being born vaginally and causing bleeding. A low-lying placenta may be spotted on a scan earlier than 20 weeks, will normally "move up" as the uterus grows: only 1 in 10 women with a low-lying placenta will go on to have placenta praevia.

Placenta praevia after 20 weeks can be dangerous due to the risk of haemorrhage. If diagnosed, you should be given lots of clear advice about how to look after yourself which may include things such as eating a wholesome iron-rich diet and avoiding sex (either wholesome or unwholesome). Depending on the position of the placenta, you may need a Caesarean section to deliver the baby and to control bleeding. Either way, you will require a bit more medical care and may need to be close to a hospital where you can get urgent treatment if you start to bleed suddenly.

'My placenta was low-lying at 34 weeks, but at 36 weeks it had moved out of the way and we had a lovely home birth two weeks ago. If it hadn't moved, they would have booked an elective C-section for around 38 weeks, which wouldn't have been so bad. I prepared myself for both eventualities – wrote two birth plans, etc. – which made me feel better.' *RunJHC*

Restless Leg Syndrome

Restless leg syndrome is a cruel trick of pregnancy. It usually creeps up in the third trimester when all that the top half of your body wants to do is rest, rest, rest. Evenings are the worst, when your legs start to feel as jittery as a tap dancer with an espresso habit. It's as if they think it might be fun to sling on some heels and go clubbing. Did no one tell them you are a Teletubby who just wants to flop in front of *EastEnders* with a ready meal?

'It feels as though a colony of ants is crawling up my legs. It's unbearable. I want to chop them off,' laments one mum.

Around 15 per cent of pregnant women suffer from restless leg syndrome (RLS), aka disco legs. Nobody knows why, although it is thought to be linked to poor circulation. It usually kicks in just as you settle down for an evening in front of the telly. There are drugs for RLS but – no surprises here – none that can be taken during pregnancy. In the meantime, there are things you can try to relieve the itchiness and feeling of pins and needles.

Things you can try

For starters, have your iron levels checked because iron deficiency can make RLS worse. Avoid becoming dehydrated as this impairs circulation. Make sure you are getting enough calcium in the form of cheese, yoghurt or milk and potassium and magnesium from bananas, or a supplement. An odd one, this: make your new nightcap a gin and tonic, but without the gin, as the quinine in tonic water may help (allegedly). 'It doesn't cure it, but it does help somewhat,' claims one sufferer. (Note: check the ingredients first to make sure that it contains quinine and is not just a soup of jolly chemicals from a physics lab.)

'I suffered from RLS from the moment I peed on the stick. I tried everything and often ended up walking around the garden in my bare feet to cool them and stop the restlessness. I also have a small fan at the end of my bed directed on to my legs and feet.' miniandme

In addition to all of the above:

- avoid caffeine, tobacco and alcohol (if you aren't already doing so), which act as stimulants
- take regular, daily exercise (not near bedtime though or that might make things worse)
- get up and go to bed at roughly the same time each day
- take time to relax before bed: a bath and a book are helpful
- stretch and massage your legs, or apply hot or cold compresses to your leg muscles.

'Help! I'm so tired. My feet won't go to sleep when I want to. I've spent my second sleepless night watching the clock tick round. I got up four times to move around, which helped, but all I want to do is sleep. How long before my feet stop dancing?' erinsmom

> If your varicose veins and elasticated trousers aren't enough to make you feel as though you are turning into your granny, RLS will: a pair of support stockings to complete the look might just stop the tingliness. Other Mumsnetter tips include putting your feet up when you can and wrapping your legs in cold flannels while watching television. Or you can try giving them a blast of cold water from the shower last thing at night to stimulate the blood flow. A few gentle stretches and light leg exercises before going to bed, or even in bed, should also help. But be warned: 'My husband used to wonder what was going on when he woke up to find my legs in the air,' confides a Mumsnetter. If that unsettles him as much as your spaghetti legs in bed, get him to give them a nightly massage. And try sleeping with your feet raised on a pillow.

'Last night I tried tonic water, a banana and bathing and massaging my legs in cold water with exfoliating gloves. Slept like a baby – no sign of restless legs! The only thing is I don't know which one helped, therefore I've got to repeat the whole process every evening before bedtime. Plus, I've got to have Gaviscon after the tonic water...' Celou

> The good news is that RLS should disappear just as fast as it arrived, usually within a few weeks of the birth.

Carpal Tunnel Syndrome (How Many More Pregnancy Syndromes Can There Be?)

The carpal tunnel is a small 'tunnel' that runs from the bottom of your wrist to your palm, through which several tendons and a nerve (responsible for movement and sensation in your hand) pass. When the space inside the carpal tunnel is reduced, the nerve is compressed and this causes feelings of pain and pins and needles (or numbness).

CTS may occur more frequently during pregnancy due to fluid retention in the wrist putting extra pressure on the carpal tunnel. Basically, your carpal tunnel is getting fat like the rest of you. The pain tends to be worse at night, making it hard to sleep. Because steroid injections or surgery aren't options during pregnancy, it's a case of finding whatever ways you can of relieving the pain, at least until after you give birth.

If you are suffering from CTS, you might experience pains shooting up your arm from your wrist and a burning sensation in your fingertips. Your hands will probably feel as though they have a life of their own. You might find it hard to grip things (so be careful when you're picking up your skinny latte), and you'll probably start moaning about the pains in your wrists and realising that this is just a foretaste of the life of an old lady.

'I can't believe how quickly it came on and got worse,' says one sufferer. 'I remember spilling red wine down myself because the pain came on so suddenly. People thought I was drunk.'

'I suffered with CTS from about week 33 with my first daughter. It was awful. My thumbs and first two fingers were completely numb, and felt all pins-and-needly. I got some splints but they didn't help at all. Shaking them a lot every few minutes relieved it a bit. I went to see a physiotherapist and an osteopath, and while neither stopped the symptoms they were able to suggest some stretching exercises. It did disappear but took its time – around ten to 12 weeks post-birth. Another one of the joys of pregnancy!' Jaysecond

If you are feeling pain in your hands or wrists, ask your GP or physiotherapist for advice (your GP can refer you to a physiotherapist, although in some places the waiting lists are rather longer than the time it will take for the baby to arrive). The first course of action is usually to try wearing splints on your wrists. Some people find that these help to ease the pain by reducing movement in the wrist. You may be advised to wear them through the night. They generally look like sturdy, hard-wearing fingerless gloves, rather than long wooden sticks wrapped in linen bandages.

'I was fine during the day but in agony during the night. I went to the GP who was unhelpful and said it would go after I had my baby (which it did but that didn't help much with months to go). So I bought a couple of wrist supports on eBay and they helped a great deal.' Haylstones

Some people swear by certain exercises or other rituals – 'hanging my hands down the side of the bed when I'm asleep'; 'clenching and unclenching my fists'; 'resting my hands in warm water' – as well as alternative therapies such as acupuncture.

'In the morning, when it is worse, I have found it is good to put a frozen wine cooler sleeve on my arm. It looks stupid, but feels lovely.' peachygirl

Sometimes a break from repetitive tasks can help. For example, if you are tapping away on Mumsnet for 12 hours a day, you might find that a few days spent watching television instead gives you some relief from the symptoms. Some people find that mouse 'wrist rests' help, although experts are dubious as to whether these really work.

The good news is that in most cases, the symptoms disappear within a few months of the birth and, in some, immediately after delivery. Post-baby you can take drastic action if necessary (such as medication or even surgery) but, for now, limit anything that causes strain on your wrists – carrying shopping, driving without power steering, peeling potatoes. You will soon have to be busy fiddling with nappies, so rest those wrists now, while you can.

Gestational Diabetes

Diabetes occurs when there is too much sugar in the blood, as a result of insufficient insulin (the hormone made by the pancreas that normally breaks down sugar). Gestational diabetes is diabetes that is first diagnosed during pregnancy in a woman who has not previously been diagnosed with the condition. During pregnancy, various hormones prevent insulin from working as it usually does, so your body needs to produce more of it to ensure that the baby gets enough glucose. If the pancreas fails to come up with the goods, blood-sugar levels shoot up. Gestational diabetes tends to occur from around week 24 of pregnancy.

If you have gestational diabetes, you are at a higher risk of developing pre-eclampsia (see p. 242). Your baby is in danger of putting on too much weight too soon (macrosomia), which could result in him being too large for a vaginal delivery, which in turn means he may need to be induced early. Your baby may also have low blood sugar (hypoglycaemia) after the birth, and there is an increased risk that he will be born with breathing problems and a slightly higher chance of stillbirth – although this is rare when the condition is diagnosed and carefully managed.

Gestational diabetes can sound terrifying, but be reassured: it is a common health problem during pregnancy and it can be successfully managed.

You are more likely to get gestational diabetes if you're overweight, older, or have a family history of Type 2 diabetes. The odds are also greater if you have had two or more pregnancies or if you've had a large baby in the past (over 10 pounds). You are also at risk if you have been diagnosed with gestational diabetes in a previous pregnancy.

Women with gestational diabetes don't normally experience any symptoms, but if any do occur they include tiredness, thirst and frequent urination. In other words, lots of the things you'd expect in a normal pregnancy. Many women only discover they have gestational diabetes after a routine urine test. Looking back, one mum says: 'I've been madly thirsty and kept waking in the night to go to the loo, so I had an inkling all wasn't quite as it should be, but I thought it was just the pregnancy.'

Your midwife will test your urine for sugar at your antenatal appointments, and refer you for further testing if any of these tests gives positive results. Women who are in a high-risk group will automatically be referred for testing. You may first be referred for a blood test, and then for an 'oral glucose tolerance test', which is done between 24 and 28 weeks (women with previous history of gestational diabetes may be offered this earlier). You will need to fast overnight and will then be given a sugary drink; blood samples will be taken over a two-hour period to assess the levels of glucose in your blood. Urine samples will also be taken.

If you do test positive for gestational diabetes, you should be given lots of information about how to manage it, but don't be afraid to ask questions. In most cases, gestational diabetes can be managed with regular exercise and a balanced diet, which means it's out with the Mars bars and in with fruit, veg and complex carbohydrates, all in careful measure. Knowing that if you continue to give in to the sweet stuff you are likely to give birth to a big baby should be a huge motivating factor. But it can still be a challenge.

'I have the oatcakes in the cupboard. They're a bit like cardboard, unless you spread half a pound of Philly on the top, which kind of defeats the whole object. I'm just trying to fill up on water and chant to myself "not hungry, not hungry", as I loiter around the fridge door looking idly inside for morsels. I'm going to get a "fridge tan" if I linger much more.' johnworf

You will have to regularly check your glucose levels with a finger-prick test which isn't painful, but can be disheartening: 'Doing the prick tests felt like failing something four times a day.' It might be a good idea to invest in a couple of good diabetic cookbooks to inspire some diversity in what might otherwise be a boring diet. As well as keeping your sugar levels in check, you might also find yourself losing weight, which is not to be sniffed at, given that most pregnant women double in size. 'I lost half a stone in the fortnight following my diagnosis, so it's not all negative,' chirps a reformed junk-food addict.

For between 10 and 20 per cent of women with gestational diabetes, diet and exercise are not enough to control the diabetes, and they will need medication for the remainder of their pregnancy – either in the form of tablets or injections of insulin. Again, it isn't as bad as it sounds. 'After the initial shock of being told I had to give myself insulin, I was fine – and I'm scared stiff of needles,' reassures one Mumsnetter. Another says: 'I know the prospect of insulin is awful, but honestly, the blood tests hurt more than the injections.' Some people find them 'totally painless'.

'I had diabetes with my second pregnancy which developed at 27 weeks. I was shocked, as I felt fine. I tried to control it by watching my diet and taking my blood-sugar readings every four hours. I lost weight, but my levels still rose! I ended up injecting insulin four times a day for the rest of my pregnancy which was strange to begin with and sometimes made me feel quite ill as the amount I was injecting was increased on a daily basis. I got used to it though and was induced at 37 weeks. My son was born weighing 9lb 3oz. My sugar levels returned to normal within an hour of delivery and I had my long-awaited Mars bar!' Happyslappy

C-section rates are often higher among women with gestational diabetes because their babies tend to be larger, but chances are that if the condition is diagnosed and controlled, you are unlikely to give birth to a bumper baby. A home or water birth will be ruled out because you might need insulin during labour, but plenty of women with gestational diabetes go on to have a full-term vaginal delivery.

When she is born, your baby may have low blood sugar, which can be fixed by breast milk or formula. Sometimes babies are given a sugar solution through a drip and will also be checked for jaundice. Six weeks after delivery, you should have a follow-up test to ensure that your blood-sugar levels are back to normal. Be aware that gestational diabetes is likely to return in future pregnancies. And some studies have shown that there is a 30 per cent chance that if you have had it during pregnancy, you will develop Type 2 diabetes in later life. But as long as you know that it is something to look out for, you can be reassured that it is something that can be dealt with.

THE BIRTH

The Labour Party – How Do You Know When It's Started, When Should You Head to Hospital and What's It Really Like?

This is it. The moment you have been waiting for. But hang on. Are you sure? How do you know if this is the real deal and not a false alarm? Maybe you are incontinent? Perhaps it is only Braxton Hicks?

One question that pops up time and again on the Mumsnet childbirth talkboard is: 'Am I in labour?' One thing's for sure: if you're able to type eloquently, the chances are that you're probably not in established labour (although there have been some notable exceptions). It is an easy call to get wrong though.

'I was in the cinema when I started to feel what I thought were mild contractions. The film had just started, but I dragged my husband out. He went marching up to tell the woman at the ticket desk, rather dramatically, and proudly, that I was about to give birth, then demanded our money back. I was mortified to have to walk past the cinema two days later, still pregnant. On the day I did give birth, we had one false start to the hospital, and were sent home. Second time around, we left it so late, I almost gave birth on the hospital steps.' custardtart

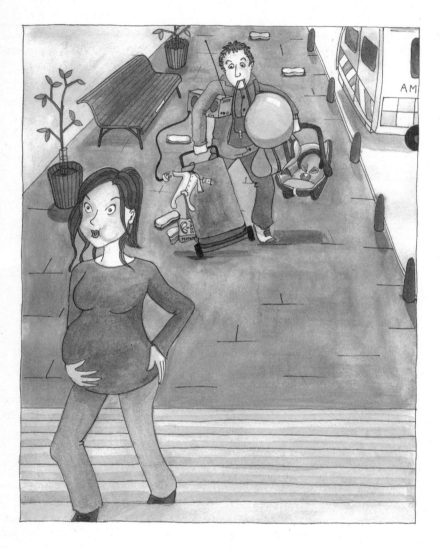

Braxton Hicks – Mother Nature's joke on mums-to-be

Many a red-faced mum-to-be has been turned away from the delivery ward thanks to Braxton Hicks (BH) contractions. These are irregular, usually painless uterine contractions that tend to occur from around the middle of your pregnancy (although they can start much earlier) and increase in frequency as you approach your due date. Essentially, they're the effects of the muscles of your womb contracting – typically for between 30 and 60 seconds at a time, but sometimes for up to two minutes or so. That's not to say that everyone feels them, and there's no need to worry if you don't.

'Mine are never painful but often extremely uncomfortable; it feels like someone has taken a sheet and wrapped it around your waist and is pulling it tight behind you. They often make me a bit breathless and can have me pacing the floor for hours. But I've never mistaken them for labour as they are never painful in the way contractions are.' Pinktulips

Experts are divided as to the purpose of BH contractions. One theory is that they help to tone the uterine muscle and promote blood flow to the placenta; another that they help soften the cervix in preparation for labour. Also known as 'practice contractions', you can use them to practise your breathing exercises. But BH differ from the real thing in that they're irregular in intensity and frequency, and their timing is unpredictable and non-rhythmic. They tend to turn up, do their erratic thing and taper off. Plus, they're usually more uncomfortable than painful. In contrast, real contractions increase in regularity, intensity and length as labour progresses, and become more and more painful.

'If you aren't sure whether they're Braxton Hicks or the real thing, have a bath or go to sleep.

Usually, if they're real contractions, neither of these things will ease them and you won't be able to sleep through them!' Ewe

While not as painful as true labour, BH can still be unpleasant. Common triggers include being active, someone touching your bump, having a full bladder, being dehydrated, or sex. 'I only ever really had them immediately after an orgasm,' one Mumsnetter confesses. Stopping what you are doing can often help; if you are lying down get up, or, conversely, if you're walking around stop and put your feet up. Equally, practising your breathing exercises (see p. 318), a warm bath and drinking a glass of water can also calm them down. If you are at all concerned, contact your doctor or midwife.

Welcome to the labour party – what to look out for

All of the following are good signs that labour is under way; if you experience any of them more than two weeks before your due date, call your midwife straight away for advice:

- Waters breaking
- Diarrhoea – this may be an early sign that things are hotting up
- Loss of mucus plug – look for a snotty, jelly-like blob or a red or brownish vaginal discharge
- Contractions – regularly spaced contractions that feel more intense than Braxton Hicks
- Lower-back pain or cramping
- Heaviness in your pelvis and the urge to push (ooops, too late)

Waters breaking: bursting your bubble

Mother Nature will give you a heads up when you are in labour, but some signs are more dramatic than others, and they don't always come in text-book order. Like everything in pregnancy, everybody's experience is different. Your waters breaking is the big Hollywood experience of labour starting (usually on the big screen it conveniently occurs about ten minutes before the baby's head appears). But despite what the movies may have you believe, fewer than 15 per cent of women start their labour this way.

'I was beginning to wonder if I should start avoiding sitting on people's sofas, but with both children my waters didn't go until I was seriously far along with the contractions. With my first, they burst open all over the hospital floor (my husband and I apologised profusely and offered to help clean up). With my second, they exploded all over the room and the midwife on my second push, but we didn't have time to even contemplate cleaning up because our daughter was out with the fifth push.' Snowstorm

The 'waters breaking' is the bursting of the amniotic sac surrounding the baby, which can happen before or after your contractions start. The water will either trickle down your leg or shoot out like a fire hose. A trickle can be disconcerting because it can feel like you have peed yourself, and you might mistake it for just the start of another fun day of female incontinence. If possible, it's important to note the colour because a brown or greenish hue could mean that your baby has opened his bowels and is in danger of being distressed.

'My waters sprung a leak in the early hours one night. I actually thought I'd wet myself and resolved to do my pelvic floors more conscientiously! A few sanitary towels later and it was time to call the midwife ...' wasabipeanut

If your contractions don't start naturally within 24 to 48 hours of you flooding the place, you may need to be induced to avoid infection. So, if you think your waters have broken, call your midwife who will advise you what to do next. Sometimes your midwife will break the membrane for you (see ARM on p. 339).

Meconium in waters – what this means

Meconium, put simply, is your baby's earliest poo. It's sticky, like tar, and normally isn't expelled until your baby is out in the big world. It lasts for a few days and will make you want to hug the person who invented baby wipes.

Sometimes, however, your baby has a bowel movement while still in the womb. This could mean that your baby is, or has been, in distress, or that his gut has reached maturity, which explains why this is more likely to happen if you are overdue. Passing of meconium while still in the womb occurs with around 12 per cent of babies, although the rate increases with the length of pregnancy. So, at 40 weeks the rate is around 30 per cent and at 42 weeks it is around 50 per cent.

Meconium in the waters increases the risk of infection during labour and delivery. But the big worry with passing of meconium is the risk of meconium aspiration syndrome (MAS). MAS occurs when meconium is inhaled by the baby and becomes trapped in the air passages, making it difficult for him to breathe. The real danger is that it can be inhaled into the lungs. Not all babies who pass meconium develop MAS – only about 10 per cent will be affected.

A sign that meconium has passed is that when your waters break, the amniotic fluid is coloured rather than clear; it will be green if it has happened recently and brownish-gold if it is older. This is why it's important to tell your doctor straight away if your waters are discoloured. If you were planning a home birth, you will generally be advised to transfer to hospital if your waters are discoloured.

The thicker the meconium and the lower the level of amniotic fluid, the more risky the situation. The baby's heart rate will also indicate whether she is still in distress. If your baby is born struggling to breathe, a tube is inserted into her mouth or

(continued)

nose to suction out the airways. Babies with MAS are likely to need special care, but the majority recover within a matter of days. 'My son was whipped down to the Special Care Baby Unit and he was hooked up to monitors. Five hours later he'd pulled out his drip and was screaming the place down. I had a phone call from the ward to go and retrieve him as his lungs had obviously recovered!' *worzella*

Losing your mucus plug – or, let's get this 'show' on the road!

Another sign that things are starting to happen is a 'show'. No, not the high-kicking chorus-line type (interrogate your partner if one of these appears) but your mucus plug coming away. This is a globule of mucus from the cervix that 'seals' your womb during pregnancy. It may look like a blob of jelly: 'It actually reminded me of a raw scallop!' remembers one mum; or it may appear as a pinkish-red or brownish vaginal discharge: 'I had a brown sticky discharge but no jelly plug,' recalls another. Although it doesn't mean the baby's arrival is imminent, it is an indication that the end (of the waiting) is nigh.

'The mucus plug is usually a clump of snot-like mucus, often blood-stained. You do get increased discharge in later pregnancy, but the "show" is often a big lump. It means your cervix is starting to thin and dilate, so is a positive sign, although labour could still be a few days away, so it's hard to predict.' Lulumama

So when *can* I go to the bloody hospital?

It's a good idea to ring your labour ward when you are pretty sure that labour has begun, so that they are prepared for your arrival in due course. They prefer a warning phone call that you are coming, rather than having you turning up unexpectedly and demanding that you see the anaesthetist *right now*. And some hospitals like to keep in touch with you and may ring you every now and then to see how you are getting on.

A very rough rule of thumb that lots of hospitals use is that you should go to the hospital when your contractions are five to seven minutes apart and lasting for one minute each time. Alternatively, if your waters have broken, they might want to admit you, regardless of whether or not you are having contractions. And, of course, if you are in too much pain to manage at home, you should give them a ring and let them know that you are coming in. If you're in too much pain to manage a phone conversation, you should definitely be off the phone and heading in.

Plenty of women turn up to the hospital only to be told to go home and labour for longer. 'Mine was a three-day labour and I was in and out of hospital like a yo-yo,' recalls one mum. 'Being turned away from hospital felt like failing an exam,' says someone who was turned away twice. It can be hard picking up your bags and heading home, but any embarrassment you might feel will quickly be forgotten in the grand scheme of things, i.e. when you have flashed your fanjo in front of half of the hospital staff.

'The time at which you should go to hospital depends on how far away you live. If it doesn't take too long to get there, I would suggest waiting till the contractions are regular – about ten minutes apart and painful. You might feel regular contractions, but not experience any discomfort: try and ignore them. As your contractions get stronger, they will make you stop what you are doing so you can breathe through them. If you have any bleeding, with or without contractions, you should go in. If your waters break, with no contractions, most hospitals advise you to go in. Many women go in with false alarms but that is not a problem. That said, it is better to avoid going in *too* early if you can – pottering about at home is much better.' (Mumsnetter midwife) mears

> There is nothing wrong with erring on the side of caution, so don't worry about going in too soon if you are concerned or in a lot of pain. Hospitals are used to false alarms and it gives them a chance to check your progress and to make sure that you are down on their list of people to expect shortly.
>
> It is also possible that you may labour quite fast and deliver quite quickly – so don't wait around at home if you have a gut feeling that things are moving along. 'My son arrived safely but was nearly born into my pants,' remembers one mum whose midwife didn't think she was in established labour. 'What I shouted to my husband will always be ingrained in my mind: "GET MY KNICKERS OFF!"'

'My midwife believed I was in labour, but wouldn't believe that I was giving birth! I said, "I think I can feel something," and she said, "Don't be silly, you were only two centimetres an hour and a half ago. Try to get some rest." I said, "No, really …" and another midwife finally looked and said: "The head is out! Don't push! Don't push!" Silly cow: it was my second, I did *vaguely* know what giving birth felt like.' princesspeahead

> Most first labours are quite long though, so try to labour at home for as long as you feel it is sensible. You can use the bath, lean on your bed or pad around on a soft carpet – at least if it is your own you are more likely to know what furniture will take your weight and you are less likely to end up with a verruca.

'The best thing you can do is not to worry about it. The signs vary so much from woman to woman (and pregnancy to pregnancy) that it's hard to follow anyone else's guidelines. First time around, I waited to go in until I was having contractions three to five minutes apart and was in screaming pain, but I didn't have the baby for another 30 hours. Second time around, I had the baby several hours after my contractions were three to five minutes apart. My neighbour had her first baby two and a half hours after she felt her very first contraction. They never got to the point where they took her breath away and she almost didn't get to the hospital in time. None of this is meant to scare you. Just to say to go to the hospital when you find that you are no longer comfortable (mentally as well as physically) with being at home.' SofiaAmes

Foetal monitoring

Although you (and your baby) are the centre of attention during labour, it can sometimes feel that you are at the end of the line when it comes to finding out the finer details of what is actually going on. Monitoring won't give your medical team all the answers they need – but it will give them some idea of what's going on in terms of your contractions and your baby's heartbeat. The last thing you want is to be poked and prodded like a car being put through its MOT – so make sure that you are aware of the different options available and the pros and cons of each.

Foetal monitoring generally falls into three categories:

1. Intermittent monitoring
2. Continuous foetal monitoring
3. Foetal scalp electrode monitoring

1. *Intermittent monitoring*

If all seems well, the only interference should be a midwife who monitors your baby's heartbeat at regular intervals using a Pinard stethoscope or a Sonicaid to keep a check on how the baby is coping. (There is a waterproof version for water birthers.) In the first stage of labour this usually happens every 15 minutes, then every five minutes in the second stage of labour, or after each contraction. 'My husband and I were more or less left alone in the labour room during the early stages, which was lovely,' writes one mum. 'The midwife popped in every 15 minutes to have a little listen to my belly with the Sonicaid. It was all very calm and peaceful.'

2. *Continuous foetal monitoring (CFM)*

If you fall into the high-risk category – if you have diabetes or pre-eclampsia, for example – it is recommended that you be continuously monitored throughout your labour using a cardiotocograph (CTG) to flag up any signs that the baby is in distress (sometimes also referred to as EFM, electronic foetal monitoring). Other reasons for electronic foetal monitoring (EFM) might be: if your pregnancy is 41 weeks plus, or less than 37 weeks; it is a multiple pregnancy; you have had a previous Caesarean; you are having an epidural; you have been induced; your baby is measuring small; it has passed meconium; it's breech; you have bled during labour; you have a high temperature; or if you have been in established labour for a long time.

If you are to be continuously monitored, then two electronic sensors – to record your contractions and your baby's heartbeat – are placed on your abdomen, usually held in place using elasticated straps (if they feel uncomfortable or too tight, let the midwife know). If possible, get into a seated position because lying down for too long can get uncomfortable and is the worst position for labouring. You may well be able to get on your feet, but being hooked up to a machine can be restricting: you won't be able to move far or have a bath.   *(continued)*

Although it used to be fairly routine, CFM is no longer recommended for low-risk pregnancies because being immobile is likely to lead to more interventions. If you do have to have CFM, discuss this with your midwife and ask whether there are ways around the lack of mobility.

'With my daughter they wanted to monitor me, but I wanted to keep moving. Fortunately, they managed to strap the monitor on while I was standing. We did lose the trace a few times, but I was able to move about a bit. I was mainly standing at the end of the bed gripping the railings during contractions.' *misdee*

3. *Foetal scalp electrode monitoring*
If your baby's heartbeat gives cause for concern, it may be recommended that a foetal scalp electrode (FSE) be clipped to his head to get a more accurate reading. This can be fairly uncomfortable for you and may also result in a little sore patch on your baby's head. In some cases, a foetal blood sample (FBS) is taken from the baby's scalp to measure the amount of oxygen in its blood. This is done by inserting a needle up your vagina and is usually more uncomfortable than painful. Low levels of oxygen may mean that they suggest you deliver promptly by Caesarean section.

'I pushed for intermittent monitoring and they were happy to do this. However, I did end up having a scalp clip attached to the baby's head as there was a problem with his heart rate dipping. But, as my waters had already broken and my pelvic pain had rendered me pretty immobile, I felt it wasn't going against my birth plan, but was rather a change in plan due to circumstances.' *LeakyDAISYcal*

Continuous monitoring – yes or no?
The Active Birth movement over the last few decades have taught us that we need to 'stand and deliver' and stay upright and moving throughout labour and birth. Keeping active is the best route to a safe and speedy delivery with as little intervention as possible. But once you are pinned to a bed with foetal monitoring straps, your hopes of an active birth go out the window, and the chances of you needing further interventions increase.

If you are healthy, have had a problem-free pregnancy and there are no indications of any problems, there is no reason why you shouldn't be left to get on with the job at hand. In the end, it is your call whether you have continuous monitoring. It is worth talking it through with your doctor or midwife until you feel comfortable with your decision. 'I put in my birth plan that I didn't want to have the belt monitor thing. I made it clear that I wanted to be as active as possible. When we got to the hospital the midwife used the belt monitor on me just to check I was fully in labour, but after that, she just used the hand-held one.' *Littlefish*

If you feel that you are pressured to have continuous foetal monitoring and can see the midwife looming with the elastic straps, then ask questions until you are sure that you understand their reasons. If there are better options, ask for them. 'My midwife said, "We are going to monitor you now," and started preparing the monitors,' writes one mum. 'I asked whether I could have intermittent monitoring instead and she just said, "Oh yes, that's fine!" Job done!'

Ever heard about Dante's nine circles of hell? Well, the good news is that there are only three stages of labour. But the bad news is that there is much more fun to be had in hell.

The first stage of labour

This is when your cervix – the neck of your womb – dilates to a rather incredible 10cm, so that your baby can squeeze its way out. It all sounds nice and easy when put like that, but this dilation occurs as a result of a process in which the womb contracts over and over again, which, as you know, is jolly uncomfortable. It can also take a wee while – typically, at least 12 hours in a first pregnancy (although it can be much longer).

This initial stage can be divided into three separate parts:

- the early phase
- the active phase
- the transition phase.

Phase 1, or the early phase of labour – also known as the latent period or pre-labour – is the very start of labour when your contractions begin, eventually causing your cervix to fully efface (or flatten) and dilate to 3–4cm in width. Typically, contractions during the early phase are mild to moderate and you can talk through them. They last about 30 to 40 seconds and are irregular, coming at anything from 5 to 20 minutes apart; they might even stop for a while. Contractions can be erratic for several days before things start in earnest. Some poor souls experience full-on contractions during the early stages, even though – particularly with first babies – there may be very little actual dilation action. On average, for first-time mothers the early phase lasts from six to eight hours, but everyone is different and timings vary wildly. It can be completely exhausting and demoralising to be in what feels like full-blown labour for days and still only be 1cm dilated. Call your midwife if you've any concerns, but try not to get too stressed: these aren't wasted contractions; they're preparing your cervix for established, active labour. And rest assured that if you dash to the hospital only to be sent home for being too hasty, you won't be the first.

'During the early phase I had very short contractions, four minutes apart for 16 hours, and got sent home from the labour ward as I was only 2cm dilated!' TotalChaos

Cervical effacement and dilation

The whole purpose of contractions is to get your cervix to efface and dilate. As you go through labour, midwives may occasionally have a rummage up there and decide how close you are to your final destination, i.e. fully effaced and 10cm dilated. Once you've reached that point, you are ready for the pushing stage, where you can push the baby out (and after the tedium of contractions, that part can almost seem fun!).

Effacement
Before labour, your cervix is like a long, firm, closed tube. As labour approaches, it softens and changes in shape to become

shorter and flatter. The contractions of the first phase of labour cause your newly softened cervix to become paper thin and drawn up into the uterus, ending up in a ring rather than tube shape, in a process known as effacement. Imagine rolling down a turtleneck jumper before pulling the neck apart so that you can shove your head through – that's effacement! It's measured in percentages, but getting from 0 per cent (not effaced at all) to 100 per cent (completely effaced and thin), can take anything from minutes to days. When your cervix is 100 per cent effaced, it is effectively just part of the wall of your uterus, and can start to dilate in order for the baby to pass through.

Dilation

Dilation is easier to understand; it refers to how wide the opening of your cervix is and is measured in centimetres. Until the third trimester, your cervix should be clamped tightly shut – in other words, 0cm dilated. The contractions of labour enable the cervix to open up, until it is 10cm in width. This is (allegedly) large enough for the baby's head to pass through – so reaching this magic number indicates that the first stage of labour is finishing, and the second stage – the birth itself – is beginning.

Things to do during the early phase

- Relax – do whatever makes you more comfortable, whether that's a warm bath or pacing around the sitting room.
- Rest – you're going to need your energy in the hours to come.
- Nibble – snack on light, low-GI snacks such as wholegrain toast or cereal, pasta, rice, dried fruit, etc., which are best for slow-release energy.
- TENS machine (see p. 307) – if you've hired one for pain relief, get wired up and whack it on now because it takes about an hour for your body to start releasing endorphins in response to the machine's electrical responses.
- Time your contractions – you don't need to sit there with a stopwatch, but it's good to have a rough idea of how you

(continued)

are progressing. If you're having a hospital birth and your contractions are coming every five minutes or so (seven if this isn't your first baby) and lasting 30 seconds or more, it's time to think about heading off.

- Check your hospital bag and pack snacks and drinks; make sure your mobile is charged.
- Ring your birth partner if they're not yet with you.
- Ring your mum so she can start getting hysterical.

Labouring with SPD (Symphysis Pubis Dysfunction, see p. 78)

(Symphysis Pubis Dysfunction, see p. 78)

If SPD has made your pregnancy a misery, then the prospect of labour can be pretty daunting, especially if you're heading into it on crutches or in a wheelchair.

Here's one Mumsnetter's SPD checklist:
'In labour:

- Don't let anyone put your legs in stirrups without first measuring how far you can open your knees painlessly.
- Don't let anyone hold your legs back to push.
- Try to stay upright or in water, as this alleviates some of the pressure.
- Wiggle your hips if your labour pains are in your back, but don't over-sway.
- Put "SPD sufferer" in your birth plan so your midwives are aware.' *hertsnessex*

If you're planning on an epidural – and let's face it, if you've been in pain for weeks or months, numbness might seem preferable – make sure those managing your labour are aware of your condition:

'Epidurals with SPD can cause permanent damage if not managed properly because you're not aware of the pelvic pain and so open your legs "too" wide, if that makes sense. So it's vital that the staff present know you have SPD and check how far you can open your legs before you have the epidural.' *Mcmudda*

Phase 2, or the active phase of labour – also called established labour is, in medical terms, when you're fully effaced (see p. 272) and about 3–4cm dilated. Typically, it lasts around six to seven hours if it's your first labour, and finishes when you're about 8cm dilated. Once active labour begins, contractions usually increase in frequency, length and intensity as the uterus revs up its efforts to open your cervix. If you have opted for no pain relief, they'll soon be too strong for you to talk through –although, strangely, you may be able to moo!

'The early phase was like wind, but stopping and starting – I laughed through contractions. But the active phase hurt a lot. I had a home birth and nothing helped. I got in the bath and out again – nothing was really of any use.' FlightAttendant

Once you're in really active labour, contractions will be coming every couple of minutes and will last around a minute each. But everyone's different, so don't get stressed if your labour is moving at a slower pace. The strength of your contractions and the position of both you and your baby have a big impact on how fast things will happen. That said, if your waters haven't already broken by this point and your labour's progressing slowly, your midwife might suggest she break them with an amniotic hook (which looks a bit like a crochet needle). It may be uncomfortable, but it shouldn't hurt. It's called an artificial rupture of membranes (ARM – see p. 339) and you will also have to have it done if your baby needs foetal scalp electrode monitoring (a tiny monitor attached to his head, see p. 270).

'I had my daughter at home, with a birthing pool. Labour was quick to establish and progressed nicely ... but the pool was so relaxing, everyone so helpful and the gas and air so effective that everything slowed down when I got to about 8cm. I demanded my waters be broken, jumped back in the pool and instantly got back to work. Stage one of labour took five hours but stage two comprised just two contractions and then my daughter was born, fit and well!'

Missingtheaction

The Escalation of Intervention (the slippery but sometimes splendid slope of drug use)

Whether or not you will need pain relief during labour is something that is impossible to determine before your contractions start to kick in. But reading up on the different methods will help you to appreciate some of the pros and cons of what is on offer: for example, how long it takes before they start working, how much you will be able to move, the extent to which you will remain lucid (or not), whether your labour will be prolonged and the after effects on you and your baby.

Pain relief comes with its own risks. If you are induced or have an epidural you are statistically more likely to have a ventouse or forceps delivery. Referred to as the Escalation of Intervention, it's the domino effect that occurs when you start to meddle with Mother Nature. However, on the other hand, there are also countless cases when pain relief is the best present a woman could ever receive, going way beyond what any man with a cold flannel could do (even George Clooney).

Ultimately, it's your choice. But before making a decision, you may want to be examined so that you know how dilated you are – you may be further along than you think. If you are having an epidural and you want it to have worn off for the second stage of labour, tell your medical team. The more informed your decision the less likely you are to have regrets. And your partner in the labour room needs to be on the ball too (just not the birthing ball).

Things to do during the active phase

- If you're having a hospital birth – go in once you're having regular contractions (usually every five to seven minutes for a first birth) or as advised by your midwife or if you want some pain relief.
- Try different positions – even if you never manage to get into a comfortable one, moving around to find one will help.
- Stay upright if possible – mobilisation and gravity will help to get your baby out so, if you're able to, squat, rock, use a birthing ball or get on all fours.
- Use your breathing techniques (see p. 318) – they can help to see you through each contraction and give you a focus.
- Request pain relief if you want it, as and when you need it – pethidine, epidural or gas and air.
- Labour in water – whether it's a bath or birthing pool, some women find that being in water can help with this stage.
- Make your demands known – don't be scared to ask for whatever you think might help you through, whether it's a back rub, lower lighting, a cold flannel or *The Archers*.
- Keep your energy levels up – current medical thinking is that, provided labour is progressing normally (and you haven't had pethidine or an epidural), you should be allowed to snack during active labour. But stick to light, non-fatty foods – banana sandwiches, low-fat yoghurts and plain biscuits are good – or nibble glucose tablets if that sounds too much.
- Keep your fluid levels up – even if you're not hungry, it's vital that you stay hydrated by drinking clear, non-fizzy beverages or sucking on ice chips. Make sure that your midwife keeps your water jug topped up.

Position of the baby and how this affects labour

The way that your baby is positioned can be crucial when it comes to lift-off. In a perfect world, it would be in an 'anterior position', meaning head down, chin tucked into chest, facing your back. The alternative is a 'posterior position' (aka 'face to pubes'), which is head down but with the back of his head against your spine, facing your tummy. If the baby is posterior (also called 'back to back'), labour tends to be longer and more painful as it turns 180 degrees. This is more likely to happen in a first pregnancy.

There are steps that you can take to encourage your little one to budge before it engages in the pelvis in this position, called 'optimal foetal positioning'. Avoid slouching and always keep your knees higher than your pelvis; get down on your hands and knees, and sway your hips. And close the curtains. (See Breech Babies, p. 327.)

During labour, try to keep upright and move around; walk upstairs sideways; get down on all fours; and sway your hips during contractions to encourage your baby to turn. Most posterior babies will turn during labour. 'My posterior baby turned in labour, and was born three and a quarter hours later with no intervention and no tearing!' reports one mum. But babies can still be born vaginally in a posterior position, although the risk of forceps or ventouse is raised.

Don't stress too much though – there are so many different experiences of labour and birth and this is just one factor among many. Lots of Mumsnetters have delivered posterior babies with no problems at all.

'I've had three posterior deliveries, and they've all been fine. My main advice would be to keep active during the labour. Lying down really, really hurts compared to standing or kneeling. There will be a big range of experiences: some people have a lot more trouble with this type of presentation but it's not 100 per cent that this will be the case. Personally, my labours weren't excessively long or painful.' *serenity*

Phase 3, or the transition phase of labour is the stage at which you dilate from around 8cm to 10cm. Contractions will be intense and you may have very little time to rest between each one. Lots of women don't actually notice this stage, but some do feel that it is somehow strangely different from what has gone before. You may feel faint, sick, wobbly, hot and sweaty or cold and chilly. Don't be surprised if you completely zone out during this phase and become unaware of your surroundings: 'My husband thought I'd fainted. I was shaking and clammy and staring into space. It was horrid,' says one Mumsnetter. This is usually the point where some mums lose the plot, decide they really can't be bothered any more and try to walk out.

'I regressed 3 billion years into primitive cavewoman during transition and tried to escape into the air vents. It was very important to me to get into those air vents, without anyone noticing, and I needed to get out of the pool, but I didn't know why. I didn't know what I wanted – I was just confused and distressed.' Joolyjoolyjoo

You may feel an intense urge to push during transition, but your midwife will advise you not to: pushing before your cervix is fully dilated can cause complications. Puffing and blowing – get your midwife to guide you – can help until you're given the green light. Transition usually lasts between 15 minutes to a few hours, so hold on. It's more likely to be quick if it isn't your first vaginal delivery. With a bit of luck, once you're fully dilated, your contractions will stop for a short while before you feel the urge to push, giving you the chance to get your breath back.

'I demanded an epidural during transition. It was pointed out that I couldn't have one as I was at home!' thisisyesterday

Things to do during the transition phase

- Take it one contraction at a time – don't worry about the next ones.
- Change position – you might find a more comfortable one.
- Don't push if advised not to – puff and blow instead.
- Apart from not pushing if advised not to, do whatever you feel like to make it feel better – shout, scream, be quiet, tell everyone to bugger off – all bets are off now, and you are in charge!

The second stage of labour – pushing out the baby

This is the most exciting part of labour. It starts once your cervix is fully dilated (10cm) and you feel an intense urge to push, and ends with the birth of your baby. The descent of your baby down the birth canal can take anything from a few minutes to a few hours. Your position, your baby's position, whether you've had any pain relief and whether this is your first vaginal birth all have a bearing on how quickly you two will get to meet for the first time.

Until now, you will have had limited control over your labour – but this is your chance to play an active part and help to push your baby out through the birth canal. Typically, contractions slow down to a couple of minutes apart. Do what feels natural and, if you feel you need help, get your midwife to guide you (especially if you've had an epidural and it hasn't worn off, as you won't have much of a clue as to when to push or how hard you're actually pushing).

It is important that you are in charge during this bit (although obviously you can take advice about pushing from your midwife if she thinks you might tear) – so get into a position that you feel is most comfortable and appropriate, push when you feel you need to and trust your body and your instincts.

The traditional image of the delivery suite in which a midwife is shouting 'Push! Push!' is one that is now felt to be outdated. Ideally, a woman needs to listen to her body rather than forcibly pushing just because a medical team has decided that 10cm is the time and place to start evicting the baby. Generally, the body will push the baby out in any case, without too much active pushing on the woman's part. 'I think "pushing" is something of a misnomer,' writes one mum. 'It's more an urge to expel, if that makes sense.'

'I "breathed" my third daughter out. As I pushed the air out of my lungs with each contraction, so she came down the birth canal. I didn't really know what I was doing, it just felt right at the time. I hadn't read a book on it or anything, I just went with what I was feeling.' Thomcat

For some women, the urge to push is very strong, regardless of instructions that might be barked at them. 'I couldn't *not* push to be honest,' says one mum, 'although being told to do so did piss me off, especially when I WAS pushing! Anyone would have thought I was crossing my legs the way I was being shouted at.'

It may feel as though you are getting nowhere, as if with each contraction your baby goes slightly further down the birth canal, only to slip back a little bit before the next one – but it's more a case of two steps forwards, one step back.

Once the top of your baby's head reaches the opening of your vagina and no longer slips back after each contraction – known as 'crowning' – you'll (unsurprisingly) feel a strong stinging sensation: 'I got the Ring of Fire with both of my babies!' remembers one mum. If you possibly can, listen to your midwife's instructions at this point, because she may want to advise you when and how to push so that your vagina has time to stretch to avoid tearing too much. If your midwife thinks either you may tear particularly badly or that your baby is in distress and needs to be born quickly, she may suggest you have an episiotomy at this point (see p. 361).

'I enjoyed this bit. It was the calmest point of my labour since 5cm. It was probably the pethidine, but I don't remember much pain, just being

calm and collected and listening to the midwife tell me what to do.' TheHedgeWitch

> Once your baby has crowned, a few more contractions are usually all that is needed before the head is fully out. The shoulders and head then naturally rotate sideways, and with a few more pushes and perhaps some guidance from your midwife, hey presto, he or she is out. Welcome to the world, little baby!

'I'd had an epidural, so my lovely midwife told me when to push, but I could feel the necessary pressure anyway. Absolutely awe-struck, I felt my daughter's head coming out and caught her under her arms and brought her up on to my chest.' Poledra

> The baby is usually delivered straight on to your tummy or into your arms. Now you will start blubbing and gibbering at your lovely baby and your partner may burst into tears. And you will feel an awesome sense of gratitude at the miracle of life and the fact that you no longer have a filing cabinet emerging from your vagina.
>
> The umbilical cord will usually be clamped and cut now (by the midwife or your partner if they fancy it) and, providing all's well, you'll finally get your first cuddle which is best done skin-to-skin (i.e. naked baby against your naked chest).

Things to do during the second stage

- Don't take labour lying down (if you can possibly avoid it) – forget everything you have learned from *Casualty*. Being flat on your back is the least effective position to labour in. Gravity is your friend. Try to remain as upright as possible whether you're squatting, standing, kneeling or down on all fours.
- Relax between contractions; there'll be another one along any minute, so rest up when you can.

- Listen to your body: Mother Nature is rather incredible, so do what feels right for you unless you're being told otherwise.
- Listen to your midwife – you won't be able to keep an eye on what's going on down there, but she'll be able to advise you when and how hard to push to minimise the chances of tearing. Your midwife might ask you to withhold some pushes to co-ordinate them with your breathing, or to breathe through some of the urges to prevent a tear in your perineum, which might happen if your baby comes out too quickly.
- Pretend you're on the loo – don't push from your upper body; instead relax your face and push from below your waist as though you're doing an enormous poo. Which you might be ...
- ... and don't worry about doing a poo; most women do at this point and midwives are used to it. They will just whisk it away with all the other rubbish and you probably won't even notice. (In a birthing pool, they will casually sift it out.)
- Don't lose hope. If you feel too exhausted to push, take a rest for a contraction or two. If you need a boost, see if you can feel your baby's head, or ask for a mirror so you can take a peek.

The third stage of labour – delivering the placenta (or 'afterbirth')

You've got your baby, you've stopped bellowing like a rutting stag and, frankly, everything else may seem completely insignificant. 'I was too busy staring in awe at my gorgeous daughter to notice this bit, to be honest,' recalls a mother. But this is the stage when you deliver the placenta – the organ that's been busy in your uterus, giving your baby oxygen and nutrients and taking out the trash, a bit like a housekeeper. Light contractions will help the placenta to break away from the uterine wall and, as it does so, the blood vessels inside the uterus will seal.

Depending on your circumstances, you can choose between 'active' or 'physiological' (or 'expectant') management of this third stage.

Active management This is where you are given an oxytocin hormone injection (which you probably won't even feel) just after the birth. It encourages a few big contractions which expel the placenta and minimise blood loss. The umbilical cord is clamped and cut soon after the birth. The midwife might apply pressure to your abdomen while keeping hold of the umbilical cord, but compared to what you have just been through, this is usually a doddle. 'I had the injection both times and didn't really think about it, just went: "Yeah, get on with it",' recalls one mum. 'Within a minute it all just came out. I was snuggling with my new baby at the time and barely noticed.'

'I didn't have active management for my second birth, and the placenta was delivered very quickly, but then I had constant pain for an hour, and bled loads, until finally I received the injection to help the uterus contract properly, rather than one hour-long contraction. Next time I will insist on the Syntocinon.' belgo

Active management is done in the majority of births because it reduces the risk of post-partum haemorrhage. For this reason, it can be seen as the 'usual approach', and, unless you request otherwise, you may find that the midwife is waving a needle towards your thigh.

'I tried for the natural route and my daughter fed straight away, but after thirty minutes of more contractions it was spoiling my first minutes with her, so I asked for the injection (and more gas and air!). My partner cut the cord, they gave me the jab and I had an enormous urge to push. It almost hit the poor midwife in the face! I think if you have had a natural birth, it is worth trying to deliver it naturally, but I had had enough after half an hour. I'd had the baby – why was I still contracting? I never considered that; it was a bit of a shock.' callmeovercautious

Some women find that the drugs used make them feel nauseous. There are also studies which suggest that active management increases the risk of retained placenta, where the placenta is not completely delivered, and surgery is then required to remove it. This is because the hormones given encourage the cervix to close, leaving a limited time for the placenta to be delivered. In a physiological third stage, there is no rush to deliver the placenta, so the risk of retained placenta may be reduced.

'In the end, I was induced and had to have the injection. They didn't cut the cord though until the blood stopped pumping (at my request). It was a compromise, but to be honest, I was spent by the end of it and just wanted it to be over.'

rebelmum1

Physiological (or 'expectant') management (no intervention)
This is where it's all done as nature intended (although you won't actually have to chew through your own cord). It involves no hormone injection, no cord clamping until it has stopped pulsating and the placenta is delivered and no cord traction (where the midwife guides the released cord and placenta out manually).

'If the cord has to be cut because it is very tight or short, or the baby needs to be resuscitated, then the oxytocin injection should be given to help the placenta to deliver. That is because the natural process has been interrupted. The cord should not be cut before it stops pulsating in a natural third stage because, again, the natural process has been interrupted. Once it has stopped pulsating it can be cut if wished.'

(Mumsnetter midwife) mears

A physiological third stage can take between fifteen minutes and an hour, and the umbilical cord will be clamped and cut only once the cord has stopped pulsating or when the placenta has been delivered: 'There is actually no need for the cord to be clamped prior to delivery of the placenta if all is well ... I had a physiological third stage, so wanted loads of skin-on-skin time, a first feed and the cord not to be cut until it had stopped pulsating,' says one mum. 'There was no rush for the placenta to be delivered.'

It is thought that the last few minutes of receiving blood from the placenta may have benefits to the baby, which is why some prefer no intervention (i.e. no clamping or cutting of the cord) during this stage.

'I had a physiological third stage. The cord was clamped after it had stopped pulsating (and my mum cut it – lovely!) and I got out of the water to deliver the placenta, which I found fascinating – I got the midwife to show me it in detail! I was amazed that my body could grow all these things properly; it's hardly ever done anything else right!' xmashampermunker

If you have had a 'natural' birth with no interventions or problems, then a physiological third stage is perhaps the logical way of managing this stage: 'If you have had a normal labour with no interventions, there is no reason that you shouldn't have a natural third stage.'

Depending on how you're doing, and what medication you have received during labour, you may have to have active management, as there are some situations where a physiological third stage is considered unsafe because of the risk of haemorrhage. 'Do keep an open mind', advises one mum, 'because if the labour didn't go according to plan, your third stage may need to be managed.'

'I had a physiological third stage, and it did take a while, but I was at home, so nice and relaxed. I would recommend deciding on the day, depending on what (if any) intervention you have had.' reikizen

Regardless of what you choose, if you are planning to breastfeed, give it a go as soon as possible. This will encourage your body to produce its own natural oxytocin, which will help this stage to go smoothly and will also help your uterus to contract.

So that's it – all done and dusted. Just the clearing up to do now, but someone else will see to that. You just lie back with your beautiful baby and wrestle that tea and toast from your partner. Well done!

Failure to progress

Labour dystocia is medical jargon for what happens when a baby's descent down the birth canal or cervical dilation stops or significantly slows down. It is known as failure to progress, abnormal labour, dysfunctional labour or difficult labour (terms all guaranteed to make a knackered mum feel like a total failure). Causes include weak, uncoordinated contractions, a poorly positioned baby, and design shortcomings (i.e. the baby's too big or mum's pelvis is too small). Pregnancies complicated by dystocia often end with assisted deliveries, including forceps, ventouse or a Caesarean section. 'I had been at 8cm for hours', recalls one mum 'and was told that nothing was happening, so I was wheeled into theatre for a C-section.'

'I went through 12 hours of very painful, continuous contractions only to find I was still only 1–2cm dilated. Exhausted, I agreed to go into hospital and have a Syntocinon drip and epidural. It turned out my son was back to back, so I ended up in theatre, having a ventouse to turn him and forceps to pull him out, and narrowly avoiding a C-section. Not at all the lovely natural home birth I had planned.' *Bumbleybee*

(continued)

Where weak contractions are the cause, your midwife might suggest an artificial rupture of membranes if your waters haven't already broken. You may also be offered an intravenous Syntocinon drip – artificial oxytocin – to stimulate the uterus and increase and strengthen your contractions. Subsequent stronger contractions can also help to turn a baby into the right position.

'I wasn't making much progress, so they stuck a drip up: cue a desperate urge to push, which I spent the next couple of hours fighting as my cervix wasn't ready. Then I was given an epidural to stop me pushing: cue nothing for several hours. Eventually my daughter was yanked out with forceps, which was OK. I was so knackered by then I didn't care if the baby was hauled out of my nostril, so long as she got born!' *Slouchy*

Failure to progress can be hard on a mum: 'I felt like a failure for failing to give birth normally' is a very common sentiment expressed by mums whose births have ended with this diagnosis. But giving birth is very much a roll of the dice, and to a large extent you get the birth you are given and there is only so much that is really within your control.

Friends may joke about you being 'too posh to push' or 'not doing it properly like the rest of us' and these comments can be very hurtful when you are feeling vulnerable and struggling with your feelings. If you feel this way, try to talk to your midwife about what happened, or ask to be referred to a counsellor with whom you can discuss your experiences. 'I spoke to a counsellor at the Birth Crisis Centre' writes one Mumsnetter. 'It really helped me get closure over my feelings of failure.'

Mumsnetters' Birth Stories (But Only the Nice Ones, OK?)

Although you'd think their options were limited (biologically speaking), somehow babies seem to have dreamt up quite a number of different ways to make an entrance into the world. Here's just a small selection of Mumsnetters' birth stories; the only thing they have in common is the happy ending.

Ventouse and forceps

'My first birth was a vaginal delivery. My son was large and got stuck towards the end. I had an episiotomy, failed ventouse, then forceps. It may sound bizarre, but the whole experience was fantastic. It was the best day of my life. My midwife was great, the doctors were close at hand, everyone listened and I was involved every step of the way. I always felt in control, despite the high level of intervention. My episiotomy healed without problems and I breastfed straight away. My husband got the raw end of the deal, as he watched what was happening to me. It all passed me by, thanks to the gas and air.' *Rosetip*

'I ended up having a ventouse, as my son was beginning to show signs of distress, even though he was nearly out. It was one quick pull and out he popped. I didn't feel a thing (due to fab epidural, which was kindly topped up by midwife, just before he emerged) and was cracking jokes with the doctor and midwife as he was born. I had no tearing or episiotomy. He did have a slight bump on his head for a few days, but it soon disappeared.' *SoMuchToBits*

'Forceps, stirrups and an episiotomy all featured during the birth of my son. But at that point I really couldn't have cared less – at least they were getting him out and the end was in sight. It can't have been that bad though as I went on to have two more children! My first baby was born with a bruised, elongated head and I blamed his poor sleeping on the forceps, but my second and third turned out to be just as bad and had normal deliveries. My attitude before labour was, "It can't go on for ever" – and it doesn't.' *miggy*

Water birth

'I was in the pool in the hospital's birth centre before they'd even turned the taps on. I stayed there for the rest of my labour and birthed my daughter into the pool. I'm sure it helped relax me and speed things up. I wanted the water really hot so they kept topping it up. It was fantastic. The only thing that slightly freaked my husband out was the colour of the water post-birth.' *Bellabambina*

'My daughter was born underwater. I was on my knees when she came out, then I turned over to a sitting position to pick her up from the bottom of the pool. As her head broke the water she took her first breath. It was the most amazing thing I've ever seen. It was such a wonderful experience.' *carol3*

'Water births rock. I gave birth to my second daughter in water, at home, with precious little preparation. She shot out like a champagne cork. Four pushes in total. VOOM. It still amazes me.' *motherinferior*

Caesarean

'I had to have an emergency Caesarean with my son who got stuck. I was up, walking to the loo, and having a shower less than 24 hours later. I didn't suffer any pain from the stitches, even when they were removed. The aftercare in the hospital was crap, but the operation itself was a blessed relief and the surgical team were lovely.' *DecafArabica*

'I had a 40-hour labour ending in an unplanned C-section, but I still think of it as a positive birth story. It helped that I was prepared beforehand (factually and emotionally) for what might happen. The staff were good at communicating, so I was sure at each stage that what was happening was the best thing under the circumstances. Labour doesn't need to be quick and "easy" to be positive.' *lemonaid*

'I ended up having a Caesarean section with my son. It was semi-planned. I was two weeks overdue, had a failed induction and a huge baby whose head wasn't engaged. Although I was nervous it was fine. The hospital staff did everything possible to make it special for me and my hubby. My son was 9lb 6oz, so I'm glad I didn't push him out. I was able to (very gingerly) get in the bath the next day and was home three days later. My wound felt numb for weeks, so I didn't feel a huge amount of pain. It was fine and I'd do it again.' *Amanda*

Planned Caesarean

'I had an elective Caesarean and it was magical. The hospital staff informed me of everything as it happened, even covered me with warm blankets while waiting for the fluids to go in. I was worried about being naked and cold on the table and they were unbelievably respectful. They automatically quietened down when my son was delivered and commented on how gorgeous and alert he was. I know, they say that for every baby, but it meant a lot to my husband and me at the time.' *Highlander*

'I have had three C-sections. My first was elective due to a breech baby, second an emergency due to a distressed baby and third an elective. Being able to plan your childcare is brilliant, stock your freezer, and get your partner to book time off work. I found the recovery from the first section the hardest but it got easier with each one. I hate staying in hospital for long but, other than that, I love sections, and would have another in an instant.' *nutcracker*

Vaginal birth after Caesarean (VBAC)

'I had a VBAC almost three years after an emergency C-section. I went into labour naturally and had my daughter in hospital after five hours with gas and air. It was a wonderful birth and it really put to rest a lot of "issues" I had after my (horrible) first birth.' *cupcakes*

'I was very happy with my two VBACs, even though my daughter was born with a bit of help from the ventouse and I tore. My second son was born at home in water with barely a word from the midwives and it was the most wonderful experience of my life, although I won't deny that it still hurt like hell and was pretty messy. I felt like I'd conquered the world. An elective C-section is going to be less stressful, but I think if you can try to labour naturally, it does at least send a warning signal to the baby that it's time to be born.' *wilbur*

'I had a lovely VBAC. My labour started with my waters breaking which had meconium in them. I was monitored periodically, but was still able to walk around and have a bath. I dilated very slowly so was put on a drip to speed things up. When it became very painful, I asked for an epidural, which was agreed, but I ended up not having one as things started moving very quickly at this point. My son was born after nine hours of labour. No stitches, no tearing, and a very happy mummy!' *surprisenumber3*

Home birth

'My home birth was a wonderful experience. It's still crystal clear in my mind. I went into labour a week earlier than expected. I was in a state of denial in the early stages, but as soon as full-blown labour began, I really calmed down and focused. The two attending midwives (who I had never met before) were wonderful – really supportive and respectful. I had a 15-hour labour, with TENS and a little gas and air. I had a small tear but no stitches. I ate jam sandwiches and sipped cold orange juice throughout and, in between contractions, listened to my husband talking to the midwives. Afterwards, the midwives ran me a bath and cleared up. My husband and I climbed into bed with our beautiful daughter and stayed there for the next two days. I felt like Superwoman.' *Marjean*

'I had my daughter at home while watching Trinny and Susannah. It was quick and really calm. It didn't hurt enough for me to need pain relief and I didn't tear. An hour after the midwives arrived, I was tucked up in bed with my beautiful daughter sipping champagne. No mess, no fuss, everyone healthy and happy.' *trice*

'I have had four babies, all born at home with no pain relief and no stitches. Two were born in water; two laboured in water but were "dry births". They were the best experiences of my life. It hurt like hell but was wonderful.' *beetroot*

Home birth to hospital birth

'I had a terrible hospital experience with my first daughter and went for a home birth for my second. My mother-in-law spent the whole of my pregnancy trying to bully and scare me into changing my mind. As it happens, I ended up being transferred to hospital at the last minute, but I didn't care. I was far more relaxed and happy labouring at home than I would have been in hospital, even if it went a little off plan (big baby in awkward position and pressing on my sciatic nerve). Even the uncomfortable hospital journey at 10cm, pushing, while strapped to an ambulance bed, was worth it.' *Stripymouse*

'Although my home birth didn't work out for me in the end (due to prolonged rupture of the membranes), I was glad I'd planned it. You have all the comforts of home; you aren't worried about going in to hospital, then being turned away for not being in labour yet; the midwife comes to you to assess the situation and will either come back later, if necessary, or stay. And you can always change your mind later down the line if you want.' *Racers*

'I knew that I would feel more confident and relaxed if I gave birth at home, and that I would have expert help on hand – two qualified experienced midwives – and a hospital near by. So, I planned a home birth for my first baby and laboured quite happily at home without any pain relief, except a TENS machine and the pool. But after I'd been pushing for some considerable time, I had to be taken to hospital, as my son was OP [occipito-posterior, or in a posterior position, see p. 278] and stuck. He was born with ventouse assistance. The obstetrician said that had I been labouring in hospital my son would have been born by C-section "hours ago". Yet he never showed signs of stress, was born with an Apgar score of 9 and I avoided a serious abdominal operation.' *Blu*

Epidural

'I'd put in my birth plan: "No epidural, no pethidine, no TENS – just gas and air please." But when it came to it, I was induced and pleading for an epidural. It was fantastic. It meant I was on the bed, but having gone from 0 to 8cm in an hour, it was wonderful to be pain-free. I had quite a few stitches, so the epidural also helped with that. My son was nearly 10 pounds and in posterior position, so, in hindsight, it was the right decision.' *musica*

'I hadn't planned on pain relief until I had to be induced. By the time the doctor arrived I was promising to snog him if he took the pain away. It was the best thing I could have done. The epidural was controlled in such a way that I could feel what was happening, but the overwhelming pain had gone. My advice is to go with the flow. At the end of the day it's a truly miraculous thing, however you go about it.' *lucy5*

'With my second son I knew I wanted an epidural for the second stage when things got really painful, so I asked in plenty of time and I only endured two or three scarily painful contractions.

By the time it came to pushing about four hours later it was wearing off (I'd asked not to be topped up) and so I could feel enough to push him out with ease. I'd recommend it.' *BigBertha*

Inductions

'I was induced, then my baby was in distress. I had to ditch the water birth and stay on the bed being monitored. I had to have an epidural, episiotomy and ventouse. But it was brilliant! The TENS really helped the first few hours, and I was racing my husband up the stairs at hospital to try and get things moving along. When the epidural kicked in, I had the laziest birth. I slept and was woken up to give a few pushes, then there was a beautiful baby. I felt a bit of a "silent partner" in the whole affair, but it was more brilliant than I ever imagined it would be.' *Quootiepie*

'I was induced at 36+6 weeks and in labour for almost 24 hours. It was the best experience of my life and I'd do it all again tomorrow. Gas and air are wonderful things especially teamed with an epidural. At one point I was laughing so much from the gas and air I started to pee, but couldn't stop laughing to tell anyone, so there was my partner and mother, both reading newspapers and the midwife, writing her notes, all sitting at the foot of my bed. All of a sudden the midwife looked up and said: "Can you hear running water?" It was only when she looked at me literally wetting myself laughing that the penny dropped as to what the running water sound was!' *ginmummy*

'I was given a prostaglandin pessary when I was nine days overdue. The pessary was inserted at 6.30 p.m. By 8.30 p.m., I was having powerful contractions in the bath on the antenatal ward, one and a half minutes apart. I was examined and found to be 5cm dilated. At 10 p.m., I was taken down to the labour suite, and my daughter was born at quarter past midnight. Yes, it was sore, especially as I went straight into established labour with no early labour contractions, but I did the whole thing on gas and air (not because I was trying to be brave), which I discarded for the pushing stage because it became a distraction. I had a lovely, supportive midwife, a speedy straightforward labour, a couple of stitches afterwards and a beautiful baby daughter at the end. Can't complain!' *lazyemma*

Free-range organic

'I had a fab first-time birth. I laboured for two and a half days at home and only made it to the hospital with seven minutes to spare. I had no pain relief and no tears or stitches with a 7lb 15oz daughter. It wasn't planned that way, but I believed the midwife in the hospital who told me I couldn't possibly be in "real" labour as I appeared too calm and in control. I was so mellow before labour; I had spent days chilling in the sun with flasks of raspberry leaf tea and a hypnobirthing CD. I look back on my labour as the best thing I've ever done. It gave me so much confidence. Be positive and believe you can do it.' *weeonion*

'My waters broke on the loo at 8 a.m. By 4 p.m., it was beginning to feel pretty painful so I went to the hospital. My son shot out at 5.45 p.m. after four big pushes. No pain relief, no stitches and only slight grazing. I sneezed a few days later and didn't even wet myself. Doesn't get much better than that.' *amisuchabadmummy*

'I had an accidental home birth with my second daughter. I had used the TENS for a couple of hours, by which time I was ready to push. My husband phoned 999 and flapped like a maestro, while our neighbour came in to look after our first child. Amid some worry, but mainly disbelief, our second daughter entered the world. Our neighbour wiped bits of me off her, while my husband made me a tuna sandwich and we waited for the midwife. An hour later, the baby was fed and asleep and I was showered and dressed, reading our eldest stories on my lap. My husband had gone down to the river "to get his head round all this". It was a very positive, wonderful, hilarious and manic experience.' *jaynehater*

Gas and air

'I got through on TENS and gas and air. I coped by taking a very business-like approach: this will be unpleasant, but it has to be done, so I might as well get on with it. I was very focused. The hardest part was being monitored, which stopped me moving. I also used the gas wrong, so the whole place stank of it. I must have been the least high person there! Labour pain is not the worst thing in the world because: a) it doesn't hurt between contractions, so you can take one at a time; b) you know it has to stop some time; and c) you can keep in mind that you're doing something amazing and important. It's not like being ill when you feel that the world has screwed you over. It's a privilege, really.' *Kif*

Mumsnetiquette: The truth about giving birth – what you should know about childbirth ... that no one ever tells you

'That at some point you may make bellowing noises that you would never dream of in any other situation, but no one will bat an eyelid. And that for weeks after you have given birth, people will still be asking you when it is due.' *Romy7*

'That there's no point buying a really nice nightie or pyjamas because they will be ruined!' *RiojaLover75*

'That you may turn into an exhibitionist. I am normally quite modest, but in all three labours I have felt the need to be completely naked, and couldn't seem to give two flying figs who might be unfortunate enough to have to witness the sight of my end-of-gestation body. I was even wheeled naked down a corridor in a wheelchair (with a blanket thrown over me by the midwife) and I cared not a jot.' *Joolyjoolyjoo*

'That contractions are painful, but not completely unbearable. It doesn't necessarily get any worse than the pain of a contraction; the contractions just get closer together and last longer. I was terrified once the contractions started. I thought if this is what a contraction feels like, how on earth am I going to cope later on in labour. In truth, that was as bad as it got.' *WriggleJiggle*

'That in between contractions it doesn't actually hurt.' *Funnypeculiar*

'That pethidine will render your brain totally useless. You may have planned an active birth but you will be unable to form enough of a coherent thought in your head to actually do it.

Instead you will lie on the bed whimpering in the position you swore blind you wouldn't give birth in.' *EyeballsintheSky*

'That bloody deep breathing, water birth and active birth positions are not enough; people have drugs because it hurts. If you have a drug-free labour you are lucky – not good at giving birth.' *MrsPickles*

'That when you push you have to push out of your bum so that it feels like you're trying to do the biggest poo ever, while simultaneously hoping that you don't do the biggest poo ever.' *CatIsSleepy*

'That the baby's head crowning really does feel like someone's opened your legs and aimed a blow torch at your fanjo.' *Findtheriver*

'That you can feel the baby go back up sometimes when you're pushing, but it will eventually stay down and come out.' *choufleur*

'That once the head is out, it's only one more push and you've got your baby. You will feel superhuman and not believe what you have just done.' *Twosofar*

'That it's OK to not feel an immediate rush of love for your baby and that it does come eventually.' *Muppetgirl*

'That it would be the most painful thing I'd ever do and yet the most amazing thing I'd ever do. I was on such a high for days afterwards.' *macaco*

'That your placenta is enormous and it's quite cool to see it.' *Turniphead1*

'That it's quick and easy compared to nine long miserable months of pregnancy. Mine was not half as scary as I thought it would be.' *Glucose*

'That the tea and toast straight after is the best meal you will ever eat!' *slinkiemalinki*

(continued)

'That you'll wake up on Day 3 with puppies that would make Jordan look as if she's on her first training bra.' *Hobnobfanatic*

'That you will wonder why you obsessed so much over how you were going to get the baby out, only to realise when the baby *was* out, you hadn't read the next chapters in the book on how to actually look after one.' *Cookiemonstress*

'Just how miraculous the whole bloody thing is, however many you've had or seen.' *smellyeli*

Pain Relief (Now You're Talking) – What Works?

'Our NCT teacher asked us to describe a time when we had been in extreme pain. When it came to my turn, I talked about how I'd set off to work that morning in a new pair of shoes. By midday I was in agony. The pain was so piercing I could hardly walk to the station to get my train home. I felt like collapsing on the spot. It was only after describing my day of torture that the teacher smiled knowingly and asked us what we thought giving birth might feel like. Of course, I didn't have a clue. Looking back, it's probably a good thing.' NoodlePip

As a pregnant woman, you are a sitting target for been-there-ouch-felt-that mothers who like nothing better than to settle down with a glass of wine and scare the bejesus out of you with terrifying tales of lazy midwives, stubborn cervixes, babies with shoulders like shelves and umbilical cords tangled up like skipping ropes. However horrifying, you find yourself hanging on to every shriek and yelp, desperate to know more about what it actually feels like to pass a baby through a hole better suited to birthing a jelly baby. Each story is different but they all inevitably involve blood and pain. It's enough to make you want to call the whole thing off.

'I had gas and air. And pethidine. And diamorphine. And an epidural. And a general anaesthetic.' ionesmum

But the point is – yes, that old chestnut – most mums do go on to have more than one child. Every day, at least 200,000 women give birth. And there are legions of women merrily pushing buggies along the street, rather than sitting on the pavement gibbering in horror at the things they have seen. Plus, you have to believe there are a lot of good birth stories out there, but perhaps those mums don't need the therapy of telling their experiences to everyone and anyone who will listen.

'It's not good to frighten the living daylights out of first-time mums with all the horror stories going, but rose-tinting the experience of childbirth by telling them they can (and should) simply "breathe through the pain" is not helpful either, as it creates false expectations and makes women feel like failures when they do ask for medication. Childbirth is not a competition and every woman is different in what she needs and wants. That should be respected.' Rochwen

Being aware of your options is a crucial part of being able to make informed and sensible decisions about your care during labour and birth. But it's also important not to plan too much or to fantasise about a dream birth 'experience'. Lady Luck plays an enormous part when it comes to giving birth. So go in with an open mind and just cross your fingers (not legs) for a positive outcome.

'My best tip for coping with labour: don't think about it before it happens and forget about it as quickly as possible when it's over.' liquidclocks

What do contractions feel like?

'Like being squeezed round the middle by a psychotic sumo wrestler who really doesn't like you.' *FrannyandZooey*

'Things like "the worst period ever" just trivialise it for me. I felt like my tummy was being crushed by a lorry.' *liquidclocks*

'Like being kicked by a horse.' *Blueshoes*

'I think a lot of the weirdness of it is because it's a huge muscular effort happening completely involuntarily. If you got that feeling in your arms when bench-pressing 30kg in the gym, you'd think "fair enough", but when it's happening in your belly without you doing anything to provoke it, it's downright odd.' *CarolinaMao*

'Like severe cramps from salmonella food poisoning.' *Bugsy2*

'Similar to having someone blow up a balloon in your insides and not stopping even when your skin was about to split.' *mimitwo*

'Like someone is cutting you in half with a rusty hacksaw every couple of minutes.' *Sweetkitty*

'My contractions made me want to curl up and want my mummy to make it go away. I haven't wanted my mother for 25 years. Nuff said really.' *arfishymeau*

'On a par with someone cutting my leg off with a chainsaw.' *TuttiFrutti*

'Like I was having my insides cut out with a red-hot blunt knife.' *cupcakes*

'Similar to what I imagine being on a bucking bronco to be like: you can't really do anything while it's happening – you just hold on for dear life and wait for it to be over.' *FrannyandZooey*

'Mild period pains, a slight burning then a baby. But I think I was very lucky ... ' *PifflinePankhurst*

Unleash your inner hippy

Homeopathy, aromatherapy, acupuncture, reflexology, massage, music, and low lighting help some women soften the birth experience. Screaming obscenities is another option. Positive thinking is the best springboard – although a grim sense of foreboding will possibly get you just as far. First off in the drug-free stakes are a few low-maintenance options.

Breathing Controlled, deep breathing (see p. 318) can help to relax your muscles, slow your heart rate and focus your mind. And even if it doesn't help with childbirth it's good practice for when your two-year-old starts screaming in the vegetable aisle at Asda.

'I was completely shocked to discover that the breathing techniques and positions I'd learnt at NCT classes were utterly useless (for me).'
SoupDragon

Visualisation This can (apparently) be a powerful weapon in the fight against pain: 'My contractions hurt, but they were completely manageable,' writes one mum. 'Ride them like waves: they build, peak, then wane. Each one is one contraction nearer to seeing your baby. I found counting my way through helped hugely. Try to focus on what your body is doing, rather than fearing the pain. Also try to imagine your cervix opening with each contraction; each and every one has a purpose.' Think loose, soft mouth equals loose, soft vagina. Then swear that you'll never get yourself into this mess again.

Eye contact Some women say keeping eye contact with their partner made an enormous difference, but maybe that was with him in a headlock.

Water Even if you haven't signed up for a water birth, you might want to spend the first part of your labour in a bath. 'It was the only place that I felt comfortable,' says one first-timer. (See p. 322.)

Positioning If you are happier on dry land, crouch, squat on a bucket, lean into a bean bag, get down on all fours, or bounce on a birthing ball (an exercise ball will do). Keep moving and keep upright. 'Standing by the bed, with my hands flat on it, circling my hips got me through the worst contractions,' advises one belly-dancing mum.

'I didn't use my birthing ball much before the labour, only to sit on when my back was playing up. But during my labour, you couldn't get me off it. I took it to hospital and my waters broke while I was on it. I was told afterwards that it probably helped my cervix dilate quicker, as in that position your pelvis is more open.' Corky

If none of this sounds quite enough for you, but you still want to try some 'alternative' therapies, here's the lowdown on some of the more popular options.

Homoeopathy While they certainly won't wipe away the pain, a number of homeopathic remedies are said to help during childbirth. Kali carb, for example is recommended for pain relief in the lumbar region, so it's supposed to be good for 'back-to-back' labours. Homeopathy must be treated with respect – far better to see a registered practitioner with experience of treating women during labour than to self-treat blindly. You may be able to arrange for your homeopath to attend to you during the birth; at the very least, a decent practitioner should be able to provide a tailor-made birthing kit for you and advise you and your partner on which remedies to use in which instance.

It's worth stating in your birth plan that you intend to use homeopathy. Some doctors and midwives support the use of homeopathic remedies, while others don't, so it's a good idea to flag up your intentions before you get to the labour suite.

'I made specific reference in my birth plan to the homoeopathic remedies I would possibly need to use and gave express permission to my birth partners to administer them to me. In the end, I took Caulophyllum to help me reach that magic 10cm, as it had taken hours for me to get to just 3cm, Kali phos towards the end, when I was exhausted and needed a boost, Arnica 200c, just before and a couple of hours after delivery and Arnica 30c for a few days either side of my due date to help the healing process.' MamaTama

Aromatherapy Not pain relief as such, but certain aromatherapy oils can help you relax during labour. Fear and pain are closely linked, so anything that helps promote a calming atmosphere is good in our book. (Check you like the smell of each of the oils before you go into labour though.) If your hospital won't let you use an oil burner/diffuser, you can get a similar effect by adding a few drops of your chosen oils to a bowl of hot water. (Whatever you do, don't drink the stuff.)

Oils that may help in a warm compress include:

- clary sage – has analgesic and sedative properties, but don't use if you're also using gas and air
- neroli – good if you're feeling very scared or nervous
- ylang ylang – calming
- lavender – calming and good for aching backs and limbs (try a warm compress) and a great antiseptic.

In fact, lavender is a hospital bag is essential, if only because you can put a few drops in the bath afterwards to help heal your bits.

'My midwives were trained in aromatherapy. (An NHS unit! Blimey!) And despite a 44-hour labour, I didn't need anything beyond rose and lavender oil (by diffuser and massage) until the last hour. I've had three children, and it was by far the most relaxed birth I have had, even though it was also by far the longest.' PeachyClairHasBAdHair

Hypnotherapy Some studies suggest that self-hypnosis during childbirth may ease some of the pain of labour, decrease anxiety and fear, lower the risk of medical complications and reduce the need for surgery. Quite impressive stuff, really. You can buy numerous books and CDs on the topic, but your best bet is probably to see a registered practitioner who specialises in teaching self-hypnosis during childbirth or offers traditional hypnosis with post-hypnotic suggestion: essentially they hypnotise you during your sessions and you are then taught triggers to get you back into that state during your labour.

One method that gets a regular thumbs-up is natal hypnotherapy, developed by UK hypnotherapist Maggie Howell. You can either attend classes or listen to CDs at home in preparation.

'I used the natal hypnotherapy birth preparation CD and found it fab. I'm convinced it was the reason that I got through my entire labour on two paracetamol only! In fact, I didn't even realise I was in labour until I was fully dilated, as I kept thinking, "Surely labour is more painful than this?"' Sterny

> **Hypnobirthing** Hypnobirthing is billed as a 'complete birth education programme' that 'teaches simple but specific self-hypnosis, relaxation and breathing techniques for a better birth'. Exponents believe it reduces the need for intervention and medication, shortens labour and makes for an all-round more positive birth. You can use the techniques at home, in hospital, in a birthing pool – wherever, essentially. There's a book you can buy if you fancy teaching yourself; alternatively classes are now run across the UK. Pass the lentils.

'I used hypnobirthing. It helped me to relax and cope, but it certainly wasn't this miracle pain remover, as there was NO WAY it was pain-free. (I have had to remind my partner of this when he says to others: "Oh, she used hypnobirthing and sailed through it all." He certainly wasn't experiencing the pains I was.)' weeonion

'Hypnobirthing worked brilliantly for me. The birth was exactly as I'd hoped and while it wasn't pain-free, I never felt I couldn't manage it. The only thing I would say is to make sure you call the midwife/go into hospital in plenty of time. I was so relaxed, I left it really late and the midwife arrived ten minutes before my son was born. Apparently, midwives are warned to take hypnobirthing mothers-to-be seriously when they say they are in labour as they're probably about to pop!' Seabird

And if all else fails ...

Set the scene Yep, it's a bit hippy-dippy, but the right sounds and calm lighting can help to put you at ease. So dim those lights and prime that iPod, although be prepared to rethink your playlists.

'I spent ages compiling a bag of CDs that I thought would help me relax. They did the trick early on, but once I was in established labour everything sounded like nails down a blackboard. I ended up screaming at my poor husband, who was frantically trying to DJ effectively: "Just turn the ******* thing off.' AbbyMN

Vocalise If you want to swear, scream, grunt or babble in tongues, then do so. Better out than in, say we.

'I screamed my head off! I never thought I would, but it felt really good – I think it scared my partner.' Lauraloola

'I found that vocalising – OK, mooing – rather than screaming, helped me manage the pain of contractions, and, while perhaps not serene, didn't stop me feeling calm.' Dramasequalzero

Hippy stuff

Pros
- No harmful effects on baby
- May relax you, which is really positive for labouring – especially during the early stages
- You can stay mobile
- Labour is a good excuse to persuade your husband to massage you – hurrah!

Cons
- None! Go for it.

TENS machine

A TENS (Transcutaneous Electrical Nerve Stimulation) machine is the gadget-lover's answer to combating labour pains. A hand-held device that can be bought or hired, it is most effective in the early stages of labour when it can be more of a distraction than anything else. In fact, a Nintendo DS might work just as well. 'When you are pushing that little button you feel like it's really helping, but my battery went dead and it took me an hour to notice.' By turning a dial, you send an electrical current via electrodes attached to your back (with small adhesive pads) to block pain messages and crack open the endorphins, the body's natural painkillers. Some women swear by it, but others find it annoying at best: 'I felt like I had ants all over my back.' Or as one Mumsnetter puts it, slightly more bluntly: 'TENS does nothing apart from make you want to shove it into the wall or your husband's face.'

TENS machine

Pros
- No harmful effects on baby
- May help you cope with early labour
- You can stay mobile

Cons
- A bit rubbish according to some
- Might be annoying
- Can't use in water birth unless you fancy being electrocuted. (Note: if you do fancy being electrocuted, please share these feelings with your midwife rather than just jumping in with it turned up to MAX.)

Paracetamol

You may be advised to take a paracetamol. Try to be polite, rather than sarcastic.

'I took our (childless) antenatal teacher's advice and took a paracetamol. A PARACETAMOL! Oooh yes, that *really* helped …' arfishymeau

Paracetamol

Pros
- Won't harm the baby

Cons
- It's rubbish (like using a pin to crack a boulder springs to mind)

Entonox (gas and air)

Entonox, aka gas and air, is women's number-one choice when it comes to choosing the sort of pain relief they will pick from the labour-ward menu. It's definitely recommended as a starter, although you might want to move on to something more substantial for the main course.

You inhale a mix of nitrous oxide and oxygen through a mouthpiece and are transformed into the 21st-century equivalent of Oscar Wilde. 'I thought I was the bee's knees while on the gas and air, cracking jokes, telling stories, reciting poems,' says an otherwise shy and retiring mum. 'Then I glanced over at my husband and the midwife who were sitting by my bed, totally po-faced.' It takes roughly 20 seconds to start working, and the idea is that you inhale just before the start of each contraction.

Entonox doesn't block out the pain completely, but you will feel so squiffy that you might not register it in the same way. And it won't affect your baby or your contractions. Should it make you feel sick, or odd in a not-good way, you can stop using it straight away and the effects should quickly wear off. 'I loved gas and air,' raves a mum. 'They had to gently wrestle it from me, saying, "Your baby is born, you can stop using it now."' Sadly though, it doesn't work for everyone: 'I never really got to grips with it. I knew I was supposed to time my inhalation with the contraction, but couldn't remember how and just got cross with my husband for not remembering how to do it either.' Beware also of birth partners who want to try it:

'I was obviously having such a good time on it that my husband thought he'd have a go. Unfortunately, he was also chewing gum at the time. This is not recommended. He had more nurses round him than I did.' BigBertha

In summary, you can either think of nothing better than to feel drunk and out of control after nine months on the wagon, or it can come as an unwelcome shock.

'Gas and air is great for sucking on – it gives you something to do instead of the howling.' Sweetkitty

Entonox (gas and air)

Pros

- Won't harm the baby
- You can stay reasonably mobile
- Might provide entertainment for your husband (but don't let him try it if he's chewing gum)

Cons

- You might not enjoy the feeling of being 'off your face'
- May make you feel nauseous or sick

Pethidine, diamorphine and Meptid

If the gas and air doesn't cut it and you are begging for more drugs, you might want to turn to the big hitters: pethidine, diamorphine and Meptid. There is no guarantee that they will work, but the idea is to at least dull the pain during a long labour and allow you to get some rest. Bear in mind that not all hospitals or units offer these drugs, so check in advance by asking your midwife for a copy of the menu before you make you choice too far in advance.

Pethidine is a usually given by an injection into the muscle of your leg or bottom (yes, there are still muscles there). It takes about 20 minutes to work and is effective for about three hours. The idea is that it relaxes you so that you don't feel the pain of the contractions with quite so much, ahem, clarity. As one mum recalls: 'I had pethidine and loved it. My husband, however, thought I'd gone mad. I was talking absolute gibberish. My baby was very sleepy for the next four days.'

'I ended up with pethidine and found it great. It sent me to sleep for two hours while my contractions continued. I woke up to be told I could start pushing. I was wide awake through the rest of my labour. My son arrived and was very alert. I had no problems feeding him afterwards.' megg

Unfortunately, pethidine has its downsides. If you don't like feeling spaced out then it probably isn't for you, plus there can be side effects. These include feeling shaky and light-headed and vomiting (you should be given an anti-emetic to relieve the latter). The main disadvantage though is that it also crosses the placenta, so can make your baby drowsy, and given too close to the baby's arrival, it may lead to breathing problems. Although these can be counteracted by using other drugs, some women feel that the risks to the baby outweigh the pain relief that the drug may bring.

'I would rather do it without drugs next time, so I can remember clearly what it was like to see my son's wee face for the first time. He was a bit groggy and wouldn't latch on for a good 24 hours, and I had to rely on my partner to tell me all the details of my labour.' Mumanon

One important thing to know about pethidine is that you don't have to go the whole hog to start with – you can ask for a half dose, and see how you get on with that. If you are worried about side effects or how you might feel, but feel that you need something to keep the monsters at bay, a half dose might be a good compromise.

Diamorphine is similar to pethidine but – and this is where it gets a bit *Trainspotting* – it is actually the medical name for heroin. This is handy because if your unit runs out, they can go to the chap behind the bus station and buy a load more on the cheap. (Note: this is not really how the NHS procurement system works.)

Some women find diamorphine slightly more intense than pethidine, offering a deeper pain-relieving sensation of relaxation: 'It certainly calmed me down and helped me get through the next few hours.' Others find that, like pethidine, the feelings it creates of dissociation are distressing and unpleasant.

'Not long after I was given diamorphine, I felt awful, sleepy and not in charge any more; they gave me the second injection of it and I just felt worse – more sleepy, less in control. I wish I hadn't had it as it didn't take the pain away, just distanced me from it, which was fine, but I also felt distanced from the birth experience as well.' Demented

As with pethidine, diamorphine can result in breathing difficulties and floppiness in a newborn baby. An antidote called Narcan can be given in extreme cases.

Meptid, or meptazinol, is similar to pethidine but usually causes fewer side effects in both mum and baby. Like pethidine, it is usually administered via injection. The main side effects for you are nausea and vomiting. Meptid doesn't cross the placenta in quite the same way that pethidine does, so is less likely to affect the baby or cause breathing difficulties (although this is not unheard of). It doesn't make you feel quite as sleepy as pethidine does.

As with all drugs, it will work for some but not for others: 'I had Meptid and it was the most useless pain relief I have ever tried!' laments one mum. 'I looked at the midwife and said, "When can I have something else?" and she looked a bit crestfallen and said, "Ooh, about X hours!"' Another mum warns: 'Don't be fooled in to thinking that Meptid will make you stop feeling the contractions: it doesn't. But it does take a considerable edge off them for a while.'

Not all hospitals offer Meptid, largely because it is a more expensive drug than pethidine. Check that it is available in your hospital before you set your heart on it and remember that, like pethidine, it takes a while to kick in (about 15 to 20 minutes).

Pethidine, diamorphine and Meptid

Pros

- Should provide some pain relief and feelings of detachment from pain
- You can stay mobile

Cons

- Can affect the baby – particularly pethidine and diamorphine
- Baby might need additional drugs to assist breathing when born
- Baby might be sleepy when born and for the first 24 to 48 hours or so

Epidurals

More than one in three women plumps for an epidural, which speaks volumes considering it involves a very big needle. An epidural can be administered once labour is properly established; a hollow needle is inserted in between the vertebrae of your back and into the space outside the coverings that surround your spinal cord; a fine tube is then passed through the needle and the needle is removed. You need to keep very still while this happens (which isn't as easy as it sounds in full-blown labour). The tube is then left in your spine (usually taped to your shoulder) and the anaesthetic is injected through it. The anaesthetic can be 'topped up' as necessary. An anaesthetist is required to set up an epidural and it takes around 20 minutes to administer. (And possibly a lot longer to find an anaesthetist!) Epidural numbs the pain signals from your uterus and cervix (those contractions) and usually numbs your lower body too. Your anaesthetist might have a cold spray that he or she will squirt on various parts of your body asking, 'Can you feel this?' to ascertain how well (or not) the anaesthetic is working.

'My epidural was brilliant – no problems whatsoever – and I hope so much that I can have another successful one at my next baby's birth. I have to say that my birth experience was incredibly serene and chilled out.' Georgiasmum

You will probably need a urinary catheter, which will restrict your mobility, although the fact that you can't feel your legs is likely to have a similar effect. You will also need constant foetal monitoring, usually with a small monitor attached to your belly with a big elasticated strap. But, hey, with a bit of luck it should block out the pain. It allows you to remain lucid and shouldn't affect your baby as much as pethidine and diamorphine.

'I have mixed feelings about epidurals. In my first labour, it was fantastic and just what I needed at the time. I even went to sleep for a couple of hours, completely pain-free. In my second labour, I had high hopes but the damned thing didn't work; I was just left with a numb bottom and one leg that didn't move, but still lots and lots of back pain. It had no impact on the pain of the contractions and my advice would be don't get one straight away; see how you feel in labour.' tunise

Epidurals sound fabbie, and it is easy to think of them as the last miraculous resort if everything gets too much. But around 10 per cent of epidurals do not offer the magical dead-from-the-waist-down experience: 'Don't assume that an epidural will provide you with a blissful pain-free birth experience. Like all forms of pain relief during labour, it might help, or it might not,' warns one mum.

'My epidural only worked on one side! What's the point of that?! I remember one midwife reassuring me that I was only feeling windows of pain – not the kind of consolation they'd give to someone in theatre having their legs removed, is it? "Oh don't worry, it's just windows of pain ..."' Stephanie1974

Headaches are also a side effect from epidurals for some women, as one mum remembers: 'I suffered blinding headaches for my whole stay in hospital. I wasn't able to stand up on my own. I couldn't lift my daughter out of her crib. I couldn't go to the toilet.'

Some hospitals offer a low dose or 'mobile epidural' which, while dulling the pain, is intended to leave you more mobile with movement in your legs and (hopefully) the feeling of being able to push. But these things are often more art than science, and moving around can still be tricky. 'I had a mobile epidural but any time I wanted to move it was a major undertaking to navigate all the tubes and wires,' recalls one mum.

Unless the epidural wears off towards the end of your labour, which is what some women want so that they get to feel those final contractions, it can be hard to know when to push – although your midwife should be able to tell you.

'You can ask for a low-dose epidural. I did this with my second labour and it meant that I could still feel some pain (but a bearable amount), but also could feel to push when the time came. With my first baby, I couldn't feel a thing for at least an hour (when the epidural began to wear off) when it came to pushing, which meant I was relying on the midwife to tell me when to do it and it was much trickier trying to get the baby out.' Oblong

There is also an increased risk of an assisted delivery by ventouse or forceps after an epidural. Its critics would say that without sensation, you are essentially a back-seat driver and that's when events start to spiral out of control. As one mum explains: 'My primary reason for not wanting an epidural was because I didn't want to increase the likelihood of further intervention. The empowerment I felt at giving birth naturally was a huge bonus, and was an important factor in going without an epidural for my subsequent vaginal birth. But the safety factor was definitely the driving force first time round.'

'Fantastic if you can do without an epidural, but so blooming what if you can't? We all have different pain thresholds and, more importantly, we all have different labours. I had an epidural after 24 hours, most of which was spent stuck at four centimetres. Yes, the pain was bloody awful but, more importantly, I was shattered and had been told that I had at least another 12 hours ahead of me. I don't think I have "failed" in any way or that I'm weaker than those who managed to go without. Comparisons are only valid when they are on a like-for-like basis. Use them when trying to select a package holiday, a new car or a mobile-phone tariff. Don't waste your time trying to apply them to something so fundamentally unique as giving birth.' willow2

Epidurals

Pros

- May provide complete or almost complete relief from pain of contractions – hurrah!
- Can be helpful giving you a bit of time to rest or even sleep during a long labour

Cons

- More likely to result in assisted birth (forceps, ventouse, episiotomy)
- May not work, or may work only partially
- You will probably be immobile
- May not be able to feel any 'pushing' sensations
- May result in headaches
- You might not be able to walk for a few hours afterwards

Spinal block

A spinal block is a mix of an anaesthetic and a narcotic drug which is injected once into the spinal fluid. The effects are pretty instant and last for a few hours. A spinal block is not usually offered to labouring women because the feelings of numbness can be quite drastic (feeling completely numb from the chest down is normal); it is usually reserved for Caesarean sections because it gives pain relief, but allows the mum to stay 'awake' during delivery, rather than being completely zonked out by a general anaesthetic.

Mumsnetiquette: Top gas-and-air hits

'After being deathly quiet for five hours while having contractions, I had my first puff of gas and air. I immediately went "Woooo!" so loudly that people in the car park outside the window started laughing. Then I proceeded to sing "Rocket Man", emphasising the line, "I'm gonna be high as kite", at the top of my lungs. I started to insist that we go Christmas shopping right this second and I had to be dragged back from the corridor as I used the going-for-a-wee ruse to try to make my escape. I had my handbag, but was naked apart from my bra.' *Kylah*

'After a little too much gas and air I turned to my husband and asked: "Am I having a pedicure?"' *NineUnlikelyTales*

'After 30 hours of labour and being told I would need help to get the baby out by a timid doctor, I was shouting, "Whatever! Am I bovered?" Catherine Tate style. Then, apparently, laughing hysterically when the stroppy midwife bashed her head accidently on a low overhead light while she tried to wrestle the gas and air from me.' *missymum*

'I kept saying: "Luke, I am your father," in between puffs of gas and air. What can I say? The noise of the gas and air reminded me of Darth Vader.' *bigbumhole*

'I was in the bath on all fours at home when the baby started to crown. High on gas and air, I was convinced the baby was coming down the wrong chute. I stage-whispered to the midwife: "The baby is coming out of my bum. Honestly. It really is. I can feel it." She said calmly: "Well, we've never had that before ..."' *annieapple7*

Breathing That Baby Out

'Don't forget to breathe' might sound like the most obvious piece of advice you can give someone, but using special breathing techniques during labour can really help get you through each contraction, stop you pushing at the wrong time and go some way to ensuring a smoother labour.

If you've booked into antenatal classes, you should expect to cover breathing techniques at some point. The good news is you can use these techniques anywhere you choose to give birth – home, hospital, birthing pool, Waitrose car park – and they won't have anything but a positive effect on your baby.

The downside is that, to be effective, practice makes perfect, and you can feel like a complete numpty puffing away at home when the only thing going on is the washing machine. But it's really worth doing your homework, so here are a few things to try.

And... breathe...

It's not exactly rocket science: just breathe slowly in and out through each contraction. Try to keep to a regular rhythm and keep the 'out' breath as long, if not slightly longer, than the 'in' breath.

It can help to count your way through each breath – so breathe in for three and out for four – and to breathe in through your nose and out through your mouth.

Breathing for active labour

As each contraction starts, give out a long 'sighing' breath and then try to keep to the slow, regular breathing above – in through your nose and out through your mouth.

As the contraction builds up, you might feel the need to take faster, lighter breaths; just don't overdo it.

At the contraction's peak it can help to pant – like a dog! – in and out through your mouth, interspersed with a deeper breath every few breaths or so.

As the contraction ebbs, slow your breathing back down, so that you're back to breathing slowly and regularly by the end of it.

'The breathing techniques I learnt at my NCT classes were amazing; I managed to fully dilate without too much pain at all when I focused on them.' charlotte121

Breathing during transition

As you near or reach transition, you may feel a desperate urge to push ... which you desperately need to resist until your midwife gives you the green light. (If you're not fully dilated you can do yourself a great disservice by trying to get your baby out early.)

Your midwife will undoubtedly ask you not to push and probably advise on how best to breathe at this point – but panting and blowing out on your 'out' breath can help hugely ... as can getting on all fours and sticking your bum in the air (nobody said labour was glamorous).

To practise this at home – the breathing, not the bum bit – try a 'pant, pant, blow' routine. (*Strictly Come Dancing* fans might like to think of this as 'quick, quick, slow'.) When you blow out, imagine you're trying to almost, but not quite, blow a candle out.

Breathing during delivery

Unless your midwife tells you otherwise, try not to hold your breath while you're pushing. It's easy to burst a facial blood vessel, which won't look great for those first pictures of you and your baby.

As each contraction starts, breathe in and out gently, and then, when you feel the urge to push, take a deep breath in, tuck your chin into your chest and breathe or blow out slowly as you bear down.

Try to be led by what your body's telling you to do. Unless you have an epidural, then your body will actually push on its own, regardless of how you're breathing.

Keeping your pelvic floor as relaxed as possible, push from between your legs, rather than holding the tension in your throat, neck or face. (Yes, we know this appears stupidly obvious, but, in reality, it can be much harder than it sounds.) You'll probably want to push about four times per contraction – so don't forget to take a big breath in before each push.

Some women do small, frequent pushes. They should be spontaneous rather than organised with big breaths – unless you have an epidural and can't feel to push.

As your baby crowns you may be told to stop pushing and just pant – this will help slow things down a bit and can help to prevent you tearing.

'My son was almost born in the hospital car park, so I did it with no pain relief. The really painful bit was in the 40-minute journey to hospital. It sounds clichéd, but I made myself breathe to deal with it and it really worked.' Whistlejacket

Getting help with breathing during labour

Giving birth can be frightening, and when you're scared your breathing rate speeds up and becomes erratic and inefficient at getting oxygen into your lungs. Your baby needs oxygen – and so do you. And if you don't get enough you will feel wobbly and tire quickly, just when you need as much energy as possible. Holding your breath for a long time will have a similar effect. This is where your birth partner can help by breathing with you during your labour. If in doubt, ask your midwife to show you what to do.

You need eye-to-eye and physical contact for this to work well, so have your partner face you and hold your hands (or they can put their hands on your shoulders and lean forward gently on them) and have them breathe in through their nose and blow out gently on to your face. Following the pattern of these breaths will help you to focus on regulating and slowing your own breathing back down.

Your partner can also help by counting for you as you breathe – this will help you keep your breathing speed under control – or by reminding you to 'pant, pant, blow' and so on.

'Breathing helped me, although I've no idea whether it was just because I was concentrating on it rather than the pain or whether it was a more physiological reason ... or perhaps a bit of both. I used the word "relax" to help me: I breathed in to "re" and out on "lax". It worked really well until my partner kept asking, "Are you having a contraction?" and expecting me to answer! (I'm breathing deeply and swaying around like a cow with a grimace on my face ... what do you think dumbass?!)' TillyScoutsmum

> Co-breathing/counting can also work well with the other styles of breathing mentioned above, so take time out to practise together with your birth partner before you go into labour. You want them to feel prepared and confident about helping you if you need it: if you both understand what's going to work best, and when, you'll have a much better chance of co-breathing working for you. Admittedly, you'll probably both feel rather daft doing this at home (we know we did), but during labour it can give you a massive boost.

'At the start I found that using gas and air helped me focus on my breathing. Then things started moving up a gear and I remember groaning as the urge to push got stronger. Meanwhile, my husband was being an absolute star and counting my breathing in and out, so I didn't lose focus. There was one brief point, which I guess was transition, where I felt I was losing it, but he got very stern about the breathing and brought me back into control. I could feel the baby moving down and was overawed at the realisation that there were actually two of us involved in this experience, it was just so amazing.' Milkycheeks

Water Babies – What Are Water Births Really Like?

'Fabulous.' 'Fantastic.' 'Amazing.' 'The best thing ever.' What on earth are Mumsnetters so excited about? A Marc Jacobs for Primark maternity range? Giving birth in your sleep? Jelly-belly firming cream? Nope. 'Water births rock!'

'Just had my first baby in a hospital pool. It was an amazing experience. I was four centimetres dilated when I got in. I had the urge to push an hour later and delivered 15 minutes after that. No tears; no pain relief. The sight of my baby swimming up to the surface still brings tears to my eyes. My midwife was very handy with the sieve and I delivered the placenta into a bowl so the water was very clean at the end. You retain a lot more privacy and therefore dignity under the water and, because it is more difficult to examine you, the midwives are more hands off which was what I wanted.' Jocesar

Some women find that with water supporting the bump, the pain of the contractions is eased. This is the main attraction of labouring in water. The warmth and buoyancy of the water can also be soothing for women who have back pain.

Experts tend to be divided on whether giving birth in water is best for babies; but it is something that has been done for thousands of years – there are even hieroglyphs on the temples in Egypt depicting women giving birth in the River Nile. Some hospital labour wards and midwife-led units have birthing pool suites but you can't guarantee that they won't be in use. If you fancy giving it a go, write in your birth plan that you want a water birth but also make sure that your birth partner tells the hospital when they telephone to let them know that you are coming in. Some hospitals ask that you attend an induction session in advance to learn more about giving birth in water and there may be some health checks:

'I'd set my heart on a water birth and dutifully attended the hospital session explaining it all, but there were concerns about my iron levels, so they weren't keen on letting me use it. I managed to get my iron levels up in the end to a reasonable level, so it's worth getting checked out as early as possible in your pregnancy if you think you might want to use the pool, to make sure you're eligible.' Munchpot

It is recommended that you don't get into the pool too early – before you are 5 centimetres dilated, as being too relaxed at this stage may slow down the contractions. Immersed, fans say they feel in a world of their own. Because of the water bearing your weight, you should feel more mobile and able to try out different positions, whether this is squatting, kneeling or floating. 'The stillness gives you a great sense of calm and helps your concentration levels, so that you can focus on the job in hand,' says a water birth veteran. 'It gives you a new lease of life when you need it.' It can also reduce tearing.

But bear in mind that, aside from gas and air, you will not be allowed any other forms of pain relief while you are in the pool. 'I had a "perfect water birth", but it was still agony. I can

only conclude that all vaginal births are horrific!' chirps one
optimistic mum.

'After about five hours of labouring in hospital I
had had enough and wanted stronger pain relief
as I was in agony, but the midwife suggested
I try the birthing pool. It was not something I
had considered before as I was aiming for hard
drugs, but gave it a go. She said if I didn't like
it I could get out and move on to pethidine, but
that once I had pethidine I couldn't use the pool.
Once I got into the pool the relief was enormous.
I still had gas and air and spent the next five
hours in there and it was fab. I was still in a lot
of pain but the water was very relaxing and I do
think it helped me. In the end I had to get out
for the last hour as my son's head was stuck so I
needed a bit of help. I would really recommend
it. My advice would be to keep an open mind
about labour, see how you feel, use the birthing
pool if you can.' Lovelybird

One thing that puts some people off water births is the fact that
you tend to open your bowels when you are in the second stage
of labour. This is quite normal and at the time you are unlikely
to be worried about it. 'I pooed in the birthing pool!' one mum
cheerfully confesses. 'But I also wet myself in the lift on the way to
the delivery suite!' If you are labouring on land, the midwife will
whip the gunk away with expert ease, and in a pool, she will sift
any floaters out with practised discretion. 'Don't be embarrassed
about pooing in the pool,' reassures one hardened parent. 'They
are ready prepared and won't bat an eyelid. And if your husband is
flagging, you can threaten him with sieve duties to perk him up.'

'I had my third child in a birthing pool which was fab, apart from the bit where I thought I was pushing him out and instead, up floated a nice big poo – which was swiftly scooped out by the midwife using a plastic sieve. I didn't find it funny at the time ...' CillaField

Getting naked is another sticking point. It's hard to imagine, but labour is a very animal experience, and lots of women find that having any clothes on is horribly uncomfortable. So, even the most prudish lady might find herself throwing her knickers across the labour room and parading around, while mooing loudly without a care in the world. As one mum says, 'I was going to wear a tankini top, as I didn't want to be naked, but somehow, dignity goes out of the window and you just don't care. I was much more comfy with no clothes on. My advice is to let yourself go and just do whatever it takes to get through the labour.'

Having your business end under water can be a relief for women who may feel inhibited and exposed labouring on dry land. Some women like to have their partners join them in the pool to provide moral and physical support. Others balk at the idea; for some, a big part of the attraction is that they are pretty much left to their own devices, without being prodded and poked.

To anyone who isn't pregnant, or Hugh Hefner, the thought of installing and filling an enormous paddling pool in their front room might seem faintly ridiculous. But for a number of women who have set their hearts on a home water birth it is cause for great excitement. Weeks even before their first contraction, some are neck high in water, enjoying a nightly wallow in their front room. 'I hired the pool for a month and it was wonderful in the last few weeks to spend the evening lying in a warm pool heaven,' says a contented water-baby mum.

You can rent or buy birthing pools; some are assembled with nuts and bolts, others have to be inflated. They can be filled by a garden hose attached to your warm water tap, and topped up with water from the kettle to maintain a nice toasty temperature.

Even if you don't use your pool beforehand it might be a good idea to practise putting it up to avoid any Frank Spencer-style accidents. Especially important is to note how long it takes to fill and how you empty it. (Most have a valve at the bottom to which you can attach a hose to siphon off the water.) This involves gravity, of course, so don't fill it in your cellar unless you have a handy drain near by. 'We had a pond pump which we used to pump out the water down the drain,' recalls one resourceful mum, adding that this was 'after my husband had used the sieve'!

If you are having a home birth and sourcing a pool to use at home, you will have to decide on a suitable size and shape (oval, hexagonal or round). Think about whether you will need extra room for your partner, what positions you might labour in and, of course, how much space you have to accommodate it. One Mumsnetter who gave birth in the summer chose to set up her pool in the garden. (This might not be ideal if you are overlooked by a block of flats.) Indoors, your floor will need to be able to take the weight of the pool and you may need padding underneath to give you a comfortable base.

The temperature of the water in your pool will need to be checked hourly; it can be topped up with warm water, if necessary, but it must never exceed 37 degrees Celsius (body temperature). Most pools come with a lockable cover to keep the heat in – and nosy pets out.

Clearing up is easier if you have a lining for the pool. And be prepared for the water to look as though you have shared a bath with Jaws. Your midwife and birth partner can deal with that side of things though; you will be too busy saying hello to your little one.

It is not unusual for mothers to labour in a pool then come out to deliver their baby. 'Not all midwives are confident or practised in delivering babies in water,' explains one mum. 'But even if you use the pool for pain relief it really helps, and keeps you calm as you can float about in between contractions and get into so many more positions.' You just have to go with the flow (literally) and see how things progress. 'I delivered my son's head into the birthing pool and then we discovered his shoulders were stuck,' recalls one mum. 'So I had to climb out of the pool, walk across the room and deliver the rest of him on to the bed!'

If you decide to stay in the water, you might want to 'catch' the baby as she comes out – but don't worry, she won't drown: your baby has already been swimming in water inside you. Babies have a 'diving reflex' which means that they don't take their first breath until they feel air on their skin. Your midwife will be paying lots of attention at this point, so don't feel that you have to 'do' anything. 'The pool is not so deep that you need to dive for the baby,' reassures one mum. 'I was so relieved that the birth part was over that I watched the baby floating around in the water,' recalls another. 'I was vaguely aware of some sort of instruction from the midwife, but I shouted, "Pick her up for me!" because I was too shocked to move!'

'I heard the midwife say, "Catch her", so I reached down and she swam up into my arms. It was the best feeling in the world and I'm crying typing it. She is perfect. And a girl and ohhhh, the world is just wonderful. No stitches, no grazing, nothing, just bliss. I'm in love and so lucky and everything is great.' Thomcat

Generally, you will be asked to get out of the tub to deliver the placenta, so your midwife can check for tearing and blood loss. Don't panic when you step out of the tub and appear to deposit several hundred gallons of blood on to the floor – the water makes it look much worse than it really is. If you need stitches, you should be offered a local anaesthetic beforehand. As with all births, for any major repair work you might need to be transferred to the hospital (if you are at home) or to the theatre (if you are in hospital).

Not everybody gets the hot-tub experience they had hoped for. 'I really didn't like it,' says one mum who scrambled out after five minutes. 'I felt out of control.' But unlike an epidural or pethidine, you can always try it, then change your mind.

Breech Babies – The Baby's Not For Turning?

Your baby isn't even born yet and you are already struggling to get it to do what you want. For goodness sake, you just want him to turn over! It's not as if you are asking him to tidy up his amniotic sac.

It's normal for babies in utero to ferret around to find a comfortable position but, during the final weeks of your pregnancy, the way they are lying takes on a new significance because it could determine how you will give birth. Head down (cephalic) is the optimal position for a streamlined departure (or maybe that should be arrival?) but around 3 per cent of babies are 'breech'. This means that instead of coming out head first, there is a bottom or foot pointing to the exit instead. (Your baby can also be 'transverse', which is another problem whereby it lies across your abdomen rather than head down.) There's not always an obvious reason for a breech position. It is more common in twin and in premature births (because lots of babies are breech until quite late in the pregnancy). Or maybe your baby is just bloody-minded.

Upside down and back to front: types of breech

Extended breech (or frank breech): bottom down, legs above the head. Imagine a baby that's folded neatly in two. This is the most common breech presentation and accounts for about 65 per cent of all breeches.

Flexed breech (or complete breech): bottom down, cross-legged – sort of in the lotus position. Think of this as your Buddhist baby. About 25 per cent of breech babies present this way.

Footling breech: bottom down, with one or both legs down under the bottom – in a sort of awkward kneeling position. This accounts for about 10 per cent of breech presentations.

'My baby had her head rammed up against my ribs from what seemed like five months onwards. She turned herself at about 36 weeks, to my relief, though it was a rather uncomfortable night. It felt like there was some kind of wrestling match going on in there.' foodfiend

It isn't unusual for babies to be breech in early pregnancy – they tend to turn as you reach full term, in preparation for the birth. By palpating your tummy – feeling it with the flat of the hand – your midwife should be able to tell you the whereabouts of various body parts, and therefore which position your baby is lying in. If you are only 35 weeks or so and you have been told your baby is breech, don't worry – there is still lots of time for your baby to flip over.

If your midwife suspects a breech presentation, and it is getting near your due date, then you will probably be booked in for a scan so that the exact position of your baby can be determined. If it is a footling breech (or twins), you will usually be recommended for a Caesarean section. If it is a frank breech, your midwife or consultant will discuss your options with you and it will probably be left to you to decide whether to proceed with a vaginal birth or whether to opt for an elective Caesarean.

Why is a vaginal birth more risky with a breech presentation?

A breech birth is riskier than a head-down delivery, largely because they are much less common and so very few midwives have had experience in managing them. The more breech babies are delivered by Caesarean section, the more the skills of delivering a breech baby vaginally are being lost, but – understandably – no one wants to be a training ground.

Of course, the risks are also medical. A baby in breech position is not in the optimal position for a safe vaginal delivery. There is an increased risk of cord prolapse, where the umbilical cord comes out before the baby, and the pressure of the baby on the cord then cuts off the baby's oxygen supply – this can result in brain damage or even death if the baby is not delivered immediately. Brain and skull injury is another complication of a breech birth, due to the sudden compression of the baby's skull when it passes through the birth canal quite quickly (a procedure which is long and slow during a head-first delivery). There are also dangers associated with the instrumental interventions that may be required, such as damage from forceps and rough handling that might be necessary to deliver the baby safely.

What can I do to turn the baby?

If your baby doesn't turn, there are steps you can take to encourage it to budge. The best place to start is probably with 'optimal foetal positioning' exercises. Don't worry, these are not actual exercises and don't involve any sweating or effort on your part – 'they are mainly variations on getting your bum higher than your chest,' explains one mum. Optimal foetal positioning is based on the theory that a baby's position in the womb is influenced by the mother's position and movement during the final weeks of pregnancy. Your midwife should be able to advise you and provide leaflets with information on exercises. When sitting, you need to try to keep your knees lower than your bottom – so no slumping back in old armchairs. Crouching and swaying on all fours with your bottom in the air is also supposed to help. 'I spent the last few weeks of my pregnancy watching television in a mirror propped up my sofa, while kneeling against the sofa with my bum in the air,' confesses one mum. You might find that keeping active and naturally adopting these sorts of positions helps: another mum's baby turned after she spent an evening 'crawling about on the floor assembling the pushchair'.

Your midwife or consultant may suggest external cephalic version (ECV). This is where a doctor attempts to physically 'flip' your baby over by pressing on your abdomen. ECV is usually performed around 37 weeks – although you can have it as late as at the onset of labour. It works for around 50 per cent of babies (you might want to find out the success rate of the obstetrician carrying out the procedure), but it isn't an option if yours is a multiple pregnancy or if you have placenta praevia (see p. 250).

ECVs are far safer than they used to be due to advances in scanning and monitoring techniques. They used to be done 'blind', but now the position of your baby, the placenta and the cord are checked, and your baby's heartbeat is monitored before and after the procedure to check that he isn't under stress. You will have various ultrasound scans and may be given a drug to relax the muscles in the uterus. A doctor will then attempt to shift your baby by gently pushing on your abdomen to lift your baby out of the pelvis and encourage him to do a 'forward roll' so that he is head down. 'Although it was uncomfortable and felt very strange it was all over very quickly,' says a mother whose ECV was successful.

'I had ECV at 37 weeks after all the alternative stuff failed. There are a lot of horror stories about ECV, mainly put about by people who've never had one. For me it was uncomfortable but not agony – and it was effective. Once the baby has been turned you have as much chance of a natural delivery as anybody else.' Frogs

Some women do find ECV painful, but make sure you make your concerns known at the time – you may be offered gas and air, or your doctor can stop during the procedure. Even if it is successful, there is a chance that your baby might turn back again, which is beyond frustrating, but you can always wait a few days and have another go.

There are a number of less invasive 'alternative' treatments for turning babies. Some swear by the Webster Technique, whereby a trained chiropractor makes a few adjustments to your pelvis, hopefully giving your baby the room it needs to get into the correct position. Others recommend moxibustion, a traditional Chinese technique which involves holding lit sticks, made from a herb called mugwort, above acupuncture points on your feet. The idea is that the muscles in the uterus relax, allowing your baby to turn. 'I've been taught to do it at home, but my husband has been complaining about the smell,' warns one mum-to-be; 'he made me finish the treatment in the greenhouse.' Or, you may need to rope in a friend to help:

'I spent an afternoon kneeling at my pregnant friend's feet holding the sticks for her. Her bump was so large she couldn't manage to hold the sticks easily (or even safely) herself and her husband thought it was a lot of mumbo jumbo so wasn't much use. I can also vouch for the stink – we did it in the garden. The good news is it

worked for her and the baby turned in time for the birth.' Hollee

Some put their trust in reflexology: 'A friend was giving me fortnightly reflexology sessions and I mentioned the position of the baby to her. After the session I felt a lot of wriggling around, and – hey presto! – at my next check the baby had gone head down.' Homeopathy fans may suggest Pulsatilla, and at least one Mumsnetter is convinced that this worked for her: 'I was getting so worried he wasn't going to turn and I think it was the Pulsatilla and cold orange juice in the end.'

There is a theory that babies gravitate away from cold, and many a concerned mum has spent an evening or two with a packet of frozen peas on the top of their belly. Some get so desperate they will try almost anything, including visualising their baby with its head engaged and telling him in a firm voice to 'Turn!' Others believe that babies turn towards the light – but if the sun doesn't shine out of your business end, you can always try a torch: 'My sister turned her breech baby at 38 weeks,' says one supportive sister. 'It's a bit off the wall, but it worked for her. Go into a dark room with a torch, strip naked, kneel on all fours with your bum in the air and shine the torch where you want the baby's head to end up.'

The prize for cheekiest breech baby has to go to the daughter of a Mumsnetter who was in a breech position but then turned halfway through the planned Caesarean. She was sent straight to the naughty step.

So what should I do?

The best way to deliver a baby that won't budge from the breech position is still a grey area. Not all midwives are experienced in vaginal breech births – and it is the experience of the midwife which is the crucial factor as far as a safe delivery is concerned.

If you would rather avoid a Caesarean, find out how experienced your delivery team is at vaginal breech births and their success rate. Explore every avenue and take heart that whichever route you go down it has worked for women with babies in a similar awkward position.

'My second daughter was breech, and no amount of consultant prodding and palpating, acupuncture, moxibustion, sitting with my knees on the sofa and my elbows on the floor could get her to turn. BUT I did have a fantastic delivery. I was devastated not to be allowed the home birth I wanted, but in the end it was by far the best birth of all my children. She was a footling breech, and the midwife got a mirror so we could see her little purple foot emerging. Of course, I'd had to have an epidural (never would have countenanced one normally, but was given no choice, and thought it was marvellous in the event), so I was relaxed and focused, and it was all really peaceful and magical.' 3PRINCESSES

Midwives are usually not keen to proceed with a home birth if you have a breech presentation, because of the additional risks. You should still be allowed the choice, even if your midwife is not happy, but it is important to have a midwife in attendance who is practised and confident at delivering breech babies. 'I had an independent midwife and she also found a second midwife who was experienced in breech births,' writes one mum who had a home breech birth. 'It went very much to plan and my daughter is happy and healthy.'

In general, most consultants will recommend a Caesarean as the safest option, although some believe the best approach is to proceed as normal provided that your labour is progressing well.

'I had a C-section with my eldest child who was breech. My delivery team were fantastic, letting me go into labour normally but I did end up with a Caesarean. It was a good experience; calm, relaxed, and the staff were very supportive. The important thing was that we had discussed what would happen if I had a section just as you would for a normal birth and all our wishes were followed, right down to the music. I subsequently had two vaginal deliveries.' Philly

Should you opt for a Caesarean and your midwife or consultant thinks this is the best approach, be assured that this is a very common way of managing breech births. The important thing is that you and your baby are healthy, so however you decide to manage it, just look forward to the moment when you meet for the first time.

Being Induced – Come Out, Come Out , Wherever You Are ...

Sex, half a dozen curries, a crate-load of pineapple, long walks, gallons of raspberry leaf tea and enough nipple twiddling to give you RSI, yet still your baby isn't showing signs of turning up any time soon. OK, so nobody likes to be rushed, but come on! You feel you would do anything to get to hold your bambino in your arms, or at least to be able to sit down on a chair without fear of breaking it.

Anything, that is, except induction. Just the thought of it makes pregnant women clench their buttocks in horror – and that's no mean feat. Yet there comes a point in every pregnancy when it feels as though your options are starting to run out. Is being induced really that bad?

In an age where organic is king, the idea of artificially kick-starting your labour can seem grossly unnatural. Fluffier approaches such as acupuncture and reflexology probably sound more appealing. But beyond 42 weeks, the general line is that your baby is safer out than in because of the risk of developing serious health problems. It is not uncommon for women to leave their 41 week antenatal appointment feeling that induction is inevitable. But not everyone agrees. 'I resisted induction, despite a shedload of pressure from all angles and everything was fine,' says a determined mother who went 18 days past her due date before delivering her son. 'They can't drag you into hospital.'

Around one in five pregnant women in the UK ends up being induced, either before or after their due date. There are usually, but not always, medical reasons to hurry things along before your due date, such as pre-eclampsia or gestational diabetes (see pp. 242 and 255). And around your due date, if your waters have broken but your contractions haven't started, you and your baby may be at risk of infection. And the further you go after 42 weeks, the more the risks to your baby.

Generally, induction is not a lot of fun. 'With induction, you have no build-up to get used to the contractions,' explains one mum. 'They just start: wham!' Also, if you are induced, you are more likely to need intervention in the form of forceps and ventouse, and you may end up with a C-section. Unfortunately, it tends to be the horror stories that get passed on and give inductions a bad rap. But, as one mum writes: 'Induction is not bad for everyone. I was induced with my third and it was great. All controlled, no rushing to the hospital in the middle of the night.'

'I was induced with my first baby at 38 weeks and it was wonderful. I had prostaglandins overnight. I woke up to artificial rupture of the membranes and a pitocin drip. Twelve hours later (including only six hours of actual labour), my son was born. I didn't have any other interventions and didn't bother with an epidural as I got on fine with no medical pain relief. I found it no more or less painful than my natural, second labour.' MKG

Why can't I let my baby cook for a bit longer?

You've spent nine months obsessing about this baby, and once you are past your due date, your baby automatically feels 'late' and things can start to feel a little ominous. But there is no reason to think this way – a standard pregnancy lasts anywhere from 38 to 42 weeks. If your pregnancy is continuing normally and you have not been told otherwise, there is no need to proceed with inductions before 42 weeks.

The risks of leaving the pregnancy for longer than 42 weeks are that the placenta starts to deteriorate and this may affect the baby. You may be on the receiving end of alarmist messages from your medical team. One Mumsnetter was horrified to be told by her midwife at 40 weeks: 'You've lasted for nine months – why put your baby at risk now?' But placentas do not have a 'Best before 40 weeks' date stamped on them, so, if you are keen to avoid induction, you should be offered monitoring (scans of the baby, placenta and amniotic fluid and monitoring of the baby's heart) to assess the situation. After 42 weeks, this must be done at least twice a week.

'I would avoid induction for as long as you safely can. My induction didn't work and was really a very unpleasant experience. Fifty hours later I had a C-section which was a wonderful, positive experience.' Hulababy

If you want to know more about induction and the NHS guidelines about it, the NICE guidelines (National Institute for Health and Clinical Excellence at www.nice.org.uk) on induction of labour are a useful place to start. They are quite clear and lay out the procedures that NHS hospitals are advised to follow.

What's the problem with inductions?

The main drawback with inductions is that once you start on the treadmill, it's hard to get off – and the more interventions that you have, the more complicated the delivery is likely to be. No one daydreams of being virtually tied to a bed with a drip while giant forceps are wielded by the bulging arms of a middle-aged consultant (or if you do, it's best not to discuss this with your husband).

One experienced Mumsnet doula explains how induction interventions can escalate:

'The pessary softens and ripens the cervix, and can start it dilating without the need for any further intervention. Often though, the pessary is followed by another pessary ... and once the cervix is sufficiently dilated, the membranes are ruptured. Then, if labour is not deemed strong enough, Syntocinon is given via a drip to augment the labour.' Lulumama

Although you might be desperate to get rid of your titanic pregnancy bulk, it's really best to avoid going down the artificial induction route if you possibly can. Instead, try natural ways of encouraging labour. Mumsnetters recommend, among other things, semen, curry, pineapples and long walks (see p. 343); make sure you know exactly what it is that you are supposed to do with each of these though – unless you want to end up with a criminal record and a lifetime of embarrassing gynaecological appointments.

Semen is full of prostaglandins, so sprinkle some on your granola or have sex with your partner. Pineapple is delicious and nutritious and – allegedly – it contains an enzyme that might soften your cervix (although it's just as likely that it will cause the runs, which might trigger your uterine contractions too). Walking is highly recommended, and although a gentle stroll is what most sensible medics would advise, Mumsnetters advise upping your pace a little: 'Walk fast – at the sort of rate that makes old ladies gasp in horror!' Being upright encourages your baby to bounce around on your cervix, which might start things off – so going for a walk or gently bouncing on your birthing ball are both good.

'I've been scoffing pineapple all afternoon, off for a walk now, making a vindaloo for supper and told my husband that he's on a promise tonight ...' clemsterdarcy

Cervical sweep

Unless your waters have broken, the first medical attempt at induction is usually a 'cervical sweep' or a 'stretch and sweep'. This is about as much fun as a smear test, except to add to the sense of jollity it's a finger rather than a speculum that is inserted. As one mum puts it: 'It's just like an internal, but with extra rummaging.' The midwife or doctor inserts a finger into your vagina, easing the opening of the cervix slightly. They then 'sweep' round with their finger, rupturing the membranes from the cervix. This is supposed to encourage the release of prostaglandins and kick-start contractions. After the procedure, you will normally be sent home to see how things progress.

The downsides are that it can be uncomfortable or even painful. It may cause a little bleeding – although that shouldn't last long. The positive side is that it can work to start labour and reduces rates of chemically inducing labour by around 20 per cent. A cervical sweep is usually done (and is most effective) around week 41, and if it is going to start the action, you should see some results within 48 hours. If it doesn't work, you might want to try another sweep.

'My midwife recommended I had two sweeps before they would induce me, in case the first one didn't work. The second one caused me to have a show, then within a few hours I was in labour – such a relief, as I was booked in to be induced the next day. It is not much worse than a smear. I'd definitely have one – especially if you are coming up to your induction date.' Nickyfen

Prostaglandins

If the sweep doesn't work, next up are prostaglandins, which are hormones given as a pessary or gel in the vagina that help the cervix to soften and contractions to start. They are usually administered using a long, thin applicator. Your baby will be monitored for a while before and afterwards, to check that she is not being stressed by the induction. Some hospitals might send you out for a walk after this, so don't be surprised to find yourself, post-pessary, out on the street, looking longingly in the windows of Mothercare, as you wait for your first contraction.

You might need more than one dose, and they may not kick things off at all – but for some women, this does do the trick.

'I had two pessaries, twelve hours apart. The second one really kicked things off. However, the midwives kept telling me it was going to be ages yet (implying a drip would be needed) and it wasn't. Twenty-five-minute second stage, and out popped my son with no other intervention.' Booboobedoo

Artificial rupture of the membranes (ARM)

If your waters haven't broken, the doctor or midwife might use a small crochet-type hook to puncture the amniotic sac and release the tidal flow.

'The midwife took a small plastic implement, about 10 inches long, with a tiny hook at the top. It was very quick – she just sort of tugged at the sac and whoosh.' Pie

ARM is sometimes done to speed up a slow labour or to try to encourage labour to progress once the cervix has dilated. It is quite a controversial procedure because it generally leads to more painful contractions and often swiftly escalates into more interventions. It can also increase the risk of cord prolapse. There is also debate about whether it has much of an effect on speeding up labour. For this reason, many people believe this to be an unnecessary intervention in the course of a normal labour.

'The research shows that breaking the waters only speeds up labour by one hour, if you are lucky. It does intensify pain and it is more likely that the baby will become distressed because they are no longer cushioned. If all is well, there is absolutely no need to break the waters at all.' (Mumsnetter midwife) mears

Letting things proceed naturally if you can still move around – keeping upright and walking about – might speed things up to your midwife's satisfaction, and this, in turn, might avoid the need for interventions such as ARM. Unfortunately, if you are being constantly monitored, this may be very difficult to do.

'I had ARM in my first labour and there were no problems with the baby, and it was a pretty quick labour too. I wish I hadn't agreed, but I was keen to get everything over with and that was the angle the midwife used to persuade me. The contractions did get far worse. In retrospect, I would have preferred the midwife to have encouraged me to move around more, instead of breaking the membranes, but they were intent on me having the heart-rate monitor strapped around me (which I hated) and so I was mostly lying on a bed.' MummyPig

Oxytocin (Syntocinon or Pitocin)

If all else fails, you may be given a synthetic form of the hormone oxytocin, usually Syntocinon or Pitocin, via a drip. Once this has started, your mobility is very much restricted: you will usually be monitored quite closely and may find yourself effectively tied to the bed with drips and monitors.

Some mums say that the Syntocinon/Pitocin drip made their contractions stronger and more painful, and many choose to step up the pain relief, perhaps requesting an epidural.

'The induction caused the contractions to come quickly together. I had no chance to recharge my batteries between contractions, so it felt more painful than my first labour, which was not induced. If I could do things over again, induction or not, I would just request epidurals right at the start of labour.' TeriHatchetJob

On the upside, it might make for a speedier delivery. 'After a long day in hospital trying to get things moving, my midwife was very relaxed and didn't expect me to deliver until the next morning; fortunately, my husband only went as far as the local Tesco Metro, because suddenly it all speeded up and our baby was born within minutes of his return,' warns one mum. However, this might mean that there is no time for pain relief: 'If you want an epidural, make sure everyone knows about it as early as possible,' advises one mum. 'I asked too late and the pain was hellish.'

If all of the above fail to get things moving, then you are likely to be offered a Caesarean. Around 22 per cent of induced births will end with a Caesarean. This may be frustrating, to say the least, but as one relieved mum puts it: 'By the time we reached the stage of having a Caesarean, I'd have been happy for them to bring her out through any available orifice. I just wanted her out.'

'It's a cliché, but once you finally hold that baby in your arms, you really don't care how they got there. I suppose, once the euphoria dies down, you may have a moment's regret that you didn't get the birth you planned, but certainly in my experience, the baby makes up for all of it.' Beebee

Monitoring

Generally, with inductions you are more likely to be subjected to continuous foetal and contraction monitoring. You should be monitored before induction begins, to assess your baby's normal heart rate and then continually which, unfortunately, means being stuck in bed unable to move. As movement and remaining upright are great for encouraging labour to progress, this can be frustrating and depressing. 'Ask not to be strapped to the monitor the whole time,' advises one mum. 'I desperately wanted to move around but couldn't.'

'What I most disliked about the induction was that I spent a lot of my rather long labour (26.5 hours) strapped up to monitoring equipment. I progressed steadily, but just very slowly – even with a drip to speed things up (one of the reasons for the monitoring). A ventouse was used at the end, but it worked. That in itself didn't upset me; I just hated being so restricted in movement for so much of the time.' elkiedee

If the initial monitoring shows that you and baby are quite healthy and things are progressing normally, you might be monitored at regular intervals rather than continually. If this is the case, try to be as upright and active as possible (gentle walks, bouncing on a birthing ball) in order to encourage the labour to progress.

It can be nerve-racking turning up at the hospital with your mini-break bag, not knowing what to expect. Although you are there to speed things up, hospital time can move incredibly slowly. 'For me the whole thing was really easy and stress-free, but incredibly boring,' says a mother who took along magazines, a radio, puzzle books and board games, but still found it hard to distract herself.

Induction doesn't necessarily mean you will have a prolonged, extra-painful labour. There are plenty of positive stories from women who have been induced. 'I was induced a week early with my son and had a fab birth,' says one mother of three. 'My labour was one hour and 15 minutes from the start of contractions to delivery. He was born in a birthing pool. I would have no worries about being induced again. Out of all my births, this was the best.' Another says: 'The pain wasn't as bad as I'd expected. The midwife noticed when the contractions were getting too close and too quick and decreased the drip accordingly. I hated not being very mobile, but still insisted on being on all fours to push the baby out.'

'The most important thing when being induced is to make sure you understand everything that might happen and to make sure that staff are aware of your wishes.' Littlelamb

Discuss things with your birth partner, so that you can make choices and decisions together. And remember: whatever they have to do to get it out, hopefully it won't be too long before you are holding your gorgeous baby in your arms.

Mumsnetiquette: Bring it on (or let's get this labour started) – but how?

Sex Semen is a great source of natural prostaglandins which can 'ripen' the cervix. But don't be too harsh on your partner if he looks pale at the suggestion. And if you have been advised not to have sex, or if your waters have broken, then *down boy*.

Nipple tweaking If you are bored with daytime television, you could try playing with your nipples, which can bring on labour.

(continued)

But you have to do it for a few hours each day, so you might want to multitask and watch and tweak at the same time.

Visualisation You are opening like a flower. Your baby is moving down. Your perineum is gently tearing. Oops, sorry.

Walking A brisk stroll can be just the job – but make sure you don't go so far that you need to be air-lifted out in the event of any action – and this is a great time to enjoy a peaceful, long evening walk with your partner. Try walking sideways up and down stairs for added variety (you probably don't need a partner for this).

Housework Cleaning windows, scrubbing floors, hoovering carpets, and polishing surfaces – any of these will do. Many women feel a 'nesting instinct' which drives them to scrub like an old-fashioned housewife.

Bouncing on a birthing ball This encourages the right posture to persuade your baby to move into launch position.

Curry This might stimulate uterine contractions through hot bowel action, though it's probably not so great if you are planning a water birth in the next day or two. Make sure you have your hip flask of Gaviscon before you start down this path.

Raspberry leaf tea (Note: this is not recommended before the seventh month of pregnancy.) Raspberry leaves in tea or tablet form have a reputation for encouraging uterine contractions.

Go alternative Reflexology, acupuncture and homeopathy are all said to help.

Talk sternly to your bump Or sit yourself on the naughty step for a few hours.

Plan something important Schedule something that you really need to do before your baby arrives or invest in some new expensive knickers – sod's law says something will come along and mess things up.

Pineapple To EAT; don't insert it, for goodness sake.

What NOT to try

Herbal remedies Blue cohosh and black cohosh are often muttered about but have a bit of an underworld feel – and for good reason: there is simply not enough evidence that these are safe options for encouraging labour. So, no matter how desperate you are, avoid anyone who is peddling these herbals remedies and stick to safer tried-and-tested methods.

Castor oil Once you get to your due date your granny is likely to appear with a bottle of castor oil, telling you that it worked for her first 12 births. Castor oil triggers nausea and diarrhoea, which in turn can trigger contractions. However, there is also a risk of dehydration, and as this is not a scientifically tested method, it's best avoided.

Caesareans – What Are They Like and How Quickly Do You Recover?

Some women set their hearts on an elective Caesarean long before they become pregnant – even if they don't admit it to anyone. 'Part of me is secretly hoping the baby stays transverse, so I don't have to justify having a section,' confides one mum. Some eventually come round to the idea of a planned Caesarean after a lengthy consultation with their doctor, possibly if they are carrying twins, have previously had Caesareans, have pre-eclampsia, placenta praevia (see pp. 242 and 250) an unusually large or a breech baby (see p. 327). And some have Caesareans thrust upon them in an emergency.

It can be hard to accept the idea of a Caesarean section if your idea of pain relief is Peruvian pan pipes and you would rather eat your own placenta than go under the knife. But however strongly you feel about wanting to avoid one, a Caesarean is sometimes the best option. Over the years, emergency Caesareans have saved thousands of lives – mothers' and babies' – so it is not something to be written off lightly. Even if it doesn't feature on your birth plan, it is helpful to find out what having a C-section involves – after all, around 25 per cent of births are by Caesarean section, and of these, around 60 per cent are emergency sections, occurring after labour has begun. Forewarned is forearmed.

Being advised by your doctor that a C-section is your safest means of delivery can be devastating and terrifying at the same time. What were all those childbirth classes about? All that huffing and puffing on a bucket? There is so much pressure these days to give birth 'naturally' that you may feel you have failed your Mum exams at the first hurdle. And it may be for you – as it is for many women – your first time in an operating theatre.

The operation – what happens?

The good news is that the operation will be over relatively quickly – after just 30 to 45 minutes or so. You will usually be able to have your partner with you to hold your hand, though they will have to wear 'scrubs' (the sight of which should, at least, lighten the tension). If speed is of the essence, you will be given a general anaesthetic (and your partner may be excluded); otherwise, a local anaesthetic – a spinal block or epidural (see p. 313) – is injected into your spine, so you will be numb from the chest down but conscious throughout. The administering of the spinal block can be quite a nerve-racking experience as you will be asked to stay as still as possible. Not too tricky for an elective, but harder when you're in the middle of full-blown labour and having regular contractions. They will probably ask your birth partner to hold your hand and to talk to you to keep you calm. Just make sure that if your partner isn't that keen on injections they keep their eyes on you rather than on the improbably large needle being used on your back; the last thing you want is them collapsing at the crucial moment.

'My husband took one look at the needle, went green and said he wanted to go for a walk. I told him in the nicest possible way that he could chuffing well stay where he was. The midwife ended up making him a cup of strong, sweet tea while the spinal "took".' Munchpot

A screen will protect you from witnessing the actual surgery and although you can ask for it to be taken down this isn't recommended unless you're a particular fan of the gory bits in *ER*. If your birth partner is at all squeamish keep them at the head end, talking to you and ideally giving you updates and encouragement. You can request in advance if you'd like them to cut the umbilical cord and/or announce the sex of the baby. They can also bring the baby to you as soon as it is born:

'As soon as our daughter was ready to be held, my husband whipped off his green operating theatre top and clutched her to his bare chest. He'd never discussed this with me, but it seems he had read that skin-to-skin contact was good for the baby. He brought her to me so I could kiss her and it was one of the best moments of my life.' Biza

You feel no pain at all during the operation, but it is definitely a unique sensation, as one mum recalls: 'It's bizarre talking to people while someone is rummaging around inside you.' And another mum says, 'It feels like someone is doing the washing up in your stomach.'

Once the placenta has been removed, you will be stitched back up and taken to the recovery room where you will be able to feed your baby if she's hungry and have a good bonding session. You might want your birth partner to take photos of things like the baby being weighed or cleaned for the records, as you may not be able to see it all.

You will have a catheter fitted and it will take a few hours for the spinal/epidural to wear off so you won't be able to get out of bed for a while. NHS hospitals will normally insist on you spending at least the first night on a ward, so that you can be closely monitored. Nurses or midwives will change your sanitary pad for you and you will have your blood pressure checked so many times you'll lose count. Be aware that when you first get on your feet there may be a bit of leakage, so don't wear your best moccasins.

I've had some warning: how can I prepare for a C-section?

If you know now that that you are going to be having a Caesarean, there are steps you can take to make it an easier and more pleasant experience.

'A midwife bustled in and said: "Right love, I'm here to give you a short back and sides." I must admit that although I was in serious pain I nearly (literally) peed myself laughing.'
wasTheNightBeforeXmasOwl

It has probably been some time since you saw your bikini line but, even under the shadow of your bump, it will not have stopped growing. Rather than wait for a midwife to lunge at you with a disposable razor, do whatever it takes to cut back any undergrowth, a day or two before your delivery date, at the top of your pubic bone where the incision will be made.

You will probably be asked to remove nail polish, so don't plan an expensive trip to the nail salon before the birth. When packing your hospital bag, include clothes that won't sit on your scar: massive Granny pants, baggy pyjamas, sarongs, etc. You might want to take some Arnica to reduce bruising, tea tree and lavender to put in the bath for your scar, peppermint tea for post-op trapped wind, dried fruit for constipation, and straws to make it easier to drink until you are fully mobile.

As far as emotional preparation is concerned, now is the time to wrest back some control. Do you want music playing? Do you want to be told the sex of your baby or for your birth partner to announce it or for the baby to be handed to you first? Do you want immediate skin-to-skin contact? Do you want to try to breastfeed straight away? Do you want your birth partner to cut the cord? Do some research and find ways you can make your birth special, even if it isn't the birth you had hoped for (and indeed even if it *is*).

Emergency C-sections

There are many reasons why an emergency Caesarean becomes necessary, mainly revolving around the safety of mum and baby. It can be terrifying to discover that your baby is in distress and needs to be delivered immediately. 'Everything was going fine,' recalls one mum. 'Then I looked at the monitor and the heart-rate line was right at the bottom. I could hear the heartbeat slowing right down. Suddenly, the room was full of people and I was dashed off to theatre.' Another mum remembers how 'I was pushing away and they said they could see a head, then suddenly they said, "Stop pushing – it's a bum", and sprang into C-section action. It was all a bit rushed and panicky for a while, but they let me have a spinal rather than a general – there was no way I was going to miss this birth having come this far – and it was so lovely to be out of pain that in spite of the shock, I just felt huge relief.'

The lack of control, however, can be frightening. Things can progress very suddenly from an emergency situation that seems to be spiralling out of control to being suddenly put under a general anaesthetic. Feelings of confusion, disempowerment and even bereavement are completely normal. 'It can take time to piece it together and feel OK about it,' writes one mum. 'In the end, I decided whatever had happened I had a healthy baby and I was OK – and that may not have been the case in the days before C-sections.'

'You're going to feel tearful and shocked for a while, you know. Please be gentle with yourself and take it very, very easy. A crash section is very scary and it's obviously far from what you had hoped for the birth of your baby. But you will get over it.' Winkywinkola

Recovery

Relatively few women set out to deliver their baby by Caesarean. It is major abdominal surgery and is not a soft option. Like all major operations, it carries a risk of complications. And even without complications, recovery can be slow and painful, although this can vary greatly from one woman – even one birth – to the next:

'I've had two sections: one elective and one emergency. The emergency one was quite rough. I couldn't walk until midday the next day (the operation was done in the evening), and even then I needed a midwife holding each arm. With the elective, which was also done late evening, I had my catheter removed the next morning and got out of bed on my own and walked around the ward just after breakfast – which I know doesn't sound like much, but I was amazed by my mobility compared with the previous time! I never felt a minute's pain post-op with the elective and only needed paracetamol. A bit different from the emergency section when I was in agony post-op and needed morphine tablets!' TuttiFrutti

Recovery from a C-section usually takes longer than if you had a vaginal delivery. Prepare for it to be gradual. Post-op you will probably feel drowsy. Take painkillers, even if you don't feel like you need them at the time, because it will help you to start moving again. Ask for them if they aren't offered – they really work. You may find that you need painkillers for a couple of weeks after the section, although some mums find they don't need them at all after a few of days.

Drink plenty of water so you don't get dehydrated and also to encourage peeing: 'They want to make sure your bladder is working OK,' explains one mum.

You will be given deeply unglamorous white surgical stockings to wear until you are properly mobile to reduce your risk of developing blood clots. Once you've had your catheter removed, you'll be encouraged to start moving around. Start slowly by rolling on to your side and sitting on the edge of the bed, get your head in gear, then try to straighten up. You will instinctively clutch your scar and shuffle rather than walk, but as this is the only way you will a) get any breakfast and b) get to the loo, you will somehow manage. 'I was allowed to walk around the same evening, but had been nagging them to let me get out of bed since lunchtime!' recalls one mum. 'My partner said I appeared to be walking more easily than in the latter stages of pregnancy!'

'At first, walking is definitely uncomfortable and you may feel like you are being stretched upwards when you try and straighten up; this is fine and will get easier – and, regardless of how you feel, you will not split in two.' notjustmom

The first bowel movement is always a momentous occasion but if you keep to a healthy diet and drink plenty of water you should have no problems: 'If it helps, place a clean pad over the wound when going to the toilet. It will feel more secure for you if nothing else,' counsels a mum.

Make sure you ask for help when you need it. 'Don't feel forced to leave before you're good and ready,' advises one Mumsnetter. And once you are home, get as much rest as possible, avoid stairs (have a nappy-changing station at every level) and don't carry anything heavy (you might feel OK with your baby but avoid lugging heavy toddlers).

'Having a section is a good reminder to everybody that you need to take it easy for a few weeks and not try to do too much. You have been sawn in half you know!' fruitstick

It will be about six weeks before all your tissues are completely healed. Your scar might feel numb for several weeks or even months and you might get a strange pulling sensation when you twist.

Check your motor insurance policy to see what it says about getting back in the driving seat after a Caesarean, but it isn't usually recommended before six weeks (although many mums reported driving a lot earlier).

'I recovered quickly, but still felt winded for a few weeks, as if someone had punched me in the stomach,' says one mum. It might well take you a bit longer to feel on top form though. The important thing is to give yourself time, not expect too much and stay positive. We all take different amounts of time to heal but everyone gets there in the end.

'Before I was pregnant, I once locked myself out and had to climb over our six-foot-high garden wall. A month or two after my C-section I remember looking longingly at that wall, thinking, my body is so wrecked, I'll never be able to do anything like that again. I was wrong. I'm back to full strength now.' snowleopard

Breastfeeding after a Caesarean

If all goes well, you should be able to nurse your baby immediately. A V-shaped cushion or feeding lying down might help if it feels uncomfortable. You can also investigate the 'rugby-hold position', which is where you hold your baby with her feet heading away from your body under one arm, rather than their feet lying across your body. If you are in pain, particularly when feeding, then continue to take your pain medication: 'The painkillers they prescribe you are a real boon to get you through the initial pain of breastfeeding; I kept taking them until the very last one had been emptied out of the packet.'

If you need advice, ask the midwives for help with breastfeeding – or ask if there is a lactation consultant who can advise you. Alternatively, contact your local NCT or ABM (Association of Breastfeeding Mothers) and get advice from their helplines. Or you can, of course, log on to Mumsnet.

Everybody's experience of a C-section will be different and some women take longer than others to recover. If you are struggling with your feelings about your birth, then there should be help for you – either through discussing your birth with your midwife or doctor, or in the form of counselling. 'I only had one session with a counsellor,' writes one mum. 'But it helped to talk through everything from start to finish, and put it in its "proper place".' Ask your doctor for more information or make enquiries at your hospital.

'Ask to see your notes and ask questions – it will all take time to digest. Be prepared for there to be no clear explanation though; often a judgement call is made in an emergency in the best interests of you and your baby. Take things one day at a time.' Moopymoo

If this is your first Caesarean and you plan to give birth again, your chance of having another Caesarean is higher – but there is usually still the possibility that you will be able to have a vaginal birth in future.

Vaginal Birth After Caesarean (VBAC)

If the first time you gave birth was the Blackpool Big Dipper of disappointments, then becoming pregnant again can feel like a second bite at the cherry (although that's long gone). Now could be your opportunity to have the birth that you always wanted. If you had a Caesarean, you could try for a vaginal delivery – or maybe you had the vaginal birth from hell and have now scribbled 'CAESAREAN' all over your birth plan.

Whatever your final decision – and getting to that stage is no small task – laying the groundwork for the type of birth you would like is a road that does not always run smooth. There will be difficult decisions to make and obstacles along the way. You are going to be bombarded with mixed messages from health professionals, friends, family and that woman in the dry cleaner's, about what is best for you and your baby. Don't be surprised if you start to lose your nerve or change your mind, only to change it back again. Above all, do your research and trust your instincts.

'It's funny, in a sad sort of way, how many women who want a VBAC feel pressured into a repeat section and how many women who want a repeat section feel pressured into a VBAC.'

Stephaniefromnorwich

It is only relatively recently that doctors have countenanced the notion of a vaginal birth after Caesarean (VBAC) and moved away from the old adage 'once a Caesarean, always a Caesarean'. Now it is even possible to make the choice to try for a VBA2C (after two Caesareans) or to deliver twins vaginally after a section. But you are likely to come up against some resistance. Studies suggest that over 50 per cent of women who try for a VBAC are successful, but it can feel like a gamble, especially when alternative medical names for a VBAC include 'trial of labour' and 'trial of scar'. Plus, the fear of an emergency Caesarean is never far away.

Some women opt to try for a VBAC for practical reasons – particularly if they have a toddler to look after – to avoid major surgery and a prolonged recovery. They want to be back in the driving seat, both literally and metaphorically, as soon as possible. But there are also emotional reasons: many women are keen to exorcise ghosts from their first birth and experience something that they feel they have previously been denied.

'My VBAC was the best thing I have achieved in my life. I was ecstatic to have "given birth" to my son. No stitches, no soreness, labour was three hours and home the next day. I'm sure the reason I had post-natal depression was due to the fact that I'd felt cheated out of giving birth naturally with my daughter, and it still upsets me. It's a very personal choice but, for me, I would go for a VBAC again.' Mummyvicky

Even if you do not manage a VBAC, the feeling of having 'given it your best shot' is hugely empowering for some. One mum, who tried for a VBAC but ended up having a Caesarean, explains why she does not regret her choices:

'I am sad not to have achieved my VBAC, but I am so glad to have laboured and tried so hard to get it. If I had taken the offered elective Caesarean at 39 weeks I could have avoided lots of stress and waiting, but I would always have wondered "What if?"' pendulum

If you want to push for a VBAC, do a bit of detective work, starting with why your previous birth ended in a C-section. If the reason for your first section was a one-off situation (such as a breech presentation), you are in a good position to try for a VBAC this time. Your medical notes from the birth should give you the answers you need and you're entitled to ask for copies of these, although there may be a small charge. Talk to your doctor and midwife about how you feel, and find out if there are going to be any limitations on you having a VBAC.

Uterine rupture, which means your old wound reopening, is one of the biggest fears of a VBAC. This occurs in 35 in every 10,000 women trying for a VBAC, compared with 12 in every 10,000 women having a planned repeat Caesarean. The number of cases is rare but it happened to this VBA2Cer: 'I had done my research and assumed it would never happen to me. But I ended up with complete scar rupture and had an emergency C-section. All's well now but it goes to show how weak my scar tissue was.'

Uterine rupture is also increased if your labour is induced; the stats are 80 ruptures per 10,000 births when labour is induced with non-prostaglandins (such as oxytocin) and 240 ruptures per 10,000 births when labour is induced using prostaglandins. The angle of your C-scar will also make a difference; the more up-to-date incision across the lower part of your uterus is less likely to rupture than the old-style vertical cut through the middle.

The risk of stillbirth is also higher for women having a VBAC (about 10 per 10,000), than for those having a planned repeat section (about 1 per 10,000).

There are steps of your own that you can take to try to ensure that your VBAC goes smoothly. 'Labour at home for as long as possible and use the minimum pain relief so that you can work with your body,' says a Mumsnetter who was inspired by her own VBAC to train as a doula. Also, keep mobile if you can, although it isn't always easy if you are hooked up to a monitor.

The degree of monitoring that you will be asked to have depends on your past history and the hospital's policy. Some hospitals prefer continuous foetal monitoring (CFM, see p. 269), but others may allow intermittent monitoring.

'I had a VBAC after an elective section for placenta praevia. I had a very enlightened consultant who agreed that CFM was unnecessary. This meant that I was able to put in my birth plan that "Mr X has agreed that CFM will not be necessary in the first instance". "In the first instance" is important. I wasn't prepared to put my baby at risk, but as long as things were progressing normally, I felt much happier with intermittent monitoring, whereby a midwife checked the baby's heart every 15 minutes or so. They even had a monitor you could use under water, so I didn't have to get out of the bath until I got to the second stage. If this is important to you, get the consultant on your side now. You can't go along hoping that the midwives will be sympathetic – you're not in the best position to argue your case once you are in labour!' Ellbell

Talk to your doctor and find out what your options are. Some doctors prefer not to use epidurals alongside VBACs in case signs of a uterine rupture go unnoticed but close monitoring should prevent that.

Opting for a VBAC is a big step in itself and the risk of the unknown can be nerve-racking. It's natural to have moments of doubt – what Mumsnetters call 'the VBAC jitters' – and to question if you are doing the right thing. 'I wonder if I am just being selfish and whether I should just book an elective C-section in case it goes wrong again?' muses one anxious mother. It's at times like this that it can be reassuring to have the backing of a doula or independent midwife. 'My doula was so valuable I would recommend one to anyone, especially those trying a VBAC.'

In some cases it is possible to have a home VBAC, even in a birthing pool, if you strongly believe that it would be best for you and your baby. But you will need to have every confidence in yourself and the full backing of your medical support team. Not to mention the determination of a long-distance runner to get what you want. Hospital is certainly the safest place to be if you are going to have a uterine rupture, so you will need to weigh up the risks and come to your own decision.

'I had a C-section with my twins and went on to have two VBACs with no problems. The extra risk if you are monitored in hospital is minuscule – certainly not enough to dissuade me – and I'm really glad I had two VBACs, as I found the experience of birth and recovery preferable.'

Oblong

Ventouse and Forceps – A Little Bit of Assistance When the Going Gets Tough ...

There is that moment on every hospital tour when the doctor starts to talk about assisted deliveries. If only you had looked away. Ventouse? Forceps? Which one looked scarier? They didn't resemble bits of birthing kit, more like eye-watering instruments of the Spanish Inquisition. It is unlikely that you are planning a starring role for either in your ideal birth, but for all the worry and fear that they instil, there are thousands of mums out there who were never more grateful to see them than towards the end of a gruelling labour. 'It saved my son from worse distress and me from an emergency section,' says one. 'I think by the time you find yourself in this position, there is no way you are going to say no.'

'I have rather fond memories of my ventouse with my daughter. After 12 hours of labour and very little progression for the last seven, I was extremely happy to have her vacuumed out rather than go on for several more hours.' fennel

Around 11 per cent of births require an instrumental delivery using forceps or a ventouse – although this rises to 15 per cent with inductions. These days, most doctors prefer to use a ventouse, rather than forceps, which are now used in only around 2 per cent of births.

Forceps and ventouse are introduced in the second stage of labour, when the baby is engaged in the pelvis, but showing signs of distress or failure to descend down the birth canal. Your baby may seem stuck; you may well be exhausted; your blood pressure could be climbing. Depending on time limitations, you should either be offered an epidural or pudendal block (an anaesthetic that numbs the area between your vagina and anus). Be prepared to have your legs in stirrups – yee-ha.

You might also be given an episiotomy to prevent serious tearing, particularly if it is a forceps delivery. 'My episiotomy gave me much less trouble than the girls in my antenatal class who tore badly in their natural deliveries, and my recovery time was much less than it would have been for a C-section,' says a first-timer who had a ventouse delivery. The idea is that the baby is pulled when you push, so only when you feel a contraction. Sit up as much as possible and, if it helps, ask for a running commentary.

'I was induced at 39 weeks (I have diabetes) and ended up having both ventouse and forceps to get him out. After 26 hours in labour, I didn't care what they did as long as he came out safely. He did have a bit of a swelling on the back of his head for 24 hours and a scab which dropped off after about a week, but other than that he was absolutely fine. It did mean we had to stay in hospital for an extra night though. And yes, episiotomy and stirrups – in fact, when I write it all down it sounds traumatic, but I was so thrilled to have a purple squirmy baby on my tummy that I just forgot about the nasty bits.' hoxtonchick

What are ventouse and forceps?

A ventouse is a soft suction cap attached to the baby's head that looks a bit like something you would use to unblock a sink and which effectively vacuums out the baby. Don't be horrified if your little one is born with a cone-shaped head; a newborn's head is very malleable, so the Mr Whippy look is to be expected after a ventouse delivery and should disappear within a few days. Your baby's head may also be red and swollen but that will go away too. A word of advice from a Mumsnetter: "It's not unusual for the vacuum seal between the ventouse cap and the head to be broken, which makes the most terrible noise and sounds like something ghastly is happening, but it's nothing to worry about – they just have another go.'

'I had a ventouse delivery with my son. He was stuck and getting distressed. The doctor was fantastic and did it very quickly. My son had no problems. I had an episiotomy that gave me minor discomfort for the first few days and then healed as if by magic.' Berolina

Forceps are metal and look like something the devil would use to serve a salad. They cup around the baby's head and vary in shape for use with babies in different positions. Babies delivered by forceps sometimes have marks on the sides of their head, but again, these will soon disappear.

For some women, forceps are a definite no-no, even when up against an emergency C-section. If you are forceps phobic, discuss it with your doctor and state your fears on your birth plan. 'My baby had four pulls with the ventouse, then one pull with forceps,' says a mum who, in hindsight, would have preferred a C-section. 'He was horrifically bruised all over his head from the ventouse and on his face from the forceps. I didn't have an epidural and found the pulls excruciatingly painful, so much so I blacked out for over an hour after I gave birth. I had a big episiotomy which was left unstitched and was extremely painful. It has taken me 15 months to heal internally and externally.'

Having said that, in the heat of the moment, the important thing is to get your baby delivered safely.

'Try not to think of the baby as being "wrenched out". Ventouse and forceps just guide the baby out, assisted by your own pushing when progress is slow.' (Mumsnetter midwife) mears

What about after effects?

Some mums have a theory that assisted-delivery babies are particularly cranky during the first few months, the assumption being that they have a headache and are generally more unsettled than most newborns. In some instances mums claim that cranial osteopathy has helped their 'assisted' babies to settle down and also to sleep. But most babies, assisted or otherwise, test their parents' patience to the limit in the first few months. Witness one mother's experience: 'My first son was delivered by ventouse. It was a massive relief after pushing for what seemed like a day and a labour that had been going on for a week. Just a snip and pop, out he came like a champagne cork; no cone head and a very content, smiley baby. My second son was born at home to soothing music and essential oils. He cried for five months.'

Episiotomy and Tearing (Eeek) – Can They Be Avoided and How Long Do They Take to Heal?

Cross your legs. OK, you're pregnant, so bite your sleeve instead. Today we are going to be talking about your fanjo. No blushing because it is, after all, public property until this baby is out.

There is a chance, er, that your fanjo will, er, tear while you are giving birth, or need to be, ahem, cut to get your baby out. Just thinking about it can give the toughest of pregnant women the jitters. But take heart: the thinking about it is usually worse than the actual act. 'So much will be going on when the time comes that it won't be anything as bad as you might imagine now,' says a mum whose fanjo has lived to tell the tale.

> 'An episiotomy was my worst fear during pregnancy, but when I ended up having one, I was so busy having a contraction I didn't even know they'd done it.' thegardener

Amazing things will happen to your vagina as you give birth. What seems like a small space for a baby's head to pass through will miraculously become roomier. As your baby is born, his head will stretch the opening of your vagina, but sometimes the space just isn't big enough and you tear, either backwards towards the anus, or, more rarely, towards the clitoris. Neither is huge fun, if we are honest with you.

'After my son was born, my legs were in stirrups while the dishy consultant peered at the train wreck that used to be my fanny. He popped out and came back with another doctor. So both of them are mutter, mutter, muttering to each other about my tear and I can hardly follow the conversation, when I hear the word "SPHINCTER" clear as crystal. I just about snapped off my husband's fingers, I was so worried that my fanny and arse were now ONE.' AnnasBananas

How can I stop this terrible fate from befalling me?

Probably around 80 per cent of women will have a tear or a cut during a vaginal birth, and around 70 per cent will need stitching. There isn't a definitive way to prevent tearing, but you can take some steps that might help reduce your risk.

One thing you can try is perineal message. Around six weeks before your due date, start massaging your perineum (if you can reach it – it's the area of skin and muscle between your vagina and anus) with olive oil to soften it up. Place your thumbs inside your vagina, and gently stretch and massage your perineum using a U-shape motion. Concentrate on how it feels to relax your perineum, this will be extremely useful for helping you give birth in a more gentle way – a relaxed perineum is less likely to tear than a tense one. If you can't reach, you might like to ask your partner to do it for you. Or you might not.

'This might have been pleasant in some kind of sexual context, but not in the context of thinking, "Oh God, a massive bony head is coming out of here".' Gemmitygem

Another important point to remember is that the position that you give birth in can affect your risk of tearing: for example, giving birth on your back is more likely to result in a tear than giving birth on your side. 'Keep moving around during labour, rather than lying flat,' advises one mum. 'If you recline, you will have to push your baby uphill to get it out.' Research has shown that it can help if the midwife applies pressure to the baby's head while protecting your perineum at the same time. It is thought that the support provided by a water birth may also reduce tearing.

Another point to remember is that your vagina needs time to adjust to your baby's head emerging – so, if you can, start panting as the baby's head makes an appearance to stop it coming too fast. Try to let your body expel the baby, rather than you forcibly pushing it out: remember the mantra: 'breathe your baby out'.

The four degrees: different types of tear

Tearing is usually 'rated' in degrees, from first to fourth. The lower the degree, the less bad the tearing. Third- and fourth-degree tears are relatively rare, occurring in less than 1 per cent of births.

First-degree tear: a small tear to the skin of the vagina and perineum, but not into the muscles; usually heals quickly without stitching.

Second-degree tear: tears into the muscles underneath the skin and will require stitching back together; may take a few weeks to heal.

Third-degree tear: this is a tear in the vaginal tissue, perineal skin and the muscles that extend into the anal sphincter (your anus). Basically, you have ripped into your arse (jolly bad luck); this will require very delicate repair work in theatre.

Fourth-degree tear: a tear through the anal sphincter and into the tissue underneath it. This is really bad luck indeed and will need extensive surgery and rehabilitation. A possible complication is anal incontinence which must be dealt with by a specialist if it does not improve after the wound has healed.

Labial graze: this is a small graze or tear to the labia, which usually doesn't need stitching and should heal of its own accord.

Episiotomies – the first cut is the deepest, baby

An episiotomy is a cut made in the perineum in an attempt to avoid uncontrolled tearing and also to give a little bit more room for the baby to emerge. In the past, the majority of women in labour in the UK had episiotomies. These days, a natural tear is generally the preferred option because it is thought to heal better. An episiotomy is only usually performed if your baby is in distress, has an XXL head or is in an awkward position. An episiotomy is performed in around 13 per cent of births.

'When it came down to it, I ended up having two separate episiotomies after I'd been trying to push the head out for nearly three hours. I couldn't have cared less at the time – all I cared about was getting my son out safe and well. I didn't feel a thing and having the stitches afterwards was nothing. It's not pleasant for the next few weeks but it was nowhere near as bad as I expected.' Twinklemegan

Whether it is best to tear or to be cut is the question on every pregnant woman's lips (no pun intended), but it helps to keep your mind open about this, as with everything else. 'I really didn't want to be cut second time around,' says a mother of two who tore giving birth to her first child. 'But the midwife thought there was going to be uncontrolled tearing. Shudder. So I said "Yes", and I'm glad I did. It was fine. A good midwife will not cut unless it's for the best. That said, there is no harm in putting it in your birth plan that you would rather not have an episiotomy unless it's absolutely necessary.'

An episiotomy is usually necessary if forceps or a ventouse are to be used.

Make do and mend – how do we fix this, then?

Shortly after delivery, you will be stitched up. 'This does feel a bit like trying to put Humpty back together again!' trills one mum.

But don't fret – you will be given a local anaesthetic or have your epidural topped up. It can take time and leave you feeling like they are making a patchwork quilt down there, but the good news is that the stitches are usually dissolvable. 'I remember telling my midwife who was stitching me up that it felt like she was doing a very neat job and would she sew some curtains for me,' recalls an embarrassed Mumsnetter who had taken full advantage of the gas and air. Another mum remembers 'lying in theatre having stitches for mega tears, listening to Rod Stewart's "The First Cut is the Deepest" on the radio'.

> 'While lying in stirrups after the birth of my daughter, I heard the midwife complimenting the doctor on the nice job she was doing of stitching me back together again. The doctor replied: "Thank you, my hobby *is* cross-stitch!" I had visions of finding a cute teddy stitched into my bits …' Charliesmomuk

There are women who, having by this stage had enough of people up to their armpits in their vaginas, refuse to be stitched, but generally stitching is the recommended route, and a bit of discomfort now is well worth it in the long run. 'I gravely regret not getting my second-degree tear stitched up,' admits one mum. 'I had a water birth with no drugs. I was in agony and couldn't see any way of either lying down or getting into a comfortable position to be stitched up. But I was in pain for months afterwards and things have not healed well. For the sake of an hour of pain I could have avoided months of stress.'

Post-tear care

Recovery can be painful. Even sitting down is sometimes a struggle. Baby stores usually have a variety of products to help with the pain. You can try sitting on a rubber ring, which some women find useful for taking the pressure off stitches. (Others find it makes the pain worse, so only try this if it feels OK.) You can also buy specially made 'valley cushions' (basically, cushions with a valley in the middle to take the pressure off your poor perineum) which might help. Or you can make your own with two folded pillows to sit on.

Keeping the area clean is essential. Give it a thorough wash in the bath, using a flannel or cotton wool and your fingers to wash any dirt gently away. Or spray yourself with the shower head (not the power shower, dear). Add a few drops of lavender, rosehip or tea tree oil to your bath.

When going for a wee, you may find it more comfortable to face the loo and straddle the seat. If the urine splashes on your tear, it tends to sting, but pouring warm water on your bits while you pee will relieve the stinging sensation. You can also lean forwards on the loo to try to avoid weeing on your sore parts. Your other alternative is to pee in a shallow bath or the shower but that isn't always practical, particularly if you are out shopping or at a friend's house.

'My midwife recommended drying my stitches after a bath or shower with a hairdryer (on a cool setting). Very strange sensation but it was much better than using a towel!' stellarmum

Change your maternity pads regularly and put them in the freezer for a DIY cool pack. Or you can buy maternity pads filled with gel which can be refrigerated for the same purpose. A bag of frozen peas has the same effect, but it's a harder look to carry off. You might need painkillers to see you through the worst, but things should start to improve after two or three weeks. For something homeopathic, try Arnica. Some women find looking at the area with a mirror reassuring, so they know what is going on down there. For others, it is a horror show best avoided.

Doing a post-stitch-up poo can be a nerve-racking experience, especially if you are constipated, so plenty of liquids and a healthy diet can at least help with that. Even if you're not constipated, there's always the fear that any pushing at all will split everything open. It's extremely unlikely that this will happen, but you can always hold a maternity pad against your stitches for peace of mind and make sure you wipe from front to back.

If the wound becomes infected, get it seen to right away as you may need antibiotics. Signs of a possible infection are if the area is red, swollen, pussy (that's pus-filled – we're not being rude) or if it feels hot to the touch. And if you have a temperature you should always contact your midwife immediately.

Getting back in the saddle

Sex is another enormous hurdle for some women post-stitch-up and it can be sore to begin with. It is normal to worry that it might be painful or that you might tear again, so take your time. Heck, you might even enjoy it. Go slow, use some lube and, when you are not in bed making up for all those months of inaction, keep up those pelvic-floor exercises and it won't be long before you are right back on track.

'I had an episiotomy and I waited until six months after birth before having sex (not because I was scared, but that's just when I was "ready"). It was painful the first few times, but very soon felt normal again, although I did find that it ached after sex sometimes. Now, two and a half years later, I have a very active sex life and no problems or discomfort whatsoever.'

Stephanie1974

Don't despair if, several months later, things still don't feel right down there. Everybody heals at a different rate, and it can take time for deep tissue damage to repair itself. It is quite common to feel that you've been 'stitched up too tight'; but at the same time you shouldn't suffer in silence either. You are the best judge if something feels amiss and it's important that you get help now, even if it takes persistence. Ask your GP to refer you to a gynaecologist, as they will be able to give you a proper examination and assess the situation.

For a few people the pain can by psychological rather than something caused by physical symptoms:

'I had a traumatic birth and was convinced I would never have sex again. I was eventually diagnosed with severe vaginismus – involuntary tightening of the vagina – that was stopping me from using a tampon, let alone having sex. I only had one session with a counsellor, where we talked about the birth and she gave me some exercises, and within a week I was cured. It had taken me months to pluck up courage to talk to my GP, and I could have saved myself a lot of anxiety and pain. My advice would be to talk to your GP early on if you have any concerns at all. They won't dismiss you and they can usually help.' Beebee

Be reassured that although it might take time, you will eventually resume something like normal service. Hark this mum who underwent delicate needlework: 'My fanjo is as good as new – or so I have been told. If you end up having an episiotomy, it's not the end of the world.'

So take your sleeve out your mouth now and don't give it another thought.

Vitamin K

Since the 1960s babies have routinely been given a single injection of vitamin K on delivery, but these days, parental consent is required. It might seem like one more thing to have to think about, but, on this issue at least, you are being invited to have your say. It's just working out what you want to say that's the hard bit ...

All babies are born with low levels of vitamin K. Among other things, it is needed for their blood to be able to clot and without it babies have a tendency to bleed easily. In severe cases, this may result in vitamin K deficiency bleeding (VKDB), also known as haemorrhagic disease of the newborn (HDN). The risk of severe bleeding may be as high as 1 in 2000. Premature babies are most at risk of the condition, along with babies who have had a traumatic birth, perhaps involving forceps, a ventouse or an emergency C-section. Although extremely rare, the condition is serious enough (usually fatal) that NHS policy recommends that all babies be given a shot of vitamin K immediately after delivery.

Some parents worry about the safety of the vitamin K dose. Doubts were raised in the early 1990s after medical papers were published suggesting a link between the vitamin K injection and childhood leukaemia. But several studies carried out since then have not supported the association and this is no longer seen as a reason not to have the injection. Nevertheless, some parents remain unconvinced. 'I went with the theory that Mother Nature is very clever,' argues one mum. 'If all babies are born with low levels of vitamin K, there must be a reason for it.'

If you decide that you don't want to take a risk and want your baby to be given vitamin K, your next option is whether to go with a single injection or an oral dose. 'We chose not to give our daughter an injection as I don't see the need to traumatise an exhausted and confused but otherwise healthy newborn,' says a mother. It is hard to imagine how a tiny pin prick will upset a baby who has just been shoe-horned down your birth canal but the choice is yours. The bonus of the injection is that it is straightforward; once it is done, it is done; whereas the oral form is more drawn out and, in order for it to be effective you have to ensure that you complete the recommended course involving several doses over a period of weeks.

'Looking back, we are glad our son had the injection because you know it has gone in and stayed in,' explains a mother. 'He was a very spitty baby and I'm not sure how much of the oral would have stayed in.'

Not all babies need vitamin K, but you don't know which ones do, and therein lies the dilemma. It's the first of many decisions you'll have to make but at least you can mull over it and not suddenly be confronted by it on the big day as one mum was: 'I had no idea what vitamin K was when they asked me if I wanted my baby to have it – I felt so dumb.'

Labour Tips for Dads – How to Be a Hero

Here's something for your other half. But before you pass it over to him, consider what part he has played in your pregnancy so far. Has he held back your hair as you have emptied the entire contents of your stomach into the loo? Gained weight and moobs in sympathy, and felt nauseous too? Swapped his loo time reading from *Zoo* to *100 Best Baby Names*? No? Well, don't chuck him out just yet. Pregnancy can be a steep learning curve but the real test is yet to come.

'In the relative still of the night at my maternity hospital, while I was appreciating the calming effects of the epidural and my husband dozed in the corner, there was an almighty crash, bang, smash. The midwife put down her clipboard and popped out of the room for a few minutes. As she came back in and the door slowly closed behind her, I caught sight of an unconscious man being wheeled past the doorway in a wheelchair by two paramedics. He was the husband of the woman next door. It had all been a bit much for him.' GrumpyOldHorsewoman

If you know that your partner will struggle to cope, it's better that you discuss it with him now. If you really want him to be there, make that clear. If he is only going to get in the way – feeling faint, with a face like a placenta – maybe you would rather have a friend/mum/sister or a doula there instead, or as well. You don't want him to feel left out, but you do need a birth partner, not a birth liability.

There is another breed of male who can't get enough of this pregnancy wheeze. If your partner is the kind of father who feels your every ache, has suffered the same indigestion, and already bought out most of Mothercare, then commiserations to you too. Sometimes it can feel like overkill. You don't want to knock all the enthusiasm out of him, but it would be nice if he occasionally thought of you as more than just a baby-carrying vessel and remembered the woman you were before he got you into this uncomfortable situation.

Either way, you are the star here, so make sure your partner is clear on where the spotlight should be falling. (Because the midwife will need it to sew you up later on.)

Dads-in-training – a note to men on the frontline

No doubt you want so badly to be a hero, to do the right thing. But women in labour can be tricky beasts. At times, it might feel like you can do nothing right. This might well be the case, and no amount of back rubbing, soothing noises and offers of cold drinks will make your partner grateful for your presence. 'Just shut up and do as she tells you,' advises one mum.

What's important though is that you exude an air of calm. It's no good turning into jelly at the first sign that she might be in labour. You are her rock. In control. Attentive to her every need. You might feel like barfing into the bin and be bored senseless rubbing her back when all you really want is to watch the footie, but do try not to let your feelings show.

'I spent most of the night sitting in a hot bath. My husband was meant to be timing contractions, but was so tired he fell asleep on the floor by the bath. I would wake him at the start of each contraction so he could mark it on a piece of paper then he'd go straight back to sleep. At one stage he asked if I would let him go to bed for a bit as not much was happening. He said: "If you need anything just shout and I'll get up." After two hours, I wanted to phone the hospital, so I shouted down the hall for him. No reply. I shouted again. No answer. I couldn't get out of the bath on my own, so I yelled at the top of my voice. I eventually resorted to throwing everything I could find (soap, rubber duck, nailbrush) down the hall in the hope that he would wake up. After what seemed like a lifetime he stumbled out of bed of his own accord and wandered in saying, "How are you getting on?" GRRR!' AuntyVi

Unless you have decided on a home birth, there will be a stage in the proceedings when between you, your partner and the midwife on duty, you will have to decide when it's time to leave for the hospital (See p. 265). It is not an easy one to call. If you are the designated driver, bear this in mind and don't fall at the first hurdle by announcing that the petrol tank is empty. In the weeks leading up to your partner's due date, make sure that it is always topped up and that you have money for the car park. It's also a good idea not be to inebriated – no going over the drink–drive limit for at least the last few weeks of pregnancy (and no moaning; she's hardly been knocking it back for the past nine months). If you are going by taxi, have at least three numbers to hand.

Check your partner's list of hospital essentials (hospital bag, camera, telephone numbers) and make sure that you've got everything. Do not wait until your partner is screeching like a pterodactyl to commence ironing a shirt or preparing yourself a gourmet snack in case you get peckish at the hospital. Remember, you are in control.

'I remember gently waking my husband to tell him we needed to go to the hospital, and watching him run around like Basil Fawlty. He tried to get me into the car before I'd even had time to get dressed. Then he discovered the car doors were frozen shut, cue more Basil Fawlty behaviour, and him saying: "You'll just have to get into the boot!" Having finally defrosted the back door, and put me on the seat, in the throes of a major contraction, I caught him looking at me in the mirror. "So, do you think this might be it then?" he said. What was he thinking? That I'd dragged him out of bed at 2 a.m. for a trial run in the freezing fog?' Joolyjoolyjoo

While your partner is in labour, grunting like a wildebeest, there are some things it is important you do *not* say. A Mumsnetter who had a home birth was puffing her way through a contraction, leaning over an air-conditioning unit, as her best friend massaged the small of her back, when her partner looked on with awe and said: 'That looks like a good position. Must remember that one for after the baby.'

'My waters broke with a very loud BANG and splashed about six feet up the wall, all over the midwife and student next to her. My husband jumped out of his skin and shouted: "What the bloody hell was that?"' frazzledoldbag34

Commenting on your partner's appearance is another no-no. 'I was in the pool and my contractions were coming thick and fast,' recalls a mum. 'I'm sucking down the gas and air, trying to be brave. My husband is looking at me closely. I think he must be thinking about the pain I am in, and how well I am coping. Then he says, "You should see your hair!" and cacks himself laughing.' At least one Mumsnetter can confirm that no lady wants to hear her husband exclaim: 'Oh my God I didn't realise it could stretch that much!' And when you first clap eyes on your baby and it is covered in gunk and screaming, try to stop yourself from shouting out, 'Crikey! It's like the Exorcist!'

As well as things you should not say, there are also things you should not do. Eating her labour supply of Custard Creams, texting 'Nearly here' messages to your mates, listening to the football through earphones, and having your head stuck in a copy of *Loaded* are all genuine crimes as recorded by Mumsnetters. And suggesting that you might be in any way suffering is up there with first-degree murder. 'During my 12-hour labour my husband complained, in all seriousness, that his feet were hurting as he had been standing up for so long,' recalls a wife who is still seeking damages. Another mum mid-labour caught her husband sneakily using her TENS machine because he had a bad back.

'During my son's high-speed labour – the uterine equivalent of 0 to 60 in about 4 seconds – my husband said to me, "Breathe! Remember your breathing!" I shouted back: "I am f**king breathing! Now f*** off!" He went and read the *Guardian* for a while.' Dinosaur

There are things you can do to distract your partner from the pain. That old trick of blowing up surgical gloves and batting them around the room usually goes down well. Bouncing on the birthing ball can also be amusing. But just the once, mind. Definitely don't try the comedy routine of wresting the gas and air out of her hands so that you can try a snort. Women in labour have very short fuses. What is funny one minute will be infuriating the next. Prepare to be a punch bag – often quite literally. Do not hit back. Do not bite back. Do not break her fingers back.

'I found the best form of pain relief was actually biting hard on my husband's hand during contractions. At one point the baby was in distress and apparently my husband left the room and said he couldn't cope. Fortunately I didn't notice (or I would have whacked him) and the midwife persuaded him to go back in. Apparently I'd been biting the hand of the doctor who had been called in. He was very good and hadn't complained.' Gigi

A word of caution: should you leave the labour ward, bear in mind that on return all the rooms will look alike.

'My husband came into the labour room with a look of total horror on his face. He'd walked in on someone else in labour, had a quick shufty at the business end, decided it wasn't mine and left quickly.' jollymum

Try not to be surprised/horrified as your partner's body does things you never thought possible. There is usually a lot of water involved, as well as blood, sweat, shit and tears. She might even curse. If you are not used to this kind of unladylike behaviour, restrain yourself from telling her to stop. The gas and air might also make her a tiny bit squiffy. Don't fret – this isn't permanent.

If your partner has a Caesarean and you end up going into theatre, you will be required to wear scrubs and a pair of wellies. This is your George Clooney moment, so make the most of it and get a member of the hospital staff to take your picture. You are not a wuss for staying at the head end, and it's OK to feel squeamish; just try not to collapse like one Mumsnetter's man (or should that be mouse?): 'My husband fainted as the decision was made to take me into surgery, so they made me walk, exhausted, to the operating room and wheeled him in on my wheelchair.'

Men at the other end of the hardness scale sometimes go too far. Do not start rolling up your sleeves in the manner of a vet about to deliver a calf. Or offer backseat advice to the midwife. They *are* somewhat more experienced than you.

'At the moment that my daughter was ready to be born, the midwife asked my husband to hold my leg. When I looked up he had my leg in one hand and a cup in the other. I had to say, "Put down the bloody tea!"' hazeyjane

You might be asked to cut the umbilical cord and you have every right to decline. Your partner might even be relieved. 'The only thing I know for certain is that I definitely don't want my husband cutting the cord,' insists a mother. 'We are going to be in a building full of experts. Why get the one guy who has no clue to do it?'

It can be really hard for a man to watch his partner in labour. She may appear to be in unthinkable agony and not being able to 'fix it' for her can be frustrating, making you feel powerless and helpless. But bear in mind that your partner doesn't expect you to do a great deal (although that doesn't mean you can sit BlackBerrying your way through the whole thing). Just be attentive to her needs and remain calm, and you won't go far wrong: 'Just being there is probably enough.'

You might think that post delivery you can start to relax. But there is still plenty you could screw up at this emotionally fragile stage: 'As soon as I'd given birth to our daughter, my husband backed out of the door whimpering, "I've got to go to bed; I'm so tired!"'

Do not talk about the labour as if you were the one who did all the hard work.

'After labour, I was lying in bed with our beautiful son, and heard my husband on his phone to his mother saying: "It was so much easier this time!"' singsalot

Instinctively, one might hope, you will tell the mother of your child what a star she is. Words like 'amazing', 'wonderful', 'strong', 'brave', 'goddess' will all be appreciated at this point. Avoid saying, 'It was so much easier than I expected' or telling people within your partner's earshot that 'It was carnage! A bloodbath!' When the midwife arrives with tea and toast, it is not for you. Now is your turn to hold the baby – and no, despite how you feel, you won't drop it.

Mumsnetiquette: Top tips for dads-to-be

Things to take

'My husband seemed to find it very therapeutic to have a Game Boy to play on during labour ... ' *SarahJaneSmith*

'Pack clean clothes for you. You don't know what mess you may get into, so it's handy to have a couple of spare T-shirts. You could be sweaty, mucky, dare I say bloody or spill a drink down you and then you will look crap for those first pics. You won't want that and she will be annoyed at you too!' *tinkertinker*

'Comfortable shoes ... my feet were knackered by the end of the day(s).' *HandyTrinkett*

'A cast-iron stomach.' *aDad*

What to expect during labour

'It'll never be how you expect, so don't torture yourself by imagining different scenarios. Focus on the end result – which WILL be worth it.' *aDad*

'Be prepared for the birth plan going completely out the window during labour.' *DrDaddy*

After the birth

'Take a camera for some nice after pictures – but not during.' *Skribble*

(continued)

'If you get a chance, a tidy, clean house to come home to would probably be appreciated.' *bigwuss*

'Don't forget the car seat for the baby! A friend did this to his great embarrassment. The hospital won't let you out the door without one ...' *DrDaddy*

'Be prepared to be very supportive if she decides to breastfeed (or formula feed). Feeding is never as straightforward as it seems, and breastfeeding may take several weeks, with lots of support, hugs, tears before she (and the baby) gets the hang of it. Be prepared to tell her it's OK for her to formula feed if she wants to, but if she wants to persevere with breastfeeding, then you will be there for her/will take the baby out for walks between feeds in the evenings to give her a break/find her a breastfeeding counsellor/get her Lansinoh for sore nipples/whatever it takes.' *Notquitesotiredmum*

And, a final word from a mum:

'I don't know how I would have got through my two labours without my partner. Not only was he brilliant at getting me to relax, but his presence meant that I could concentrate on the business in hand and be sure that he wouldn't let anyone do anything that I didn't want. He made me feel really safe – he'd done his homework and knew what was going on. He was absolutely vital to me and helped to make both experiences about as good as anything so painful could be. So all you dads just remember – whatever your partner says to you in the heat of the moment, the fact that you're there and trying to help really means something.' Azzie

Giving Birth – It's a Serious Business

'My waters broke just after my partner had left for work. He wasn't answering his mobile, so I chased after him, holding my bump, dressed only in a velvet dressing gown slashed to the thigh and white flip-flops, no knickers, with water trickling down my legs. I ran down the platform and made the guard make an announcement while I stood there, waters still breaking.' *Thomcat*

'I was in full-blown labour and suddenly everything went haywire. The midwife told me to "make a fist", but all I heard her saying was, "Make a fish". I panicked, of course, because I didn't know how to make a fish.' *Pinkbubble.*

'After nearly two days of labour and not getting anywhere they agreed to a section and a registrar tried to do an internal before I went to theatre. As this was about the 20th internal, I wasn't impressed and punched him. Apparently he wasn't popular on the ward with staff or patients, so the midwives thought it was great.' *Nikkie*

'When I was in labour, I declined to remove my knickers and asked the staff to just "work around them". I am rather shy.' *moaningminnie2020*

'During the final stages of having my son, I was feeling somewhat out of it from loads of gas and air. I was kneeling on the bed, draped over the headboard, when I suddenly realised someone was trying to take my watch off. I started to fight back and screamed, "Get off you mugger!" But it was only my husband who was worried that I'd smash it against the metal bed frame.' *MegaLegs*

'My friend was being given an internal examination by the midwife and found it so painful that she clamped her legs shut, trapping the midwife, who desperately tried to reach the emergency button with her other hand but couldn't. She kept saying, "You have to open your legs and let me get my hand out."' *Wickedwaterwitch*

'The midwife (who was tiny) told me to put one foot on her hip and one foot on my husband's and push. I kicked her across the room.' *sallystrawbery*

'I remember the midwife saying, "Put the husband down." I looked down and I had him in a headlock with one hand, and a handful of hair in the other hand.' *BabyMadwithBump*

'I was quite shocked on reaching down to feel my son's head crowning when the midwife explained to me that my clit was stuck on his head. I thought it strange. I know you kind of change shape down there during labour, but I was confused as to how my bits were actually stuck to his head. My husband kindly told me she had said "clip" which was attaching the monitor to his head.' *Numptysmummy*

'I went to the toilet while I was wasted on pethidine. The light in there was broken so it was pitch black and in my delirium I decided to keep my hand down there in case the baby fell out. Mid-crouch, something came out that I could feel on the palm of my hand. I screamed "My baby!" The midwife, my mum and husband all came running, just in time for my whole waters sac to crash on to the floor and cover them in amniotic fluid. Classy.' *eternalstudent*

'A friend of mine went to a work Christmas dinner, ate like there was no tomorrow and promptly went into labour. At the hospital, she started vomiting and the midwife rang the panic button shouting, "She's bringing up clots!" All hell broke loose until she managed to get heard above the panic: "It's OK, it's the garlic mushrooms."' *ManxMum*

'My sister's son was breech so a consultant came into the room. She'd just been given pethidine and, as he peered up her fanjo, she looked down and said, "Is that your face? Or a mirror?" I cried with laughter as the doctor really did have a bum face.' *StrictMachine*

'I bit the doula's hand. I thought it was mine. She was saying, "No biting! Stop!" and I was thinking, I will bite my hand if I want to.' *FrannyandZooey*

'I was so used to everyone peering at my bits that at one point I offered my fanjo up for inspection to a very embarrassed male cleaner.' *zookeeper*

'I was so tired and in such pain, I had missed my partner getting changed into scrubs for theatre. When he sat down next to me I thought he was a doctor and I remember thinking, haven't you got a job to do? When he held my hand I snatched it back. It wasn't until he spoke that I realised who he was.' *mollysawally*

'When I was going up on to the bed to push my son out I asked if I should take my knickers off, to which the midwife replied: "Yes, unless you want baby to bungee."' *rozzyraspberry*

'I remember watching my husband struggling back from the car park after delivering me to the labour suite. My room overlooked the car park which was at the top of a hill. He was loaded up with my hospital bag, baby bag, food supplies, a stereo and a birthing ball. Suddenly, mid-contraction, I saw him lose control of the ball and watched it bounce down the hill. He launched after it, bags in tow. I laughed so much that I vomited and lost my mucus plug all at the same time.' *Dofeellikedancing*

'The midwife asked me to rate my pain between one and ten periodically. At one point I said nine and she rushed to give me some entonox. I was actually just telling my husband what the missing number was on his Sudoku.' *Rachelhill*

'I got up immediately after my home birth, offering to make the midwives a cup of tea. The only problem was I hadn't yet birthed the placenta.' *Ate*

Express Deliveries: Unplanned Home Births

It's all very well being able to fashion a sling from a large handkerchief but if your baby pops out rather unexpectedly, your first aid skills may be stretched to their limit. It's no use hunting for dock leaves now.

Whatever happens, try not to worry too much. Plenty of women give birth on their own without any assistance. A woman's body knows what to do. An oft-cited rule about attending a birth is: 'When in doubt, do nothing.' So don't feel a terrible burden of responsibility. Everything is likely to be just fine.

> 'Babies *are* capable of being born on their own – nature can be a wonderful thing.'
>
> (Mumsnetter midwife) mears

In the meantime, scream for the neighbours and call 999: this is no time to feel guilty about over-stretching the ambulance service.

'A friend of mine gave birth to her second in the car just outside Mothercare. She said: "I'm pushing" (she was kneeling on the front seat holding on to the head rest). Her husband lifted up her nightie saw the head, pulled over, ran around to her side and helped deliver it. Instead of calling 999 like a normal person, he calls directory enquiries for the number of the hospital, goes through all the automated messages and finally speaks to a midwife who talks him through it. And then instead of waiting for an ambulance to get to them, once the baby was out (and still attached with umbilical cord) he drove her to the hospital where the staff were waiting for them. Apparently he was cool hand Luke the whole way through.' JoshandJamie

Top tips for birth partners coping with an unplanned home delivery

1. Babies are very slippery when they are born. You need to prevent the baby from skidding across the floor and disappearing under the sideboard. Lay down some pillows/sheets/towels underneath mum's hips. You will get shouted at about the laundry stains later on, but don't worry just now.
2. Wash your hands. Scrub up and only touch mum and the baby. Don't stop to stroke the dog.
3. Check for crowning. This is where the baby's head can be seen in the birth canal. There may be squealing from the mother as she enjoys the sensation of a 'ring of fire'. You should see the baby's head quite clearly. There may be a membrane (the amniotic sac) over the baby's head, like a balloon emerging. You can pinch and twist this to break the amniotic sac. If the baby is born in the sack, you will need to quickly break the sack to retrieve him.
4. Gently guide the baby out by holding his head. Don't try to shove him back in, and don't yank him out: you aren't delivering a calf. The woman's body knows what to do. Just give gentle support to prevent the baby from bursting out and splitting the mother in two or smacking itself on to the floor. The baby will slowly move out with each contraction. He will also turn slightly as the head emerges – this is normal.

'My cousin gave birth in the car. They were on their way home from a restaurant and at first she thought it was indigestion. The whole thing from start to finish apparently took about 10 minutes. She was lying on the back seat and her husband who was driving heard a thud, which was the baby falling on to the floor!' TuttiFrutti

5. Once the head is out, wipe any mucus away from the mouth and nose with a clean towel. Gently stroke down the baby's nose to push out any mucus. The baby is a bluish colour at this stage. Don't panic. He will start screaming shortly and then he will get pinker.
6. It is quite common for the cord to be wrapped around the baby's neck. If possible, gently manoeuvre the cord over the baby's head. Don't yank on it though. If you can't get it off easily, remove it once the baby's body is born.
7. Guide the shoulders out, starting with the top shoulder, as baby emerges with the contractions: remember no yanking! Once the shoulders are out, the rest will slide out. Don't drop it.

'My husband delivered the baby but let it slip through his fingers, despite 20+ years of semi-professional rugby playing…' reluctantincubator

8. Newborn babies need oxygen and warmth. Make sure the airways are clear and baby is breathing. Then place baby on mum's bare chest and cover them both in a towel. That's it.

'If a baby arrives quickly – although it can be frightening for the mum – it is generally OK. The important thing to remember is to keep baby warm, put it skin to skin with mum on her chest with something like a blanket, coat or whatever is handy covering them both, and wait for help to arrive.' Helenhismadwife

9. Of course, there are other things that need doing such as the placenta being delivered and the cord being cut etc., but all of that can be left for the paramedic team.

'I had an unplanned home birth. The paramedics did a good job and when my son is bigger I'm sure he will love the pictures of him wrapped in a towel being cuddled by the paramedic! So if it all goes to pot on the day, stay calm and relax in the knowledge that the ambulance crews are great.' littleducks

> 10. If the placenta is born, place it next to the baby. Don't worry about cutting the cord or any of that faff. As long as your baby is breathing and wrapped up, everything is fine. Well, except for all that laundry.

'I made a right mess of some lovely White Company towels and the upstairs carpet looked like someone had gone mad with an axe. Our home insurance paid up for replacements and cleaning without batting an eyelid...' treacletart

'My grandmother gave birth in the local milk shop back in the 1940s. She didn't go into detail, but this was central Europe in January, so there would have been a considerable quantity of woolly underwear involved. She never told anyone until I had a very rapid birth with my son 50 years later. She is very much the grande dame, and clearly was deeply embarrassed by having done something as vulgar and *proletarian* as give birth in public. Apparently the hospital colluded with her worldview, and certified that the place of birth had in fact been the hospital.' frogs

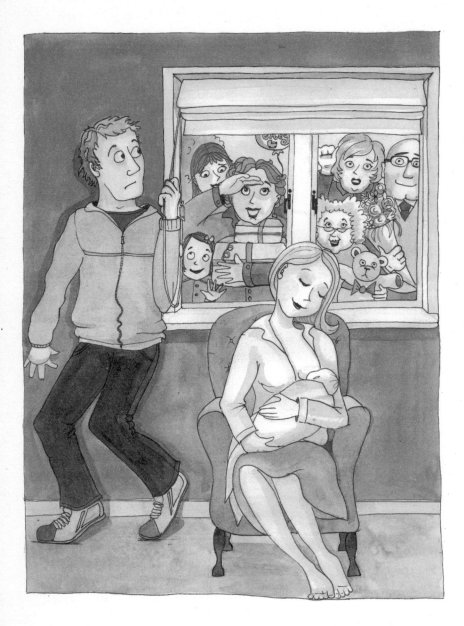

Fourth Trimester:

Life After Birth

In this chapter ...

Heading Home – The First Night (and Days) With Your New Tenant

'I remember leaving hospital with my daughter. The midwife waved us off and that feeling of being on our own was overwhelming. We were slightly hysterical. By the time we got home, and she hadn't suffered any damage, it was just exciting and not scary any more. Don't panic! You'll be fine.' wheresthehamster

> You wait for hours to get signed out, and – eventually – shuffle towards the big doors at the front of the hospital. Suddenly, you are standing on the threshold of a whole new life. What on earth is the hospital doing sending you home in charge of this baby? Waaaaaaagh! There's a screaming sound in your head, but it's not coming from your infant. What has happened to the world since you gave birth? It never looked this threatening (or filthy) before. The thought of strapping your baby into a car seat that has been fitted by your partner, in a car with your partner at the wheel, is almost too much to bear. Or as one mum said: 'I kept saying to my partner: "The hospital should never have let us out; it was harder to get the cat from the RSPCA!"'

'That first night home with my baby son was scary for me. I really couldn't get over the fact that there was a new third person in the house who was tinier than our cat. I felt we had been visited by a fairy and he might disappear in a puff of smoke. When he fell asleep in his Moses basket upstairs, I had to keep opening the door to check I wasn't dreaming him.' Tigermoth

Not all babies do as the books say and sleep soundly for the first few days. Accept now that you aren't going to get anything done for a few weeks bar feeding and changing nappies. If you are blessed with a sleeper, make the most of it: try to sleep when your baby sleeps, no matter if it is the middle of the day. More likely, he will refuse to drop off unless you are holding, rocking or feeding him; this is normal too, just more annoying. But these are very early days, and it's just a case of getting through them. It will get better, honest. Now is not the time to start flicking breathlessly through the Owner's Manual searching for the chapter on sleep training.

Don't feel pressured to meet your public. If you want privacy, head straight for your bed and camp there John-and-Yoko-style for as long as it takes. But if you were hoping for more of a celebration, invite people over and pop open some champagne; just make sure they wash their own glasses and don't let them outstay their welcome. Every set of parents needs a secret code – a fake cough or rub of the eye – to indicate to the other half that now's time to start moving guests towards the front door, so agree on one now. Otherwise, you may find yourself using the time-to-leave code of sobbing hysterically. You're not being rude, you've just had a baby.

Top ten tips for early motherhood (by Morningpaper)

1. **Eat properly and a lot – and drink a lot of water**
   Make sure you eat one or two good meals a day. Go out for lunch if you can, especially at weekends, even if you have to take turns eating and walking outside with screamy baby. Or go for lunch with parents and make them cook you a proper roast. Eat a decent breakfast. Eat lots of snacks. Keep a lot of fresh and dried fruit around. Keep your iron levels up because low iron makes you feel like death; eat a handful of apricots with orange juice once or twice a day.

2. **Go to bed early**
   Don't try and get stuff done in the evenings because you are only robbing yourself of sleep time. This stage won't last for ever, you just need to get through it and remain healthy and sane.

3. **Get out every day for a walk**

   With the pram. The car doesn't count. You need a walk in the fresh air. Walk to the park. (Watch smiling, laughing parents pushing their children on the swings, and remember that at least a few of them are wanting to scream: 'I USED TO BE A PLAYER AND NOW LOOK AT ME – I'M A SODDING SWING PUSHER!') This knowledge will cheer you up. Alternatively, put your baby in a sling or backpack and go for a walk in the woods. At the weekends, do this with your partner and make him carry the baby. Do you have a local beauty spot or similar? If so, become very familiar with it!

4. **Accept all offers of help**

   From husband/parents/relatives. This is not the time to be proud. Become a YES person. Whether they are offering to make a cup of tea or take the baby for a walk. Just say yes. And if you can get a cleaner for a couple of hours a week, *do it*.

5. **Find some friends**

   Pick a mums' group – whether it's a breastfeeding group or a mother-and-baby one – and keep going to it every week. You are not going for baby or for advice; you are just going for *you* and to be sociable. That's why *everyone* is there. Over time, you will make some friends/find people you can mix with or chat to, and that will really help.

6. **Take time for yourself and rest**

   Your body needs to recover from birth/feeding/all the changes it has had. 'Sleep when baby sleeps!' is the standard advice, but if you can't bear to do this, at least carve out a little bit of time for yourself, anyway. As soon as baby falls asleep, don't rush around with the Hoover; just sit down with a cup of tea and a biscuit. Give yourself ten minutes' peace minimum, before you start running around tackling chores. Small babies are often quite entertained and soothed by the sound of the Hoover or washing machine, so if you must do housework, leave it until she's awake. And if you *can* sleep, do.

7. **Don't gate-keep baby related jobs**

   If you have a partner, don't automatically take over certain tasks just because you do them better. He'll learn to do them just as well. Make him solely responsible for certain tasks, such as bath time. Let him do all of that, while you rest or do something else.

   (continued)

Do this now and you will avoid being bitter and twisted and in charge of everything domestic for the next 50 years.

8. **Get a paper delivered**
I think I survived the early days by just having the *Guardian* every morning. My partner would put it on the bed, so it was there for me when I woke up for the morning feed. Keeping abreast of current affairs made me feel less like a drudge/housewife and more like a normal person. And it took me out of my daily grind. Alternatively, get a stash of novels in or some light reading (maybe not fashion mags though, unless you have extremely high self-esteem ...).

9. **Know your mental-health limits**
Be aware of your mental health, but at the same time, try not to focus on it too much. Remember that *most* new mums at this stage are feeling massively shocked, emotionally and physically. Don't panic that it is past mental-health problems creeping back or an inevitable decline into postnatal depression. Feeling terrible is normal. But if you think your mental health is worsening or becoming a major problem, speak to your health visitor or GP.

10. **Look at your baby every day ...**
... and tell yourself how fabulous and amazing you are for growing this wonderful person.

Breastfeeding – How to Get Going

Unless you've been living on another planet during your pregnancy, you can't have failed to notice that 'Breast is Best'. You will already know that breast milk is the most nutritionally superior food you can give your baby and that it has a positive effect on your baby's health (and your own) that cannot be duplicated by formula milk. That's why both the Department of Health and the World Health Organisation recommend that you exclusively breastfeed your baby for the first six months. This is not to say that formula milk is worthless. It's a perfectly adequate substitute for breast milk, but *not* an equally good alternative.

'I think we need to be absolutely honest with mothers and not patronise them by sugar-coating the facts. Just because formula-feeding is more common, it doesn't mean it's normal. Breastfeeding is, biologically, the default position.' princessglitter

Breast milk is packed full of antibodies to protect your baby from infection and reduce the chances of her contracting all sorts of diseases from asthma to eczema. Babies who are breastfed are less likely to become obese or get diabetes. Breastfeeding mothers are less likely to develop breast cancer or suffer from brittle bones when they are older. As long as you don't reach for a king-size Mars bar at every feed, it might even help you to lose some of that extra padding gained during pregnancy. Now, if that isn't reason enough to whip out your jugglies, what is? 'I did it because it meant I could leave the house at a moment's notice without all the hassle of measuring, sterilising and carrying bottles around with me,' says one mum. 'It was hard and painful for the first few days, but once you get the hang of it, it's wonderful.'

Mind you, just because breastfeeding is natural, it doesn't mean that doing it comes naturally. For every mother who's lactating like a fountain and loving it, there's another who's wincing at the prospect of a small mouth clamping down on her nipple yet again, or as one mum puts it: 'For the first couple of months, I felt like I was trying to attach myself to a stapler every two hours.' And, frankly, there's no telling which type of mother you're going to turn out to be. Whether you give your baby breast milk or formula (or a combination of both) is an entirely personal choice. Seven out of ten British mums start out breastfeeding, but six weeks later, half of them will have stopped. There are lots of different reasons, but at the root of them all (well, almost all) is that breastfeeding isn't how most women imagine it to be.

'I do think many women expect breastfeeding to be easy from day one, and forget that it's

something mum and baby need to learn together.' Shazronnie

So before you even try on your nursing bra, it's wise to make sure that your expectations are properly adjusted.

'My midwife said I should allow six weeks to get breastfeeding right, which sounded like a shocking amount of time. Then she said: "What's six weeks out of your life?" And I thought, "Yes, it's not long really". That thought has stayed with me – and helped.' NoBiggy

Mumsnetter Hunkermunker's top five things you need to know about breastfeeding

1. **It takes a bit of getting used to**
   It can come as quite a shock to discover that once the birth's over you have to learn a new skill – with a pupil who is minutes old and doesn't appear to have read the *How to Suckle* manual.

2. **It's always worth giving it a try**
   Even if you're not really sure you want to do it for long – or at all. It's far easier, physically, to switch from breastfeeding to formula-feeding than the other way round. And, if you don't try it, you'll never know if it was going to be straightforward for you. Even if you're pretty sure breastfeeding's not for you, consider giving the first feed (or first few feeds) because your milk (or colostrum, as it's called at this stage) will be jam-packed with antibodies and all sorts of goodies that help to stabilise your baby's blood sugars, line her gut and generally ease her introduction into the world.

3. **It pays to do your homework**
   Many hospitals have policies that actively support breastfeeding mothers, but the shift changes and inclinations of individual midwives may mean your own breastfeeding support is not as effective as it could be. Far better that you've spent a little time

thinking and learning about it beforehand; you'll feel more empowered and capable (and if there's anything you need to feel just after you've had a baby it's empowered and capable). The NCT runs breastfeeding classes, so perhaps attend one of those before the birth. Their breastfeeding counsellors can be useful post-birth too, as are drop-in groups, midwives and health visitors. The Association of Breastfeeding Mothers (ABM) runs local groups around the country, including the magnificently named Breastfeeding Advocacy and Peer Support Group (aka BAPS). And don't forget online support. Many a mum has found that breastfeeding has clicked once she asked for advice on Mumsnet – and even if it hasn't, she's found support and empathy. Also, make a note of the helpline numbers of the various breastfeeding charities, and find out, too, if there are breastfeeding drop-in clinics or baby groups near you and on which days they run.

4. **It's good to talk**

   Ask other women you know about their experiences of breastfeeding. It'll help you to get a picture of what it's like. But don't imagine you'll have a carbon copy of your mum/sister/auntie/grandma/best friend's experience. Remember, your baby's never been born before and you've never breastfed before. Your breastfeeding relationship with your baby is unique and you will work it out between you, learning as you go.

5. **It gets easier**

   Breastfeeding can be hard, especially in the early weeks when you're recovering from the birth and have the pretty relentless task of building your supply by feeding regularly. But it's OK and perfectly normal for it to be hard, as long as you can access decent support to make it easier for you. Many women would say that if you can manage the first six weeks of breastfeeding, the following weeks/months/years are a comparative doddle.

Bottle-Feeding – Advice for Those Who Can't or Don't Want to Breastfeed

You've been lugging them around them like two life rafts throughout your pregnancy. But when you actually need them, the damn things don't work. Or maybe the whole business of breastfeeding is so off-putting that you don't even want to try. Meanwhile, all around you, wholesome mums are whipping out their organic knockers everywhere you go, fortifying their babies against asthma, eczema, hay fever, obesity, idiocy ... the list goes on. Frustrated? Feeling guilty? Well, stop it! It certainly is not an offence to bottle-feed your baby, but it is a violation to feel guilty about it, as if it somehow makes you a bad mother.

'I wished it could have been different but it has turned out fine – an allergy-free (fingers crossed) healthy, happy and bright little girl. For my next child (fingers crossed) I will give breastfeeding another go, but will be far less hard on myself if it fails again, and definitely won't allow anyone to push me around. I know one girl who used to hide her bottles away when her midwife and health visitor came round to see her.' JayTree

Bring a bottle – how to make up formula

There is something almost Willy Wonka-ish about making up your first bottle. And it's terrifying – doing it incorrectly or carelessly could make your baby ill. But it won't be long before you can do it with your eyes shut, which is just as well given how tired you'll be. The only safe alternative to breast milk for babies under one year is infant formula. This has been produced commercially for nearly 150 years. Most formulas are made from processed cow's milk. Of course, it is not an exact replica of breast milk, but it's the best substitute for breastfeeding that has been developed to date.

The official guidelines for making up bottles of formula are subject to change, so don't rely on what your mum/sister/best friend says, even if they insist it never did their babies any harm. Always make up formula according to the manufacturer's instructions.

The rules for storing formula have also changed in recent years. You now have to make up each feed as you need it, rather than making up a day's (or night's) batch and keeping it in the fridge until you need it, as your parents may have done in days of yore.

There are shortcuts that are safe, though. You can buy ready-made-up formula in cartons (these are sterile). Or, to help you at night, you could go up to bed with a flask of boiling water, a pre-measured portion of powder (you can buy special containers for this) and a bowl of cold water. When your baby cries, put the boiling water and powder into a sterile bottle and place the bottle in bowl of cold water to cool it to drinkable temperature (or run it under a cold tap). It shouldn't take long to make and, more importantly, it is safe.

It is worth investing in six bottles and teats. The choice of teats on offer can be bewildering and it may be tempting to switch to a different one if your baby isn't feeding well. But don't be too hasty – they might just need settling-in time. All bottles and teats must be sterilised until your baby's first birthday, by which time they will be eating Cheerios off the kitchen floor anyway, so it starts to feel a bit pointless. Microwave and electric sterilisers will save the time and effort of boiling pans of water, but if you're strapped for cash, boiling it all up for 10 minutes in a pan you keep solely for this purpose will still work. Before sterilising, clean the bottles, teats and rings with hot, soapy water and a bottle brush.

To make up a feed, start by wiping down the work surface and washing your hands. Boil some fresh tap water in the kettle (not bottled water because its mineral content isn't always suitable for babies) and let it cool for up to half an hour before pouring the correct amount into a sterilised bottle. Measure the exact amount of powder, add it to the bottle, screw on the cap and shake until the powder has dissolved.

Always check the temperature before you give your baby the go-ahead by dripping some formula on the inside of your wrist.

Don't keep it warm for more than 20 minutes before the feed as germs will start to breed. Throw away what is left at the end of a feed.

Keep a carton of ready-made formula handy for emergencies.

Some bottle-feeding no-no's

- Never leave a baby with a bottle propped up in her mouth in case she chokes.
- Never put anything else in the bottle with her milk, such as a rusk. (Even if Granny swears it will make her sleep till next Wednesday.) You should also ignore her helpful suggestions of adding brandy for the same reasons.
- Don't encourage a baby to finish each bottle. 'Feeding up' a small baby (especially a low-birthweight one) is associated with a higher risk of childhood obesity.
- Don't give a baby 'follow-on' milk before she's six months old (if at all), no matter how big she is. Her digestive system just won't be able to cope with it.

How to get that formula into your baby

Getting your baby to drink formula milk out of a bottle may not be as 'technically' demanding as getting her to drink breast milk from your breast can be, but that's not to say you can just shove a teat in roughly the right direction and be done with it.

When it comes to actually putting teat to mouth, your midwife/health visitor should be able to help and advise you. You may have to ask quite loudly though, as the drive to encourage more women to breastfeed does mean that information about formula-feeding is not routinely given out. Rightly or wrongly, this can mean that some formula-feeding mothers can miss out on knowing stuff that would come in really useful, such as when to change bottles and teats for new ones, or that ... :

'... despite all the various health claims on the tins, the difference between brands of formula is probably very small.' tiktok

When it's time for a feed, get into a comfortable position and don't forget to protect your back. Settle down and make this your time together. Try not to rush the feed, but savour it as a chance to bond. Breastfeeding mums don't have the monopoly on bonding and cuddles at feeding time. You are 100 per cent mother and your baby knows that, so don't let it get in the way of your enjoyment – or their dinner.

I Love Being Pregnant Because ...

'... I feel whole, complete, sexy and fab; I love it. I mean sure, the acid heartburn is a pain, the leg cramps waking me up, the pins and needles and so on are all pretty unpleasant, but on the whole, yeah man, being pregnant rocks.' *Thomcat*

'... I love having radiant skin and really thick, shiny hair, the camaraderie between pregnant women and the fact you make new friends. The best bit is going on maternity leave – especially the bit before the baby comes – lots of shopping, swimming and lazing around. I liked getting a seat on the Tube, although I have to say it didn't always happen. I was fortunate that I didn't get stretch marks, varicose veins, piles or morning sickness and, although my son was 8lb 13oz, with a large head, I had a straightforward delivery with no stitches. (I loved the epidural!) All the flowers, pressies and cards you get are great, of course, and I'm lighter now than before I was pregnant.' *Flippa*

'... of the way everyone assumes you're a lovely person just because you're going to have a baby (which of course I am).' *skidaddle*

'... of buying new clothes, being offered the last piece of cake, having an excuse to nap in the afternoons.' *MrsBadger*

'... I'm able to eat loads without being told off because I'm allowed to eat for two (I know that's not strictly true, but I'm upholding it!).' *PurpleLostPrincess*

'... I like shopping for baby stuff, decorating the nursery and making sure the house is really tidy – something I previously felt completely unmotivated to do; seeing the scan pictures, watching big, healthy limbs squirming and jutting around your tummy; wondering what sex it is and what you'll call it.' *Bobbins*

'... I loved dreaming about what my son or daughter would look like; sitting in meetings at work and never getting bored because I can always feel my bump and get kicks to wake me up; the excitement when you feel the first kick, or waiting outside the radiographer's room for your first-ever scan, then being told all is well. I was even excited when I realised I was in labour. I knew that I would see my baby soon and I was so ready for it (or so I thought!).' *Mum2toby*

'... I loved all the check-ups where I got to listen to the heartbeat; I loved that sound.' *Choochie*

'... I can wear tight tops stretched over my tummy, for once in my life!' *Philippat*

'... I can balance a plate on the bump, while slouching in front of the TV. Oh, and no periods.' *Doormat*

'... I've just discovered my favourite bit. I've started maternity leave, the weather is beautiful and I can sit outside in the sunshine with a huge glass of orange juice and tickle my baby's feet. She loves it and chases my hands around, sticking her feet out further and further. It's the first proper interaction I've had with my unborn child, and I know it's going to be over so soon, but for these last couple of days, it's just me and her in the garden, enjoying the peace.' *ShowOfHands*

'... of feeling a life inside you, everyone smiles and is nice to you, it's a good excuse to eat more cakes, a good excuse to do less housework, wondering what it's going to be and, finally, having a cleavage (though maybe that's countered by the hideous maternity bras!).' *Ninja*

'... I love feeling the little person who will be such a huge part of the rest of my life wriggling away!' *Hunkermunker*

'... I just loved the feeling of completeness ... I can't really explain, but being all blooming and rotund and people complimenting me on it. Just that glowing feeling. Being pregnant can be so sexy too!' *Winnie1*

'... I liked knowing the due date is approaching and feeling like me and my partner were in a lovely bubble of expectation. It was so romantic going for walks, picnics and meals out together ... talking about the future and feeling so close and happy.' *rubles*

'... I can eat ginger biscuits in bed first thing in the morning and not get moaned at about the crumbs!' *Badjelly*

'... of the ultimate thing for me, which (although obviously I was not pregnant any more) is bringing the new bundle home to meet the world.' *mrsjaffabiffa*

'... I love smiling secretly to myself in meetings when no one else knows; the look on my parents' faces when we tell them; rubbing my tummy absent-mindedly all the time; quitting work a full 11 weeks before the birth and watching the *ER* double episode every day, while eating crushed ice and ice lollies; bizarre dreams; hiccups in the womb; decorating the nursery and spontaneously bursting into tears of joy when everything was finished at the sheer excitement; the first images on the screen at the scan, and walking around all afternoon saying, "Oh my GOD! Oh my GOD!"; the labour and the birth being all OK and hearing the words, "You have a beautiful girl"; seeing her face for the first time and thinking she looked familiar already ... I can't wait to do it again.' *Snickers*

'... you don't need to worry about looking fat.' *Grommit*

I Will Never Get Pregnant Again Because ...

'... at three weeks postnatal, I wrote a list to stop me if I ever feel like trying for child number four. The list includes: night sweats, sore boobs, piles, the head coming out, indigestion, talking about your body and internals with almost anyone, thrush and piles cream.' *Edgarcat*

'... of stretch marks, "deflated" boobs, varicose veins, sickness, no sleep (before or after), puffy ankles, feeling emotional all the time ... not to mention no booze or Stilton.' *Sb34*

'... day sweats in a summer pregnancy, carpal tunnel syndrome – I had that pleasure with my second – and the extra two stone in weight left behind by the other two children.' *Iota*

'... of rib pain; spending a fortune on large bottles of Gaviscon, which I had to lug around in my handbag; people staring at me as if I was a mutant in the gym; worrying over not feeling foetal movement; losing my own identity and becoming a walking uterus/grandchild provider; and being given "advice" all the time.' *Flippa*

'... of not being able to get into a comfy position when sleeping; waking up constantly during the night to pee; people automatically putting their hands on your bump to feel (without asking); walking with non-pregnant people – and not keeping up; seeing people on the train/tube/bus, hide behind their books or papers pretending they didn't see you, so they don't have to give up their seat. *Metrobaby*

'... I can't afford it – in terms of health, time, money or sanity.' *Griffy*

'... I'm rubbish at it! I spend the first (at least) 12 weeks ridiculously anxious, the next eight desperate to feel movement, then my pelvis goes at around 20 weeks. The last six weeks, I just want to sleep and people either tell me how tired I'm looking, or they say stuff like, "You're looking a lot better," which makes me wonder how bad I was looking last week!' *tassisssss*

'... of leaking breasts – most embarrassing in public; the feeling when the head was coming out – ouch; and piles – ouch, ouch.' *Doormat*

'... a C-section scar that itches all the time; a flabby tummy that hangs over said scar; stretch marks on my boobs and hips (they never told me about those).' *DebL*

'... of being repulsed at the thought of losing your dignity while giving birth and being determined not to, then going and throwing all those good ideas out the window as soon as the first cramp hits, then regretting the loss of dignity afterwards. Then there's the lack of bladder control, which they say will probably continue for the rest of my life.' *Meanmum*

'... of resembling Elizabeth I for months after each baby because of spectacular hair-loss and then effectively having a "mullet" for another five months while it grows back; episiotomy and tearing (sitting on the cheek of one buttock for five weeks because of too-tight stitching); sciatica; Symphysis Pubis Dysfunction; insomnia from 34 weeks; chronic sleep deprivation; the whole breasts-containing-milk thing; having to wear wire-free bras while breastfeeding; breast pads showing through T-shirts; looking fat, not pregnant, from three to six months.' *Molly1*

'... of the headaches, ooh the headaches – agony for the first 16 weeks.' *Chiccadum*

'... I had insomnia from 20 weeks because of chronic restless leg syndrome. The only thing that stopped it at night (for about 20–30 minutes at a time) was a really hot bath. By 37 weeks, I was having six hot baths during the night every night. *Griffy*

'... I don't get any sympathy. My husband keeps worrying about how we will cope with a toddler and a baby, and when I say it will be a piece of cake compared to being pregnant, he thinks I am mad or just making it up. I think I would feel so much better if he could just understand what it is like. I also get frustrated by the fact that if a non-pregnant person was that ill for so long people would expect them to stay in bed until they felt better, but if you are pregnant you just have to get on with it.' *CookieMonster2*

'... I have so little energy and I feel I really lose a huge part of who I am. I'm normally cheerful and contented, but when I feel utterly drained and exhausted after a day that I know wasn't really too demanding workwise, I just turn into a miserable grump. I hate it!' *miffin*

'... of the progression into a demented, fuzzy-haired, tiny-eyed monster with no sense of humour and serious chocolate addiction. And it says something about the sleep deprivation that it took me two months to figure out that I felt like death because I had an infection and wasn't just exhausted.' *Gizmo*

'... of too much time given over to worrying; puking over yourself while driving to work (perhaps that was only me); a complete inability to concentrate on anything important; a constant need to pee; a constant need to eat; a constant need to sleep; a constant need to puke and worry about where you're going to do it; going off chocolate, bread and cereal and feeling ill from the smell of deodorant, perfume and cooking; waddling; the fact you're not allowed to lift anything; midwives taking pints and pints of your blood (well, it felt like it); finding suitable pots to pee in (and carry to work for most of the day before your appointment); being constantly kicked in the ribs/cervix/lungs; crying at sentimental songs spun by Terry Wogan. (But maybe I will do it again one day ...)' *Philippat*

'... I hated being told that it would all be worse when the baby came. Just open the oven door for me to stick my head in, why don't you? It was better once the baby came, horribly tired though I was, I didn't have the sick fluey exhaustion I had all through pregnancy.' *Cicatrice*

'... I had one child, then twins – I know I would have triplets if I went on.' *Custardo*

'... it's exhausting. Someone once told me that a pregnant woman is putting in the same amount of physical effort when she is sitting on the sofa as a bloke when he is climbing a very steep hill. I have no idea if this is true or not, but it did silence my husband.' *FruitfulOfFruit*

'... everything that can go wrong probably will and you will never quite feel good. Actually that's not quite true – I had four hours last week when I felt fecking marvellous, but this turned out to be delirium, as I was promptly hospitalised for dehydration. It's a myth that every woman blooms; I don't bloom, I fester. But the good news is, that it does end eventually, and you get a baby out of it. Otherwise, it's just a shocking pain in the arse in every possible sense.' *whomovedmychocolate*

'[fingers in ears] ... la la la la ... not listening ... la la la la ... I will have another ... I don't care how awful pregnancy and birth were with my son ... I won't listen ... I refuse to remember ... la la la la la ...' *Ghosty*

Appendices

APPENDIX 1: Your Pregnancy Development Calendar

Note: this guide tells you how your baby is developing week by week. But remember, not all babies develop exactly like each other, so this can only be a general guide: you should ask your doctor or midwife for any specific information about your pregnancy.

We all know babies come in two flavours, but, for clarity – as many of you won't know what flavour you're getting – we'll refer to your baby here as 'she'.

Weeks 3 to 8

How your baby is growing

Your pregnancy is actually counted from the first day of your last period. So, when sperm meets egg, you're already counted as being two weeks pregnant! (Which is why this calendar starts at week three, not week one.)

Your baby (well, she's actually officially still an embryo till eight weeks, but we'll gloss over that) starts off as a flat disc of cells and not, as you might imagine, a cute jellybean.

These cells divide continuously to form three layers called the ectoderm, mesoderm and endoderm. This may be more information than you need, but what your baby does with these layers is deeply impressive. She somehow manages to grow specific parts of her body from each layer. So, the endoderm layer develops into the brain, nervous system, hair, nails, enamel in teeth, sweat glands and the linings of the ear, nose, throat and eye; the mesoderm layer develops into your baby's head and its muscles, bone, heart, arteries, veins and kidneys; and the endoderm layer develops into the lining of the body, such as the cells lining the gut, lungs and bladder.

From around four weeks on, your baby's flat disc shape starts folding to form a head and a temporary thin tail. By the beginning of the fifth week, your baby is developing paddle-shaped buds that will become arms and legs. By the sixth week, these paddles flatten at their ends and grooves appear in them that will eventually grow into fingers and toes.

Your baby's looking a bit top-heavy (for now) because her head is growing so fast. She's also starting to develop little outgrowths that will become ears, as well as areas for her nose and eyes.

And there are other things happening too: she's starting to develop muscles and, during the sixth week, may twitch her body and arms. (The legs develop a little after the arms.) Her heart is developing and dividing into chambers; it is beating and beginning to push blood through the blood vessels that are growing around her body.

Despite all these achievements though, your baby is still very tiny. From the top of the head to the middle of her buttocks (what doctors call the crown–rump length), your baby measures a minuscule 10–14mm (about the size of a small bean). She's surrounded by a thin, but tough, 'bag' (called the amniotic sac) that's full of fluid to cushion her and keep her safe and she's joined to you, her mum, through the umbilical cord, which will do the job of sending in food and taking out waste products.

How your body is changing

Some women feel the effects of being pregnant quite dramatically. Others feel a bit nauseous and wonder what all the fuss is about. It's a very individual thing, determined partly by your body's response to the increase in hormones. But you can expect to have some degree of morning sickness and/or nausea, tiredness, spots, tender breasts and moments of faintness/dizziness.

Weeks 9 to 12

How your baby is growing

In the ninth week, your baby loses her funny little tail and becomes altogether more baby-like (and, officially, a foetus, rather than an embryo). Think jelly baby with an oversized head.

Your baby's face is broad, with eyes widely separated and shut tight (eyelids are fused together until 27 weeks), and her brain will be forming brain cells at a rate of 250,000 a minute.

The rest of her body is catching up fast, though: by the end of the 12th week, she will have doubled in length to about 5.4cm. By then, her arms will no longer look like short flippers but will be in proportion with the rest of her body. Her legs take longer to develop and her thighs will stay slightly stumpy for a while.

By the end of the ninth week, all babies look pretty much the same but, a mere three weeks later, some will look a lot more like little boy babies, while others will look more like girls. Everything's still quite immature, though, and it's unlikely that, if you had an ultrasound now, anyone would commit themselves to the sex of your baby.

Muscles and joints are also growing fast now. At eight weeks, your baby can make some movements but, by 12 weeks, these will seem more purposeful. She's now developed the sorts of muscles we use to walk and run and which she can use to move her limbs and stretch her legs, body and neck.

It's thought that babies move in response to movements in the amniotic fluid that surrounds them – ripples in their own swimming pool. Ultrasound studies show that foetuses move a lot around ten weeks and then start slowing down, as they get bigger and your womb gets less roomy.

Your baby's internal organs, such as her liver and pancreas, are also coming along nicely. The intestines part of her gut is starting to develop specialist cells: some will have protective, immune roles, some will produce enzymes to break down food and some will grow into the nerves that stimulate the intestine into churning up food and pushing it through the system. Your baby's intestines are already a hollow tube, through which the amniotic fluid is moving, and from which protein is digested every day.

Your baby's spinal cord – the long column of nerves that runs down the length of her spine – can just about be seen now. And her diaphragm is developing too. This is a sheet of muscle, shaped like a leaf, which separates the chest from the abdomen, dividing the area into a space for lungs, stomach and bowels, respectively. Once this happens, your baby can get hiccups if her diaphragm is irritated in some way. You won't notice them now but, when she is bigger, her hiccups will take over your life – or at least wake you up as soon as you drop off to sleep.

How your body is changing

You will have missed your second period by now, so pregnancy may be becoming even more real. You may be really tired (yes, even more tired than last month), sick and headachy (bed rest does help for this). Your breasts will still be tender and they will definitely be bigger. Don't try to cram them into your usual bra and, when you buy new ones, bear in mind that the size your breasts are now will not be the same as their size at the end of the pregnancy. Nowhere near.

Weeks 13 to 16

How your baby is growing

Your baby is starting to look more and more like a little human. This is because her face is sorting itself out and her body's growth rate has speeded up to catch up with her head. By now, she will be around 14cm long and weigh around 200g.

Your baby's eyes, which have been a bit to the side, now take up their rightful place looking straight ahead. Although closed, they'll be moving slowly under her eyelids. Meanwhile, her ears, which started as little buds, are now standing out a little. She's also grown a proper neck, which means her chin is no longer touching her chest.

Her body and head are covered from now until birth with a fine, wispy layer of hair called lanugo (from a Latin word meaning down); this is thought to help insulate babies and keep them warm.

By 16 weeks, your baby's legs have got longer and she's also starting to grow nails on her fingers and toes. And, all the time, her limbs are developing proper hard bones: the first bone that is formed is actually the clavicle (collar bone); the second is the femur (thigh bone).

If you have an ultrasound around now, you may be able to get the ultrasound operator to tell you the sex of your baby, as genitalia are well formed. But babies are notorious for refusing to co-operate in this respect, so unless your ultrasound operator can get a clear view, they are unlikely to want to commit themselves.

Your baby's moving around quite a bit now, kicking, flailing her arms and grasping with her hands. She has bursts of activity, stretching her legs and arms. Her muscles are continuing to develop, as are the nerves that make them work, and it's thought this activity is practice for the outside world, so that each group of baby muscles knows what it's meant to do when it grows up.

Your baby's skin doesn't look much like it will do at birth – it is thin enough to be able to see blood vessels in places – and because she doesn't have any fat yet, she looks vaguely pink and skinny.

All the organs in your baby's body, including her stomach and bowels, are continuing to grow. Her pancreas will be producing insulin, which is needed to control levels of sugar in the blood, and her liver is making bile. Her lungs are also growing and she will be practising how to breathe. She doesn't need to breathe 'properly' in your womb because her blood largely bypasses the lungs and gets the oxygen it needs through the umbilical cord. But, as soon as she's born, the umbilical cord and placenta will be history and she'll need to breathe to get oxygen from the air around her, so wisely, she has a gentle try-out before birth. Because she's surrounded by amniotic fluid, this means she's effectively breathing underwater.

Meanwhile, your baby's heart has stormed ahead development-wise, folding itself from a hollow muscular tube into a small, fist-like muscle with four chambers. It pumps around six gallons of blood a day. If you hear its heartbeat (through a Doppler machine, see p. 10) it can sound alarmingly fast – like a mad galloping pony. This is normal. Your baby's heartbeat is around twice as fast as yours.

How your body is changing

If you've been feeling sick, the waves of nausea might be fading away by now (but we can't promise!). You'll probably notice a change in your body shape: that bulge is actually your womb rising out of the pelvis to occupy part of your lower abdomen. You can just about feel it and it may make sleeping on your tummy uncomfortable. You could find that you're getting constipated, too, one of the side effects of pregnancy hormones being a more sluggish bowel.

The good news is that most women start to feel less exhausted around this time, although, unfortunately, this is a temporary state and you will feel even more tired later on (and more tired still, after the baby is born).

Weeks 17 to 20

How your baby is growing

Your baby doesn't grow as quickly now, but builds on what she's done already. Over these four weeks, she'll grow about 50mm to 15–19cm, weighing between 250g and 450g, and her arms and legs will reach their final size in relation to the rest of her body. Her neck gets stronger too, and she'll hold her head up more and more.

She moves more strongly now, and her kicking will become more and more forceful (as you may well come to rue). Incidentally, it's worth making a note of the day you feel that first kick: one study looked at the relationship between when you first feel your baby move and when you give birth and found that the average time between feeling the first kick and having your baby was 147 days.

There are some downsides to being in an amniotic fluid bath for nine months and, during these four weeks, your baby develops some protection in the form of a cheesy, white cream that covers her whole body and head. Called vernix, it's made by her sebaceous glands (the ones that make oily fluid to protect our skin) and acts as a waterproof layer to protect her delicate skin from getting chafed. It's said to make your baby pass through the birth canal more easily – it certainly can make babies feel rather slippery when they come out – and you'll see the remnants of it on her skin at birth.

Your baby also develops some thermal insulation now by forming a special kind of fat called brown fat. Found around the kidneys and under the skin at the base of the neck, it produces heat, when needed, during the newborn period. Her body is also busy insulating developing nerves with a covering layer called myelin that makes the electrical impulses that travel down the nerves go faster and more smoothly.

Meanwhile, the pads on your baby's fingers and toes are beginning to develop patterns of whorls and swirls. Hopefully, she will never get fingerprinted in later life, but this is where these unique identifiers begin. Also, her eyebrows and hair are now sufficiently bushy to be seen on ultrasound scan, and little buds are developed for milk teeth (and, behind them, already, tooth buds for grown-up teeth).

If you're carrying a girl, her womb will have grown and her vagina will now start developing. If you're carrying a boy, his testes will start moving down from where they develop inside his abdomen, quite high up on the back wall, to their eventual home in the scrotum.

Your baby's lungs are becoming more mature, with tiny air sacs called alveoli that provide a huge area for the lungs to take in oxygen and get rid of carbon dioxide once your baby's born. She will also have a fine set of vocal cords, which she may exercise, obviously silently, ready for her big moment. She won't be breathing fully because she is essentially underwater in her amniotic bath, but she does have a go. It is this that can give her hiccups, which, early on, can feel like little flutters but, later, may be seismic movements that make your belly shake.

You'll no doubt be thrilled to learn that your baby has also managed to get together her first bowel movement. Meconium, as this is called, is made up of amniotic fluid and bits of old cells and other debris from the lining of the bowels. It is green, black and tarry. It is incredibly sticky and difficult to get off so it's worth remembering, as you lovingly cuddle your newborn baby, to get a nappy on her as soon as possible.

Your baby's heart is growing stronger. And, as time goes on, won't beat quite as fast as it did earlier on in its development. And her brain is going through a highly specialised growth phase, developing the senses of taste, smell, hearing and sight.

How your body is changing

As your womb grows and rises up and out of your pelvis, it stretches the ligaments that fix it in place. This is obviously necessary but, unfortunately, it can really hurt. You may find you get a brief stabbing pain below your bikini line; sometimes it can be a dull, achy pain, particularly if you have been on your feet all day. If it stays, gets worse or you have any other problems like cramps, spotting or sickness, you need to see a doctor or midwife. Other things you may notice include bleeding gums (flossing is your friend), nosebleeds and, possibly, a touch (or more than a touch) of heartburn.

Weeks 21 to 24

How your baby is growing

By now, your baby will be around 23cm long and weigh between 500g and 620g. She looks lean but already more babyish; she will start seriously putting on weight between 24 and 37 weeks, at a rate of around 15g a day.

Most of your baby's organs are formed now, but they'll need to develop more before they work properly. At 24 weeks, a premature baby has a chance of surviving, although a few babies have actually done so earlier because medicine and technology advance every day.

Her cheeks are filling out slightly and her skin is becoming more red than pink, and less translucent. Her lips and tongue are formed and she will be getting used to them, licking her lips and maybe sucking her thumb if she bumps into it. Her eyes may just have opened and they move quickly – she will blink if startled by a loud noise near your abdomen. Her hair and nails continue to grow. Nails can get quite long and need to be cut soon after birth to avoid your baby randomly scratching her (or your) face.

Your baby's immune system is getting going as she starts making white blood cells, which specifically attack bacteria and other infections, but perhaps the most important thing that happens to your baby at 24 weeks is that her lungs become more properly developed. They are still immature, but their air tubes are like a tree and they keep separating into smaller and smaller branches until they form tiny air sacs. At 24 weeks, there are quite a few little air sacs. The cells that make up the walls of these sacs start producing a fluid that is essential to your baby's survival. The fluid is a fatty layer of liquid called surfactant and it keeps the tiny little airways open. These airways need to be open when your baby is born, so that she can breathe in enough oxygen. The blood vessels around the lungs are also developing now, so they can pick up the oxygen the lungs have brought and take it round her body.

Your baby now has the same sleep patterns as she will have when she is born. She will spend around six hours awake and 18 asleep – and will sleep in set positions. There is some debate among researchers as to what being awake really means. Certainly, there are times when your baby will respond to things happening on the outside – to you perhaps – if you are startled by a loud noise, for example. Some researchers think your baby isn't really awake because while it is developing the activity of her brain and nervous system is kept quiet by hormones produced by the placenta.

Your baby can hear in the womb and her hearing is getting better as time goes on. She prefers lower, intense sounds to start with. There is some research to suggest that newborn babies respond to sounds they have become familiar with in the womb. Certainly, newborn babies prefer the sound of their mother's voice and are calmed by it. There has been a trend to play babies classical music, read them great works of literature and take them to plays while still in the womb. These are all worthwhile activities but, however smart your unborn child is, she's unlikely to gain an enormous intellectual advantage from them. You'd have to suspect she would prefer you watched *CBeebies*.

How your body is changing

You may be blooming. The spots of early pregnancy will have gone and your skin should be glowing from those female hormones coursing through your body. You will feel vigorous and alive. After 6 p.m. it is a different story, but enjoy it while it lasts. You may find you have an overwhelming urge to scratch your abdomen and other parts of your body (a side effect of the increased blood flow around your body), but do try not to, as scratching only makes you want to scratch more and you can break the skin. Wearing light, loose cotton can help, as can taking your clothes off (in the privacy of your own home). If you feel the itching is really bad, and/or you think your skin is looking yellow, see your doctor or midwife.

You may notice you aren't as mentally quick as you were before you got this pregnant. It is as though a fog descends into your brain, making thinking a bit of a struggle sometimes. It's hormonal and patchy, and it does lift.

Weeks 25 to 28

How your baby is growing

Your baby will be up to 27cm long now and weigh between 900g and 1300g. You will feel her movements more strongly – a well-aimed, unexpected kick (and they are always unexpected) can make you jump.

This is a period when the brain develops rapidly and becomes able to control some of the things we do all the time, such as beginning to breathe in a regular way. She'll be able to open and close her eyelids and will be sensitive to bright light, especially if it's close to your body. This is because the retina – the part of the eye that responds to light – is now developing.

Your baby's spine (which has 150 joints and is incredibly supple for a column of bones) is getting stronger, as the joints, ligaments and bones that protect the spinal column with all its nerves are developing more fully.

During these next few weeks, your baby's lungs will develop rapidly too – to the extent that, if she were born now, she would be able to bring in oxygen through her lungs and breathe out carbon dioxide. This ability to exchange gases through the lungs is still immature and premature babies often need help to do it, but your baby is now definitely getting the hang of breathing. In fact, lungs take ages to develop properly and your baby's lungs will continue to do so well into childhood.

She will also be developing proper swallowing reflexes – swallowing, for example, when something gets to the back of her throat, rather than just swallowing because she can. She will be able to open her nostrils if she wants and make a fist. (Obviously, she uses her hand to do this – not her nostrils.)

Your baby's spleen is busy making red blood cells to carry oxygen around her body, and white blood cells to fight infection. Later on, her long bones, particularly those in her legs, will make red blood cells.

Your baby will be getting more and more cuddly and less like a prune, as she continues to store fat under her skin. At this stage, less than 4 per cent of her body weight will be made up of fat. Her head will now be more or less in proportion to her body.

How your body is changing

If you're lucky, you will be feeling well, patting your bump fondly, and you won't be too physically inconvenienced. But carrying a growing baby inside your womb – one that kicks your bladder and bowels and increasingly presses up against your ribcage and lungs – can mean you start to get leg cramps, back pain (be careful with those stilettos) and piles (sorry!).

You may also be anxious – not only about giving birth but also that your baby will be healthy. Talking to other women can be very helpful, but be warned that some women like to tell horror stories about giving birth, so divide the horror factor by at least half. The odds of having a healthy baby are overwhelmingly in most women's favour, but we all know that's not guaranteed, which is why we feel a little anxious. This anxiety for your child will last for the rest of your life – even once she is married with a baby of her own.

Weeks 29 to 32

How your baby is growing

Your baby's weight is now increasing much faster than her height. Between the 24th and 37th weeks she will pile on the grams, at a rate of 15 a day (soon, fat will make up 8 per cent of her weight). She will be around 28–30cm long and weigh 1400g–2100g.

She will look pink and develop body contours that will give her her baby shape. She will be ditching the downy hair on her head and growing her first proper baby hair: this will have colour although, like babies' eyes, it can change after birth.

Your baby's brain is still hard at work, with nerve cells reaching out to meet other nerve cells to form the intricate systems of wiring that determine who we are and what our potential is and control what our body can do. Increasingly, your baby's brain will be able to control her breathing and temperature. The complex wiring and connections that the brain has to grow mean that it takes a while for the developing baby to co-ordinate all the control mechanisms the brain performs. How fast you breathe for example, can change depending on how hot you are – and wiring your brain up to deal with that is something of an intra-uterine challenge.

Your baby will be able to move her eyeballs, although there isn't much to see in your womb, so she probably won't be doing it much. And, even though she now has the right nerve cells to distinguish colours, these won't work until she is born so, to her, everything in the womb is monochrome. All five of her senses will be in working order.

She will still turn the odd somersault but, increasingly, it will get crowded in your womb, so her movements will be restricted. They will be more forceful, though, and you can sometimes see what looks like a foot or fist sticking up through your abdominal wall.

Your baby's bones will be storing calcium and other minerals that make them hard and strong, and they will now be the main supplier to the body of red blood cells, which carry oxygen and nutrients around the body. Her lungs will still be developing, and each week they get better at breathing.

How your body is changing

You may find you need to eat little and often, because you don't physically feel you can eat a full meal at one sitting. You may also be getting less sleep because of getting up at night to go the toilet – your baby is now pressing on your bladder and you will feel like passing urine more often. Your belly button will probably have popped out by now, too. You may find you get restless legs, heartburn (or worse heartburn than that you've had so far!) and/or that you've acquired some varicose veins (they should disappear after the birth).

You may also start to feel quite lonely. The changes your body goes through, the extraordinary process of growing a baby inside you, can make you feel separate at times. You may feel preoccupied with being pregnant and the physical changes it brings. Some women also feel strange that their partner or friends (who haven't had kids) have no real idea of what they're going through. Try to talk to your partner and concentrate a bit on your relationship.

Weeks 33 to 37

How your baby is growing

Your baby is now putting the finishing touches on her development. She's still gaining weight, but not so rapidly, as she realises space is at a premium. She will measure between 31cm and 34cm and weigh between 2200g and 2900g.

She will have a firm handshake and would already be able to look you in the eye, although she needs to learn how to adjust the lens to focus on near and far objects properly. (She'll do this once she's out of the womb.)

By now, your baby is likely to have shifted to lie in the head-down position (her head in your pelvis and her legs up against your ribs). This tends to happen earlier on in first pregnancies when you still have abdominal muscles to give some direction to your baby – in subsequent pregnancies, she may be swimming around for slightly longer.

Your baby's lungs continue to develop. The number of tiny air sacs (essential for oxygen to get into the body via the lungs) is increasing all the time. Their walls are getting thinner, so the oxygen can get through faster, and there is less of a gap between the walls of the air sacs and the tiny blood vessels that carry the oxygen around the body. As your baby practises breathing in your womb, she breathes in amniotic fluid (which is full of protein, chloride and surfactant – see p. 416); this helps the lungs develop and gives the muscles in the chest, which will do all the breathing when your baby is born, something to do. When your baby is born, her breathing will squeeze this fluid out of her lungs and through her mouth and also into the blood vessels of the lungs where it will be absorbed.

The amniotic fluid your baby swallows also helps develop her gut and bowels: it contains up to 10–15 per cent of the protein she needs for growing them. Her bowels will take a while to develop.

Other organs, such as the liver, also take a while to mature. At birth, your baby's liver may struggle to break down a substance called bilirubin (some of which the body makes naturally – it's the stuff that in high levels makes babies look a bit yellow). Most bilirubin is disposed of through the placenta.

Your baby has learnt to suck – something she will rely on for months after she is born – and her sucking ability is already incredibly strong. Meanwhile, her heart rate has been slowing down from its original gallop in the 20th week to a more sedate average of 142 beats a minute. It speeds up when she moves her arms or legs and seems to peak between 8 a.m. and 10 a.m. and slow down between 2 a.m. and 6 a.m.

How your body is changing

You may still be luxuriating in the perfect pregnancy and not suffering from any of the side effects of carrying a baby in your womb, or you may be cream-crackered and wincing with permanent backache and swollen feet. You may notice some Braxton Hicks contractions (tightening across your abdomen, see p. 261): despite the name, they are not the start of labour because they do not become more frequent and regular and they do not get worse. Having said that, sometimes they can be strong enough to make you stop what you are doing. There is nothing that is known to really stop them, although having a bath may help.

Weeks 38 to 40

How your baby is growing

Your baby is getting ready to start life in the real world. She will be around 36cm long and weigh around 3400g, but this is only a guide as some babies can be very long and some can weigh a lot. Generally, boy babies weigh more than girls and are often longer. By the time she is born, your baby will have lots of fat to keep her warm and make her cuddly. About 16 per cent of her body will be made up of fat.

Babies have characteristics you can easily overlook. They have little chests that seem to stick out and tiny breast buds. Some are born with a complete hairstyle; others are practically bald. If your baby's eyes are blue, they may darken as pigment develops over the first few months. If your baby has brown eyes, they won't get lighter. Pigment is only added, not removed.

Your baby will have been developing her own routine. This, of course, is nothing like yours. In the last six weeks in the womb, your baby is either active or quiet. She will be in an active state for up to 70 per cent of the time. The quiet moments last from between 15 to just over 20 minutes. Her eyes will be open when she is awake and shut when asleep. While your baby is active, she will be moving her legs and arms, her heart rate will go up and she will be making breathing movements. When she is quiet, she won't be doing any of these things and her heart rate will stay the same. Who knows what she's doing when she is quiet?

The first breath is a big shock for your baby and she will be practising for this moment right up until birth. She will hiccup a lot around this time, as the amniotic fluid she is breathing in will sometimes tickle her throat. She is learning how to co-ordinate sucking, swallowing and breathing.

Your baby's bones are getting harder, but some of her skull bones will stay soft to help her get down the birth canal. Her gums will be quite hard when she's born yet, remarkably, her tooth buds will soon push teeth through them.

Your immunity to various infections will have been transferred, as antibodies, through the placenta to your baby, and if you go on to breastfeed your baby then your milk gives her more of these.

There is less and less room for your baby to move in your womb now. The amniotic fluid that has been cushioning her has fallen from 800ml at 32 weeks to 500ml.

After 40 weeks, your baby has done all the work and is now ready to live without your womb and the life support your body has been providing. But don't expect her to be happy about it. Many babies are pretty miserable until they get used to having to do all the things for themselves that you did. That includes eating, going to the toilet (both sorts), regulating body temperature and breathing. So be patient. Don't expect her to be grateful to you for having her for at least, oh, 20 years.

How your body is changing

You can be short of breath late on in pregnancy because your diaphragm is pushed up and your lungs have less room to suck air in. This can mean you take more shallow breaths and feel breathless. You can't do much about this except try to relax: you are getting enough breath in, and if you start breathing faster you will feel dizzy. You may also feel that everything in the lower part of your body is trying to escape. Leaking urine when you laugh or strain, or even if you get up and walk, is quite common at this stage of pregnancy, but it's annoying and can be a real problem if it happens a lot. Since the problem is caused by the baby inside your (large) womb pressing on your bladder, things should become a lot, er, drier, once the baby's out.

APPENDIX 2: Dads-to-Be: Bootcamp for Beginners

Well done, chaps, you have knocked her up. Jolly good work ... But this is just the beginning.

'I feel like my life's in limbo, just waiting and waiting for the baby to come along. I'm going to be glad when this whole pregnancy thing is over.' Markedwards

For your partner, the nine months of pregnancy are to grow and nurture your baby and prepare herself for the birth; for you, they are to master the technique of getting the infant car seat in and out of the car.

The best thing you can do during your partner's pregnancy is to appear interested, even if you don't feel particularly so. It isn't your body going through all these changes, so it is not surprising that you aren't as obsessed as she is. But make the right noises: talk about the baby, attend antenatal appointments and scans and classes, read a book about parenthood, place a hand on her stomach when she says the baby is kicking, be sympathetic about her tiredness and nausea – and, of course, memorise the infant car-seat manual.

Your lovely partner is now a giant human host organism. Don't be annoyed if she goes to bed at 6.30 p.m. Sympathise with how she is feeling: she isn't *ill*, but she *is* vomiting into a bucket, so sympathy and a cuddle are in order (once she's wiped off the solid bits). Morning sickness is not to be treated lightly. Feeling like you have got a hangover 24/7 is *not* being fussy.

'There are so many things that I just can't face eating any more. My husband doesn't seem to understand this at all. He demands to know at 9 a.m. what I want for my tea that evening. I've tried to explain that it's best to wait and see, and nearer the time I'll know what I'll feel up to eating. He told me that I am "just being fussy". The other night I decided to have a jacket potato, cheese and salad, as I knew I would be able to eat that. Fine – then he dumps a load of overcooked broccoli on my plate, the smell of which makes me heave.' Chequers

Your partner's hormone levels are shooting through the roof – during pregnancy, her oestrogen will climb to nearly 1,000 times its normal levels. If you thought PMT was bad, it's time to start digging out that old air-raid shelter at the back of the garden. She may well become *even* more 'crazy and irrational' (your words, not ours) than usual. She may start listening to Bryan Adams and weeping over washing powder commercials. Be reassured that this is hormonal, and won't last for ever.

'For my husband, the biggest challenge was my mood swings, but he became very good at tuning in quickly to them. A good example was when I smashed the lid from the crock pot on the floor – he was dying to laugh but didn't, because he didn't know if I'd laugh or cry myself, so he tried his best to keep a straight face. The hormones hopefully won't last for ever. My husband has become very good at the phrase, "Yes, dear".' Munz

Mumsnetiquette: Useful things dads-to-be can actually *do*

Master the car seat Put it in. Take it out. Repeat.

Refill the car Petrol fumes will probably make her gag and are not good for the baby. Make sure the car is topped up, so that she doesn't have to vomit or faint on the forecourt.

Take charge of shopping and cooking If she's nauseous and can't face cooking, take over any cooking and food shopping jobs that she usually does. Microwavable ready meals may be a good solution if she retches at the sight of an onion.

Clean the bathroom No one wants to kneel down to a messy toilet bowl. Scrape off the bad stuff and keep it sparkling for your princess.

Manly practical stuff Put up shelves. Paint the nursery with those hazardous toxic paints. Fill in ponds. Fit child locks on cupboards containing bleach or high-quality Scandinavian porn.

Attend her antenatal appointments and classes It's crap being the one in class who has to pair up with the teacher. Turn up and support her.

Spend time with a mate who is a father Try to spend some time at the coalface if you can. Accompany a friend and his children to the park. Ask questions. Find out which end is which.

Sex and pregnancy

Right. Now that we have persuaded you that the way forward is to be Mr Sensitive And Interested Metrosexual, we will cut to the chase. Yes, you can have sex during pregnancy (with your partner, not Claire in HR), but it's not compulsory. Some women don't feel like it, and lots of men don't either. Usually, one of you will be gagging for it and the other will be recoiling in horror.

Some worries are somewhat intangible: a vague feeling that sex with a pregnant woman is somehow 'just not right' is common, along with the feeling that 'the baby is watching'. If you are the sort who can't possibly get naked if the dog is in the room, then pregnant sex might not be your bag.

One common man-worry is a fear of hurting the baby, but rest assured: your todger may well be of impressive proportions (and yes, we do say that to everyone), but your baby won't actually get concussion if you have sex. You may also worry that your vast schlong might pierce the sac of waters, which will pop all over the both of you and then you'll be forever impotent with the horror of it all. Again, this is unlikely. And, if it does happen, at least you'll have a tale to entertain dinner party guests with for years to come.

'We did ask the doctor what the natural protection was in her body for when the baby got bigger – just to reassure ourselves. He told us there was nothing to worry about unless you were medically abnormally large in that area. I wasn't sure whether I fell into that bracket and was unzipping my fly to whap it out on the table for the doc's opinion, but the wife was very definite that I shouldn't worry for some reason ...' EricL

Although these fears are largely irrational, they are all quite understandable. If either one of you doesn't fancy the full monty, find other ways to 'marital intimacy' that are non-penetrative. Unlock the Scandinavian porn cupboard for ideas. Just don't forget to shut the dog out of the room.

What to say to a pregnant lady

A fast route to your lady's heart and an easy life is to remember to compliment her and make her feel good about her rapidly melting body. Most women have hang-ups about their bodies, and these can be amplified during pregnancy, when she is piling on the pounds like never before. You might see her belly as a magnificent torpedo-like testimony to her youth and fertility, but she just wants to cry as her weight climbs to previously unimaginable figures. Jokes such as, 'I'm not sure whether to make you a cup of tea or throw you a fish,' while undoubtedly funny, are probably best avoided. If possible, break the bathroom scales (she may already have done this herself), and tell her on a regular basis that you still find her attractive. Try to do this without actually Jack-Russelling her while she is unloading the dishwasher.

'My husband says that my arse has not so much got bigger, but spread higher up my back. WTF? Don't you blokes realise yet that when asked THE questions, you know the ones: Am I fatter than I used to be? Do you fancy me more than Angelina Jolie? etc., you are meant to LIE FOR GOD'S SAKE! We know the answers already.'

Foosfan

Now, obviously during pregnancy there may be a mismatch of libidos, but try to be discreet about your surreptitious one-in-a-bed sessions. A pregnant lady scorned is a devious enemy.

'When I was pregnant I was an absolute whale. One day I found some porn mags in my ex-husband's wardrobe. I was distraught. Then I had a brainwave and replaced them with *Practical Parenting*. It was never mentioned.' Lilibet

Try to be positive, even when actually, she is rather hysterical and, frankly, a bit pathetic. 'Give positive feedback,' begs one mum. 'In the first hard few weeks, often my husband putting his arm round me and telling me what a brilliant thing I was doing really kept me going.'

And whatever you do, don't make the same mistake as one Mumsnetter's husband, who bought her an exercise bike as a giving-birth present. For a start, she'll probably have to have the saddle surgically extracted. Or you might. (Which may be even worse.)

'Don't ever start a sentence with: "Well, my mum says ..." Unless it ends with " ... you're doing fantastic work!"' StealthPolarBear

Labour

Labour is a funny thing for chaps, because you don't really *do* much. This can be quite frustrating if you are the sort who runs to the tool box in a crisis. It is mainly a matter of standing around, possibly watching the golf, while your partner goes through the seven circles of hell somewhere near by. Lots of women don't even want their partners to do much, and prefer to labour pretty much on their own.

Labour is a very animal experience, and your partner will not be her usual calm, rational self.

'Stick up for her if she doesn't want or does want something; if you side with the midwife, then consider where you will be living for the next few months.' Skribble

Your main job is really to be your partner's advocate. 'You have to act as translator between her and the rest of the world, as she will be off her head,' advises one mum. Be positive and reassuring, but 'don't sound like a cheerleader shouting, "Come on! Great! Great!" or she will want to hit you.'

'Don't be afraid to piss off the hospital staff,' writes one dad. They may be annoyingly blasé and tell you that everything is fine, but while they are experts at delivery, you are the expert when it comes to knowing your partner. Your partner might not be in a position to be arsey, but you are.

'Don't wear new clothes to the hospital, don't try to reach for the gas and air and don't crack jokes in the maternity unit.' Munz

In terms of what actually occurs in the labour room, be prepared for the birth plan to go completely out the window during labour. 'It'll never be how you expect so don't torture yourself by imagining different scenarios,' advises one Mumsnet dad. 'Focus on the end result – which WILL be worth it.'

So, the first big test: your first job as New Dad will be to act as Master Of The Car Seat. Don't forget it when you come to collect your new family from the hospital. They won't let you out of the door without it. Chances are that your missus will be too knackered, and possibly chopped into little pieces, to be man-handling a heavy car-seat-and-baby into the car. So work out how this is done beforehand. You don't want to have a full-scale domestic argument about your incompetence while standing outside the maternity unit with your midwife waiting to wave you off.

'Find out how the car seat fits into the car. Read the manual and practise. You'll get lots of brownie points if you can do this safely, speedily and possibly with your eyes closed.'
Notquitesotiredmum

Hospital man bag

You could just wander along to the hospital with nothing but a few loose coins and your house keys in your pocket, and that will be fine. But if you want to Be Prepared, give some thought to what you might need beforehand. Don't worry about what your partner might want (she probably packed a hospital bag the day after she peed on the pregnancy test), but what she doesn't want is you whining: 'Did you bring me a snack?' She might be in labour for a day or two, which is a long time without sleep and an even longer time without food. So pack yourself a man bag and you'll be ready for the long-haul.

(continued)

- **Snacks for you** Sandwiches, drinks, muesli bars, cakes – anything that will sustain you. Not Stella. 'Your relationship may be over if you leave to grab a snack (or if you take a trip to the chip shop like my cousin's husband did).' *TheArmadillo*
- **Thick skin** You will be bossed around and sworn at (hopefully just by your wife, rather than the nursing staff). Don't walk out. Let it all wash over you. Also cast-iron stomach – you may see Awful Things.
- **Camera** Maybe not for the full-on tearing-down-the-middle action shots, but it's lovely to have some pics of the minutes-old baby. By this stage you will probably be immune to the sight of bare breasts, smeared blood and floating poo, so try to cover those up a little bit when you are framing the shots, so that your workmates don't faint when they see your screensaver.
- **Clothes and shoes** You will probably get messy, so take a change of clothes; and you might be on your feet for more hours than you have ever been before – so wear comfy shoes.
- **Phone numbers of people you might need to ring** Your partner has probably got a small database of 'People To Ring' along with assorted coinage, but if there are any people you will want to call afterwards, make sure you've got their numbers there, too. She might be highly organised, but not to the point of having your HR department's direct line on her mobile.
- **Headache tablets** You may not need them, but if the labour is long and tense, in the bright lights and heat of a hospital you may well get a headache, and your partner is likely to be in no mood to share her pain relief with you.
- **Car seat** For Goodness Sake.

Finally we meet, Mr Bond

The moment comes; the baby slithers out, the panting stops, the room is a whirl of commotion and congratulations. 'Any doubts I had were obliterated the first time I saw my son,' writes one dad. Ahhh.

You may well fall in love with your child the moment it pops out, but it is equally likely that your first thought will be, 'She has given birth to a drowned ferret,' or, 'Thank feck I can go to bed now,' or perhaps, 'I wonder if I can make it home in time for *Match of the Day*?'

There is a broad spectrum of emotion around greeting your child for the first time, and any of the above is quite normal. Likewise, your wife may be hearing fireworks and music, or she might just be thinking, 'Oh dear God, where is the woman with the needle?' Either way, where babies are concerned, actions speak louder than words: you don't *have* to fall in love with your baby right away, you just have to look after her. And of course, gently wrestle her into that car seat.

Sex after birth

If pregnancy has been a bit barren on the shagging front, don't expect to leap on your other half as soon as the curtains are closed around the bed on the maternity ward. It generally takes a few months for sex to be back on the agenda, partly because of physical changes (e.g. having her genitals – or stomach – ripped in two and then sewn back together again) and partly because of exhaustion, with all the night-waking and round-the-clock childcare.

Some women also feel rather 'touched out' by the end of the day, because the fat starfish hands of a baby can be patting and grabbing at a mother pretty much all the time. Once you do start venturing into the bedroom again, take things slowly. She will probably have lost a lot of confidence in her body, and will feel very differently about things. 'Because of breastfeeding, my breasts just feel functional now,' admits one new mum; 'I may as well have two toasters strapped to my front.'

'When starting out with breastfeeding, her breasts will be very tender and swollen. These gigantic boobs are Not Sexual Playthings. And when your sex life resumes breasts may be a bit off-limits as they can be sore, tender, leaky and over-stimulated.' Sidge

'Sex is still very good after childbirth,' according to one dad, although, 'I count myself very fortunate that she still allows me to go near enough to find this out.' You both might be slightly worried that post-birth sex will be akin to 'parking a mini in an aircraft hanger' but most men report very little difference. Although one Mumsnet dad confesses: 'After two natural births my wife is definitely looser. Of course, after witnessing two births, it's entirely possible that I've shrunk.'

Cold feet

'I spent most of my wife's pregnancy bricking it,' admits one dad; 'but it's natural to fear the unknown.' Having a baby is a massive life change, and it's normal to feel nervous, or indeed terrified, at the prospect of everything changing. When you are happy and satisfied with your life and your relationship, having everyone tell you that a baby is like a hand grenade tossed into your marriage is not very reassuring. While women at least know that they will have a period of time off work to adjust, dads can have the added worry of having to stay sane (and awake) at a desk, feeling the burden of financial responsibility for the whole family.

It can be easy to stress about everything not being 'ready' for the baby, but don't get too hung up on everything being catalogue-perfect for the new arrival. 'Things will never be ready for a new baby,' writes one Mumsnetter, 'but as long as they have something to sleep in, something to wear, and something to crap in, you'll be fine.'

'Part of the problem is that for men, the negatives are easier to dwell on than the positives,' says a dad. 'That, and the fact that books on fatherhood are completely sh*te.'

'Avoid dwelling on it. I have a one-hour commute on the Tube each way, and I'd often find myself falling into a "negative mindset", dwelling on all the bad things to come (lack of sleep/sex, finances, being really responsible for another little creature, etc.). I found giving myself a mental kick in the arse whenever that occurred was helpful.' TheSelfishMan

> Some dads find that things are easier once the baby is born: 'I find it easier to deal with the here-and-now of a baby once it exists rather than speculate about what it might be like.'

'I had a wonderful, if trying, time in my three weeks' paternity leave. I had our son a lot while my wife was sleeping it off – I even took him up to the allotments on day two to meet the committee! Yes, it gets in the way of all those other things I enjoy doing at times, but life is about positive choices.' Triathlete

> It is worth mentioning here that when the baby is born, it won't be very interesting. In fact, it is pretty much just an animal with extremely high needs. 'Expectation management is important,' advises one wise Mumsnetter. 'In the first weeks, babies tend to sleep, eat and cry, and the crying can go on for a long time. They don't spend much time just being at one with the world.'

'Don't expect the first six months to be a bed of roses with lots of fun and carefree bonding all round. Expect it to be bewildering, knackering and, at times, downright boring. Expect to play an important, but ultimately peripheral supporting role.' DJ

> 'Dads can feel excluded because they can't breastfeed,' points out another veteran mum, 'and some babies will only fall asleep in the early days if "fed to sleep" (which, incidentally, despite what the books say isn't a problem in itself). This leaves them with the crying bit. In the early days there may be nothing you can "do" about the crying bit except hold the baby and wait for it to pass.'

'View the first six to 12 months as the start-up investment. You are investing your energy, your time, your sleep and a chunk of your sanity. You are investing in new skills and in your new team. Don't expect any returns until after the first year. The returns will come, though, and by God they are pure magic!' DaddyJ

When it comes to parenting, the early months can be jolly hard work, but you need to play a long game. Eventually, you will be a very, very proud dad to a very, very delightful child. 'As a dad, all I can say is that the hard parts will pass and you will bond with your baby,' says one father. 'In the early months, you have to take the rough with the smooth. Think of the long term.'

And the car seat. Please don't forget to think of the car seat.

The best of times, the worst of times

'Having a newborn is like being stranded on a desert island and having to learn to live all over again.' *Mrtribpot*

'You can be assured that now that I'm a father, I wouldn't go back for anything.' *TheSelfishMan*

'I aged ten years in the first week of my son's life.' *MrIntergalacticWalrus*

'You can kiss your weekends goodbye, likewise lie-ins, and any time you want a break for a drink. Open your wallet once a week and pour it down the drain. It's hard until they're about one year old, and then, if they are teething, it's not really much better.' *MrMunz*

'Remember that you might feel a bit useless during the early weeks, but there are things you can do. You can hold the baby in a sling, go for long walks with the baby while your wife sleeps, do baths and baby massage and, of course, change nappies. It all gets better after a few months when they are more interested in playing.' *MadamePlatypus*

'Keep talking to each other, think critically about your own experiences of being "parented", expect the unexpected, love your partner and child and don't expect life to be ever the same again.' *MetallicCerise*

'When the first child arrives, you soon understand what the word zombie actually means. But no one can describe the feeling of joy you will feel as a dad.' *DrDaddy*

APPENDIX 3: Useful Websites for Parents-to-Be

Pregnancy and Baby Gear

The Maternity Exchange (www.maternityexchange.co.uk)
Second-hand maternity clothes, shop clearance and end-of-season maternity wear.

Freecycle (www.freecycle.org)
Keeping stuff out of landfill – sign up to see what's going free in your local area.

eBay (www.ebay.co.uk)
The online auction site, good for maternity bargains and selling on your maternity wardrobe.

Travelling

The Medical Advisory Service for Travellers Abroad (www.masta.org)
Useful info if you are travelling abroad while pregnant.

Birth planning

The National Institute for Health and Clinical Excellence (www.nice.org.uk)
National guidelines for managing pregnancy, pregnancy-related conditions and birth.

Doula UK (www.doula.org.uk) and The Doula Directory (www.douladirectory.co.uk)
Information about hiring and finding a doula.

Independent Midwives UK (www.independentmidwives.org.uk)
Information about hiring an independent midwife. Includes a searchable directory.

Csections (www.csections.org)
Information about Caesarean sections.

Action on Pre-eclampsia (www.apec.org.uk) and the
Pre-eclampsia Foundation (www.preeclampsia.org)
Information about pre-eclampsia.

Breastfeeding

Association of Breastfeeding Mothers (www.abm.me.uk)
A charity run by mothers for mothers, committed to giving
friendly support and supplying the right information to all
women wishing to breastfeed.

La Leche League UK (www.laleche.org.uk)
Breastfeeding support from pregnancy through to weaning.

Kellymom (www.kellymom.com)
Information and advice about all aspects of breastfeeding and
parenting.

Health

NHS Direct (www.nhsdirect.nhs.uk)
Official website for the NHS 24-hour telephone helpline, NHS
Direct. A good place to start when you or your baby is poorly.
Information about health problems and how to keep healthy,
and advice on when to call for help.

BBC Health (www.bbc.co.uk/health)
Health news, health guides, and a searchable conditions database.

Support and listening

The Miscarriage Association (www.miscarriageassociation.org.uk)
Support and information for people suffering from pregnancy
loss.

The Birth Trauma Association
(www.birthtraumaassociation.org.uk)
The BTA supports all women who have had a traumatic birth
experience.

Birth Crisis Network (www.sheilakitzinger.com/birthcrisis.htm)
The Birth Crisis Network is a helpline that women can ring if they want to talk about a traumatic birth.

Patient Advisory and Liaison Service (www.pals.nhs.uk)
PALS is there to listen to patients' experiences and to improve services based on patient feedback.

Bliss (www.bliss.org.uk)
The special care baby charity, offers support and information.

Parenting and families support

Elizabeth Pantley (www.pantley.com/elizabeth)
Information about the 'No-cry' series from Elizabeth Pantley.

Gingerbread (www.gingerbread.org.uk)
The Organisation for Lone Parent Families.

The Twins And Multiple Birth Association TAMBA (www.tamba.org.uk)
Support and information for parents of multiples.

Homestart (www.home-start.org.uk)
Parent volunteers supporting families.

Sure Start (www.surestart.gov.uk)
Government programme providing multi-disciplinary services for children, partly via local children's centres. May provide local services (or signposting to services) for children and families with special needs.

Contact a Family (www.cafamily.org.uk)
Contact a Family is good for children diagnosed with medical conditions. It lists all the support groups.

Money and savings

Department of Work and Pensions (www.dwp.gov.uk)
Government department with information about benefits as well as information for employees.

HM Revenue & Customs (www.hmrc.gov.uk/childcare)
Information and guidance about tax and National Insurance
contributions (NICs) on employer-supported childcare (childcare
vouchers).

Child Tax Credits (www.taxcredits.inlandrevenue.gov.uk)
Information about Child Tax Credits, entitlements and how much
you may get.

Entitledto (www.entitledto.com)
Calculator and information about the benefits and tax credits to
which you may be entitled.

Child Trust Fund (www.childtrustfund.gov.uk)
Information about the Child Trust Fund (CTF) savings and
investment account for children.

Working and childcare

**DirectGov Work and Families (www.direct.gov.uk/en/
Employment/Employees/WorkAndFamilies)**
Guidance on family employment rights, including your rights as a
new parent.

ChildcareLink (www.childcarelink.gov.uk)
National and local childcare information: find childcare in your
area.

Ofsted (www.ofsted.gov.uk)
The official body for inspecting childcare providers such as
nurseries and childminders. Provides links to reports and official
publications as well as a FAQ and contact details.

INDEX

A

abnormal labour 287–8
aches and pains *see* pain
Active Birth movement 111, 270
active labour, breathing techniques
    318–19
active management, delivery of
    placenta 283–5
active phase of labour 275–7
acupressure, for morning sickness 47
acupuncture
    for back pain 166
    for headaches 66
    for heartburn 157
    inducing labour 344
    for morning sickness 47
    for thrush 171
adrenalin 204
afterbirth *see* placenta
age of mother, and Down's
    syndrome 82
air travel 237–40
alcohol 6, 26–7
allergies
    hay fever 63–4
    peanuts 28
aloe vera 74, 163
alveoli 415
amniocentesis 86, 177–80
amniotic fluid
    and baby's movements 411
    and development of breathing 421
    hiccups 415, 423
    meconium in 264–5
    quantities of 423
    20-week scan 176
    waters breaking 262–5

amniotic sac 383, 410
anaemia, iron supplements 29
anaesthesia
    Caesarean section 346
    epidurals 313–16
    pudendal block 358
    spinal block 316–17, 346
anal fissures 76
anomaly pregnancy scan 85
antacids 157
antenatal care 11, 427
    booking-in appointment 10
    maternity notes 10, 11–12, 174–5
    multiple pregnancy 35
    second trimester 173–83
    tests and scans 80–6
antenatal classes 38, 108–14, 427
antenatal depression 57
anterior position, baby in labour
    278
antibiotics
    Group B streptococcus 249–50
    and thrush 169–70
    urinary tract infections 63
antibodies, in breast milk 393, 394,
    423
antihistamines 63–4
anus, tears 363
Anusol 74
anxiety 419
arms, development of 409–11, 414
Arnica 303, 348, 366
aromatherapy, in labour 98, 303–4
artificial rupture of membranes
    (ARM) 275, 288, 339–40
aspirin 22, 65
assisted delivery 358–61

blood clots
    after Caesarean section 350
    deep-vein thrombosis 239
    vitamin K and 369
blood pressure
    fainting 78
    high 241–2
    maternity notes 12
    pre-eclampsia 242–6
blood sugar levels 78
    gestational diabetes 255, 257–8
blood tests 84, 85
blue cohosh 344–5
body temperature, fever 64
bodysuits 230
bonding with baby 435, 436
bones, development of 412, 420,
    423
booking-in appointment 10
bottle-feeding 396–9
    equipment 220
bottles, for expressed milk 221
bowel movements
    after Caesarean section 351
    after tears and episiotomy 366
    constipation 159–61, 413
    diarrhoea 262
    during labour 283
    meconium 264–5, 415
    water birth 324–5
bowels, development of 411, 421
bowls, top-and-tail 227
boxes, toiletry 226
brain
    development of 410, 415, 418, 419
    memory problems 140–1, 417
brain damage, breech babies 329
bras
    breastfeeding 229
    underwired 25–6
Braxton Hicks contractions 136–7,
    261–2, 422

breaking the news 13–16
breast pads 229–30
breast pumps 220
breastfeeding 378, 392–5
    after Caesarean section 215, 352
    after labour 287
    antibodies 423
    bras 229
    expressing milk 220–1
    lactation consultants 352
    multiple births 35
    support groups 111
Breastfeeding Advocacy and Peer
    Support Group (BAPS) 395
breasts
    in first trimester 412
    sex after birth 433
    underwired bras 25–6
breathing
    development of 413, 416, 418, 421,
        423
    hypnobirthing 98
    meconium aspiration syndrome
        264–5
    as pain relief 302
    premature babies 418
    techniques in labour 318–22
    in third trimester 423
breech babies 327–34
    delivery 329
    home births 95
    risks 329
    turning 330–4
    types of breech 328
brown fat 414
buggies 222–3
    forward- or backward-facing?
        224
    for multiples 34
bump bands 138
    see also support belts
burial, after miscarriage 128, 198

co-breathing 320–2
cocaine 22
coffee 26
cohosh 344–5
colds 64–5
colon, constipation 159–61
colostrum 394
colour
  eyes 419, 422
  hair 419
colour vision 419
combined test 86
complete breech 328
complete miscarriage 116
compliments 428–9
constipation 159–61, 413
consultants 88
continuous foetal monitoring (CFM)
  269–71, 342, 356
contractions
  active phase of labour 275
  after artificial rupture of
    membranes 340
  Braxton Hicks 136–7, 261–2, 422
  breathing techniques 318–19
  delivery of placenta 283–4
  early phase of labour 271–4
  failure to progress 287–8
  induction of labour 335, 341
  miscarriage 121
  pain 296
  second stage of labour 280–2
  signs of labour 259, 262
  transition phase of labour 279–80
  water birth 101, 322
  what they feel like 300–1
  when to go to hospital 266, 274
convulsions, eclampsia 246
cooking
  and morning sickness 46
  partner's role 427
cord see umbilical cord

cot bumpers 230
cot death, smoking and 20
cots
  bedding 230
  choosing 217
  cot-beds 226–7
  for multiples 34
cotton wool balls 221
coughs 64
counselling
  breastfeeding 395
  Caesarean section 212–13, 353
  for amniocentesis 178
  for miscarriage 127
  late miscarriage 198
  problems in labour 288
  for sex problems 368
  single mothers 36, 37
cramps, leg 419
cranial osteopathy 361
cravings 21, 59–61
cremation, late miscarriage 198
crowning, baby's head 281–2, 297, 383
crying
  hormones and weepiness 56–8
  newborn babies 435
curry, inducing labour 337, 344
cushions, valley 365–6
CVS see chorionic villus sampling
cystic fibrosis 83
cystitis 63

D
dairy products, listeriosis 28
dating pregnancy 7
dating scan 85
death
  from Caesarean section 211
  stillbirth 356
  sudden infant death syndrome
    (SIDS) 20
  see also miscarriage

joints
  development of 418
  painful 167

K
Kali carb 303
Kali phos 303
ketoprofen 22
kicking *see* movements, foetal
knickers 229

L
labial graze 363
labour
  active phase 275–7
  back pain and 168–9
  birth partners 184
  birth plans 205–10
  birth stories 288–96
  breathing techniques 318–22
  doulas 184, 186–8
  early phase 271–4
  failure to progress 287–8
  first stage 271–80
  foetal monitoring 268–71
  home birth vs hospital birth
    87–102
  induction 276, 294, 334–43
  labour dystocia 287–8
  labour wards 89–90
  late miscarriage 197–8
  length of 275
  multiple births 35
  pain relief 276, 298–317
  partner's role 370–9, 430–3
  piles and 76
  position of baby 278
  positions in 277, 282, 302
  second stage 280–3
  signs of 259, 262
  third stage 283–7
  transition stage 279–80, 319

water birth 322–7
when to go to hospital 265–8,
  274
see also contractions
lactation consultants 352
lanugo 412
laparoscopy 119, 120
'late' babies, induction 334–5,
  336
latent period of labour 271
lavender oil 304, 348
legs (baby's)
  development of 409–10, 411, 414
legs (mother's)
  cramps 419
  deep-vein thrombosis (DVT) 239
  restless leg syndrome (RLS) 251–3,
    420
  sciatica 165
  varicose veins 71–3, 420
length of labour 275
length of pregnancy 7, 12, 336
leukaemia 192–3, 369
ligaments
  back pain 165
  Braxton Hicks contractions 136
  hip and pelvic pain 78, 415
  in multiple pregnancy 33
light, turning a breech baby 332
lighting, dimmer switches 217–18
linea nigra 161–2
lips, development of 416
listeriosis 28
liver (baby's)
  development of 411, 413, 421
liver (in diet)
  safety 28
liver (mother's)
  obstetric cholestasis 163–4
LMP (last monthly period) 7, 12
lochia 228
lone-parent families 36–41

lungs (baby's)
   development of 413, 415, 416, 418,
      420, 421
   meconium aspiration syndrome
      (MAS) 264–5
lungs (mother's)
   in third trimester 423

M
mackerel 28–9
malaria 240
marijuana 22
marlin 29
'mask of pregnancy' 162
massage
   during labour 99
   perineal 362
   for sleep problems 147
Maternity Allowance (MA) 105
maternity certificates 104
maternity leave 102–8
maternity notes 10, 174–5
   birth plans 207
   terminology 11–12
maternity nurses 184, 188–90
maternity pads 228, 366
maternity pay 104–5
maternity support bands *see*
   support belts
mats, changing 222
mattresses, cots 217
meat
   listeriosis 28
   toxoplasmosis 27
meconium 264–5, 415
meconium aspiration syndrome
   (MAS) 264–5
medicines *see* drugs
melanin 162
membranes
   artificial rupture of (ARM) 275,
      288, 339–40

cervical sweep 338
   waters breaking 262–5
mementoes, late miscarriage 198
memory problems 140–1, 417
mental health, after birth 392
Meptid (meptazinol) 98, 99, 312
Methotrexate 119–20
midwives
   antenatal care 11
   birth centres 92
   and birth plans 207–8
   booking-in appointment 10
   breech births 329, 332–3
   home births 95, 100
   hospital births 90
   independent midwives 184, 185–6
   midwifery units 92–3
   second stage of labour 283
   stitches 99
migraine 65
milk
   expressing 220–1
   see also bottle-feeding;
      breastfeeding
milk teeth 414
mini-pill, and ectopic pregnancy 118
miscarriage 13, 114–29
   amniocentesis 86, 178–9, 180
   bleeding 53–4
   causes 124, 199
   chorionic villus sampling and 86,
      178
   diagnosis 114–15
   emotional problems 125–9
   evacuation of retained products
      of conception (ERPC) 122–3
   late miscarriage 197–9
   medical management 123–4
   natural miscarriage 120–2
   treatment of, 120–4
   types of 116–17
   when to call doctor 115

Miscarriage Association 128–9
missed miscarriage 116–17
mitts, scratch 219
'mobile epidurals' 314
monitoring
    foetal 268–71
    induction of labour 342–3
    vaginal birth after Caesarean
        (VBAC) 356
monitors, baby 224–5
monozygotic twins 30
mood swings 426
morning sickness 42–8, 410, 425
    causes 42–3
    hyperemesis 45, 54–6
    smoking and 21
    treating 45–8
Moses baskets 34, 223, 225–6, 230
mother-and-baby groups 391
mothers, relationship with 16–19
mothers-in-law, relationship with
    16–19
mouth, bleeding gums 157–8, 415
movements, foetal
    and date of birth 414
    in first trimester 135–6, 411
    in second trimester 412–13, 414
    in third trimester 417–18, 420
moxibustion, turning a breech baby
    331–2
MRSA 88
mucus plug, signs of labour 262, 265
multiple pregnancy 30–5
    breastfeeding 35
    home births 95
    labour 35
    shopping for 34
    support for 34
muscles, development of 411, 412–13
music, during labour 306
muslin cloths 219
myelin 414

N
nail polish 348
nails (baby's)
    development of 412, 416
    scratch mitts 219
names
    choosing 193–6
    surnames 194–5
nannies, night 189–90
nappies 221–2
nappy bags 221
nappy cream 222
nappy rash 222
naproxen 22
naps, in pregnancy 147, 148
Narcan 312
natal hypnotherapy 304–5
National Childbirth Trust (NCT)
    antenatal classes 109–10, 111
    breastfeeding classes 395
    second-hand maternity wear 139
National Health Service (NHS)
    cost of Caesarean section 215
    umbilical cord blood banking
        192–3
National Institute for Health and
    Clinical Excellence (NICE) 336
National Insurance contributions
    105
natural miscarriage 120–2
nausea
    morning sickness 44, 45
    pre-eclampsia 245
NCT *see* National Childbirth Trust
neck, development of 412, 414
neroli oil 304
nerves (baby's)
    development of 414
nerves (mother's)
    carpal tunnel syndrome 253–5
nervous system, development of 411,
    412, 419

pain relief 276, 298–317
    after Caesarean section 350, 352
    after tears and episiotomy 366
    birth plans 210
    breathing techniques 318–22
    diamorphine 311–12
    drug-free methods 302–7
    entonox (gas and air) 308–9, 317
    external cephalic version 330
    in first trimester 22
    gas and air 295–6
    home births 97, 98
    and induction of labour 341
    Meptid (meptazinol) 312
    paracetamol 308
    pethidine 310–11, 312
    spinal block 316–17, 346
    for stitches 99
    TENS machines 98, 273, 307
    water birth 322, 323–4
    see also epidurals
paint, safety 22–3
pancreas, development of 411, 413
panting, in labour 318, 319, 363
pants, support 73–4
paracetamol
    for back pain 165
    for coughs and colds 64
    for headaches 65
    in labour 98, 308
    safety in pregnancy 22, 65
parasites, toxoplasmosis 27
partners 425–37
    after birth 391–2
    birth partners 184
    and birth plans 208
    bonding with baby 435, 436
    breaking the news to 13
    and Caesarean sections 346, 347
    choosing baby names 193–4
    eye contact with during labour 302
    fears 434–5

    help with breathing techniques
        320–2
    and home births 94
    hospital bag 431–2
    and miscarriage 127
    and newborn babies 434–7
    relationship with 420
    role during labour 370–9, 430–3
    sex 142–4, 427–8, 429
    sex after birth 433–4
    single mothers 36, 37–8
    20-week scan 176
    unplanned deliveries 383–5
passive smoking 21
Patau's syndrome 83
peanuts 28
pelvic-floor exercises 367
pelvic girdle pain (PGP) 78–9, 166–8,
    169
pelvic inflammatory disease (PID) 118
peppermint tea 348
perineum
    episiotomy 281, 358–9, 360, 361,
        364–5
    massage 362
    tears 281, 283, 358–9, 361–7
periods
    after miscarriage 129
    LMP (last monthly period) 7, 12
pessaries
    antifungal 170
    inducing labour 294, 337, 339
pethidine
    effects of 296–7, 310–11
    home births 98, 99
    pros and cons 312
phlebitis 73
phone numbers 234, 432
photographs 198, 432
physiological management, third
    stage of labour 285–7
physiotherapy

Statutory Maternity Pay (SMP) 104–5
stem cells, umbilical cord blood
  banking 190–3
sterilisers 220, 221
sterilising bottle-feeding equipment
  397
stethoscopes, Pinard 269
stillbirth, vaginal birth after
  Caesarean and 356
stirrups, assisted delivery 358
stitches
  Caesarean section 347
  episiotomy 362, 364–5, 366
  home birth 99
  incompetent cervix 197
  tears 362, 365, 366
stockings see support stockings
stomach, 20-week scan 176
stomach acid, heartburn 155–7
streptococcus, Group B 170, 247–50
stress, and sleep problems 148
'stretch and sweep', inducing labour
  338
stretch marks 68–71
strollers 224
sucking ability 421
sudden infant death syndrome
  (SIDS), smoking and 20
Sudocrem 75, 222
sunlight, and chloasma 162
supplements 29, 43
support
  after birth 391
  multiple pregnancy 34
  single mothers 39
support belts
  backache 166, 168
  hip and pelvic pain 79
  multiple pregnancies 33
support pants 73–4
support stockings
  after Caesarean section 350
  for fainting 78

flight socks 239
for restless legs 252
for varicose veins 72
surfactant 416, 421
surgery
  ectopic pregnancy 120
  retained placenta 285
  see also Caesarean section
surgical stockings see support
  stockings
surnames 194–5
swaddle blankets 219
swallowing reflexes 418
swimming 111
swollen hands 243, 244
swordfish 29
symphysis pubis dysfunction (SPD)
  78–9, 167–8
  in labour 274
Syntocin
  birth plans 206
  delivery of placenta 284
  failure to progress 288
  inducing labour 337, 341–2

T
tea 26
  peppermint 348
  raspberry leaf 344
tea tree oil 348
tears 361–7
  avoiding 281, 283, 362–3
  forceps and ventouse deliveries
    358–9
  recovery after 365–7
  sex after 367–8
  stitches 99, 362, 365, 366
  types of 363
teats, bottle-feeding 397, 398
teeth
  cleaning 158
  development of 414, 423
television 50

www.mumsnet.com